Movement-Driven Development

Movement-Driven Development

THE POLITICS OF HEALTH

AND DEMOCRACY IN BRAZIL

Christopher L. Gibson

Stanford University Press

Stanford, California

Stanford University Press
Stanford, California

Printed in the United States of America on acid-free, archival-quality paper

Library of Congress Cataloging-in-Publication Data

Names: Gibson, Christopher L., author.
Title: Movement-driven development : the politics of health and democracy in
    Brazil / Christopher L. Gibson.
Description: Stanford, California : Stanford University Press, 2019. | Includes
    bibliographical references and index.
Identifiers: LCCN 2018029565 (print) | LCCN 2018031504 (ebook) | ISBN 9781503607811
    (e-book) | ISBN 9781503606166 (cloth : alk. paper) | ISBN 9781503607804 (pbk. :
    alk. paper)
Subjects: LCSH: Medical policy—Brazil. | Urban health—Brazil. | Public health—
    Brazil—Citizen participation. | Civil society—Brazil. | Social movements—
    Brazil. | Democracy—Brazil. | Municipal government—Brazil.
Classification: LCC RA395.B6 (ebook) | LCC RA395.B6 G53 2018 (print) |
    DDC 362.10981—dc23
LC record available at https://lccn.loc.gov/2018029565

Typeset by Motto Publishing Services in 11/14 Adobe Garamond Pro

Cover design by Rob Ehle

To Katie

Contents

List of Tables		ix
Acknowledgments		xi
Acronyms and Abbreviations		xv
1	Subnational Democratization of Health	1
2	Pragmatist Publics in Urban Brazil	28
3	Sanitaristas and Infant Mortality Reduction	61
4	Belo Horizonte	97
5	Porto Alegre	134
6	Curitiba	171
7	Fortaleza	208
8	Movement-Driven Development in Comparative Perspective	241
	Notes	267
	References	277
	Index	293

List of Tables

Table 2.1. Types of Health Democratization in Urban Brazil 57

Table 2.2. Consequences of Health Democratization in Urban Brazil 59

Table 3.1. Data Sources Used for Scoring of Sanitarista Office-Holding Variables 66

Table 3.2. Descriptive Statistics and Sources for PCSE Model Variables 67

Table 3.3. Predictors of (Logged) Infant and Child Mortality Rates, 1995–2014 70

Table 3.4. Predictors of Primary Public Health Care Delivery, 1995–2013 73

Table 3.5. Fuzzy-Set Scores for Outcome and Causal Sets 79

Acknowledgments

The time and energy that went into researching and writing this book too often seemed unjustified, except for the fascinations they sustained and the relationships they made possible. I will never be able to repay most of these people for the knowledge they shared with me.

The project was born in Brown University's Department of Sociology and Watson Institute for International and Public Affairs, where it was molded by the guidance of many generous intellectuals. I thank Patrick Heller for deepening my passion for civil society and the beautiful messiness of politics. His selflessness, support, and insights made this project possible more than any other single person, and I'll never be able to adequately thank him. I am grateful to Gianpaolo Baiocchi, whose *carinho* in sharing comments on the first stages of this project offered useful ways to strengthen and contextualize its arguments. I thank Nitsan Chorev, who inspired me to prioritize theoretical reconstruction and clear-minded comparisons. John Logan always asked difficult and thought-provoking questions that improved the quality of analysis in the end. I also thank my other teachers and mentors at Brown University, including Phil Brown, Melani Cammett, Jose Itzigsohn, Sharon Krause, Susan Short, Rich Snyder, Patricia Sobral, Barbara Stallings, Ana Catarina Teixeira, and Michael White. I benefited greatly from the intellectual riches that Jim Green of Brown's Center for Latin American and Caribbean Studies (CLACS) and the Brazil Initiative brought to campus. During his scholarship in residence, Fernando Henrique Cardoso generously tolerated my questions and shameless monopolization of his office hours. Erin Beck, Jennifer Costanza, Esther

Hernandez-Medina, Sukriti Issar, and Celso Villegas offered encouragement and constructive suggestions. I was also fortunate to meet Jorge Alves, who continues to enrich my understanding of subnational health politics in Brazil today. The early, immensely positive influence of Michael Woolcock has made so much possible that I shudder to imagine the counterfactual of my life without having met him at Harvard. My other teachers there, especially Archon Fung, Dani Rodrik, and Roberto Unger, captured my imagination and inspired me to explore the myriad possibilities of democracy.

In Brazil, I benefited greatly from the graciousness of countless scholars, institutions, interviewees, and Municipal Health Council participants. Above all, I thank the many activists, politicians, bureaucrats, and especially sanitaristas who so graciously shared countless hours relating their mobilizational histories and knowledge of Brazil's public health sector. In São Paulo, my research affiliations with Fundação Instituto Fernando Henrique Cardoso and the Centro Brasileiro de Análise e Planejamento (CEBRAP) were instrumental for conducting fieldwork. At CEBRAP, Adrian Gurza Lavalle and Haroldo Torres generously offered helpful guidance early on. In Porto Alegre, Marcelo K. Silva and Soraya Cortes in the sociology department of the Universidade Federal do Rio Grande do Sul (UFRGS), and Claudia Fonseca in its Department of Anthropology, contributed useful feedback early on. Oscar Paniz of Porto Alegre's CMS was an especially generous resource. In Belo Horizonte, Leonardo Avritzer offered helpful reflections on health-policy-making, and the library of Instituto Cultural Brasil–Estados Unidos always offered a quiet place to write field notes and take stock. My overlapping time in the city with Brian Wampler led to many fruitful discussions. In Rio de Janeiro, many publicly minded scholars, especially Sarah Escorel of Brazil's National School of Public Health/Oswaldo Cruz Foundation (ENSP/FIOCRUZ), Sonia Fleury of the Fundação Getúlio Vargas (FGV), Regina Abreu (UNIRIO), and Guilherme Franco Netto (Health Ministry) have made a treasure trove of interviews with sanitaristas and other archival resources publicly accessible in convenient online formats.

Generous funding from several sources made possible the over two years of fieldwork I undertook for this project. These include support from a National Science Foundation (NSF) grant, a Fulbright Commission of Brazil/International Institute for Education (IIE) research award, and an Inter-American Foundation Fellowship. The American Council of Learned

Societies (ACLS) and the Mellon Foundation provided a generous fellowship. I was also very fortunate that Duke University's Center for Latin American Studies hosted my fellowship in Durham as John French convened a Brazil Working Group that included Alexandre Fortes and Cristiani Vieira Machado, who were giving of their time and thoughts. Brown's Center for Latin American and Caribbean Studies (CLACS), Watson Institute, and NSF-funded Graduate Program in Development (GDP) supported my early fieldwork. Follow-up research and conference travel was funded by Simon Fraser University and Canada's Social Science and Humanities Research Council (SSHRC).

For their feedback on portions of the manuscript and related work, I thank Rebecca Abers, Salo Vinocur Coslovsky, Tulia Falleti, John-Paul Ferguson, Agustina Giraudy, Amir Goldberg, Lucas González, Joseph Harris, Wendy Hunter, Margaret Keck, Matthew Lange, James Mahoney, Ann Mische, Al Montero, Jennifer Pribble, Aruna Ranganathan, Kenneth Roberts, Andrew Shrank, Sarah Soule, Celina Souza, Jocelyn Viterna, and Wendy Wolford. I also benefited from comments on presentations of early findings at Boston University's Department of International Relations, Indiana University's Department of International Studies, McGill University's Department of Sociology, and Stanford University's Graduate School of Business. At Simon Fraser University, many thoughtful colleagues in the School for International Studies encouraged me and read earlier portions of the manuscript, including Onur Bakiner, Jeffrey Checkel, Elizabeth Cooper, Alec Dawson, John Harriss, Andrew Mack, Tamir Moustafa, and Gerardo Otero. Tanner Boisjolie, Anthony Pereira-Costa, and Raied Yahya provided able research assistance. Any errors are mine alone. Portions of chapters 3 and 8 appear in my articles, "The Consequences of Movement Office-Holding for Health Policy Implementation and Social Development in Urban Brazil" (*Social Forces* 96, no. 2: 751–78) and "Programmatic Configurations for the Twenty-First Century Developmental State" (*Sociology of Development*, 42, no. 2: 169–90).

I am extremely grateful for the support and patience that Kate Wahl and Marcela Maxfield, my editors at Stanford University Press, showed for this project. I also thank Olivia Bartz, who helped produce the book. My debt of gratitude to the book's two reviewers, Peter Evans and Sam Cohn, for their extensive and challenging comments is too deep to ever adequately repay. Both generously un-blinded themselves to invite deeper discussions about the book's arguments. Peter returned to Brown after I had left Providence, but his lifetime of rich scholarship inspired the arguments in this book as much as any other single person, and his incisive comments on the manuscript helpfully pushed me to defend and fortify its theoretical claims. And beyond just his infectious passion for the sociology of development, I greatly appreciate Sam's incisive suggestions and entreaty to let the findings do the talking.

I am eternally thankful for my family, who have always been there when I needed them. The love and support of my dad, Laurence, and my sisters, Shannon and Diana, transcends the miles that separate us. I'm sorry that Gayel couldn't see this book come to fruition. Finally, Kathleen Millar, a godsend from another multiverse, changed everything for the better. Her fierce intellect, deep reservoirs of courage, and indefatigable passion stretch what seems humanly possible, and this book never would have materialized without her love and support.

Acronyms and Abbreviations

ABRASCO	*Associação Brasileira de Saúde Coletiva*, Brazilian Public Health Association
ACS	*Agentes Comunitários de Saúde*, Community Health Agents
AIS	*Ações Integradas da Saúde*, Integrated Health Actions
AMC	*Associação Médica Cearense*, Ceará Medical Association
AP	*Ação Popular*, Popular Action
ARENA	*Aliança Renovadora Nacional*, National Alliance for Renewal
BF	*Bolsa Família*, "Family Allowance" Program
CCT	Conditional cash transfer
CEBES	*Centro Brasileiro de Estudos de Saúde*, Brazilian Center for Health Studies
CIMS	*Conselho Intermunicipal de Saúde*, Intermunicipal Health Commission
CLIS	*Conselho Local da Saúde*, Local Health Commission
CLT	*Consolidação das Leis do Trabalho*, Consolidation of Labor Laws
CMC	*Centro Médico Cearense*, Ceará Medical Center
CMR	Childhood mortality rate

CMS	*Conselho Municipal de Saúde*, Municipal Health Council
CNPq	*Conselho Nacional de Desenvolvimento Científico e Tecnológico*, National Council of Scientific and Technological Development
CNS	*Conselho Nacional de Saúde*, National Health Council
CONASEMS	*Conselho Nacional de Secretarias Municipais de Saúde*, National Council of Municipal Health Secretaries
CONASS	*Conselho Nacional de Secretários de Saúde*, National Council of Health Secretaries
CUT	*Central Única dos Trabalhadores*, Central Workers Union
DCE	*Diretório Central dos Estudantes*, Central Student Directorate
DDS	*Departamento de Desenvolvimento Social*, Social Development Department
DEROS	*Departamento de Educação, Recreação e Saúde*, Department of Education, Recreation, and Health
DMP	*Departamento de Medicina Preventiva*, Department of Preventative Medicine
DS	*Diretoria de Saúde*, Health Directorate
FASPES	*Federação das Associações dos Servidores Públicos Estaduais*, Federation of State Civil Servant Associations
FAURGS	*Fundação da Universidade Federal do Rio Grande do Sul*, Federal University of Rio Grande do Sul University Foundation
FCMR	*Fundação do Caetano Munhoz da Rocha*, Caetano Munhoz da Rocha Foundation
FHEMIG	*Fundação Hospitalar do Estado de Minas Gerais*, Hospital Foundation of Minas Gerais
FOPS	*Fórum Popular de Saúde*, Popular Health Forum
GERUS	*Rede Gestão do SUS*, SUS Management Network
GHC	*Grupo Hospitalar Conceição*, Conceição Hospital Group
GPLD	*Gerência do Planejamento e Desenvolvimento*, Division of Planning and Development

IDQ	*Índice de Desenvolvimento de Qualidade dos Serviços,* Index of Service Quality
IMR	Infant mortality rate
INAMPS	*Instituto Nacional de Assistência Médica da Previdência Social,* National Institute for Medical Assistance in Social Security
IPEA	*Instituto de Pesquisa Econômica Aplicada,* Institute of Applied Economic Research
IPEDASAR	*Instituto de Preparo e Pesquisas para o Desenvolvimento da Assistência Sanitária Rural,* Training and Research Institute for the Development of Rural Sanitary Care
IPPUC	*Instituto de Pesquisa e Planejamento Urbano de Curitiba,* Institute for Urban Research and Planning of Curitiba
ISC	*Instituto de Saúde Coletiva,* Public Health Institute
KSSP	*Kerala Sashtra Sahithya Parishad,* People's Science Movement of Kerala
LIBELU	*Liberdade e Luta,* Freedom and Struggle
MDB	*Movimento Democrático Brasileiro,* Brazilian Democratic Movement
MDS	*Ministro de Desenvolvimento Social,* Federal Social Development Ministry
MP	*Ministério Público,* Public Prosecutor's Office
MS	*Ministro da Saúde,* federal health ministry
MS-DAB	*Departamento de Atenção Básica do Ministro da Saúde,* Health Ministry's Basic Attention Department
MST	*Movimento dos Trabalhadores Rurais Sem Terra,* Landless Workers' Movement
NOB	*Norma Operacional Básica,* Basic Operating Norms
OP	*Orçamento Participativo,* Participatory Budgeting
OPAS	*Organização Pan-Americana de Saúde,* Pan-American Health Organization
OS	*Organização de Saúde,* Health Organization

PACS	*Programa Agentes Comunitários de Saúde,* Community Health Agents Program
PAM	*Programa da Assistencia Médica,* urgent-care units
PCB	*Partido Comunista Brasileiro,* Brazilian Communist Party
PC do B	*Partido Comunista do Brasil,* Communist Party of Brazil
PDT	*Partido Democrático Trabalhista,* Democratic Labor Party
PFL	*Partido da Frente Liberal,* Liberal Front Party
PIASS	*Programa de Interiorização das Ações de Saúde e Saneamento,* Internalization of Health and Sanitary Actions
PIQ	*Programa de Incentivo à Qualidade,* Quality Incentive Program
PMC	*Programa Mãe Curitibana,* Curitiban Mother Program
PMDB	*Partido do Movimento Democrático Brasileiro,* Brazilian Democratic Movement Party
PMS	*Partido Mineiro Sanitarista,* Mineiro Sanitarista Party
PNH	*Política Nacional de Humanização,* National Humanization Policy
PSB	*Partido Socialista Brasileiro,* Brazilian Socialist Party
PSDB	*Partido da Social Democracia Brasileira,* Brazilian Social Democracy Party
PSF	*Programa Saúde da Família,* Family Health Program
PT	*Partido dos Trabalhadores,* Workers' Party
PTB	*Partido Trabalhista Brasileiro,* Brazilian Labor Party
PUCPR	*Pontifícia Universidade Católica do Paraná,* Catholic Pontificate University of Paraná
SES	*Secretaria Estadual de Saúde,* State Health Department
SESAC	*Semanas de Estudos sobre Saúde Comunitária,* Community Health Studies Weeks
SESB	*Secretario de Saúde e Bem-Estar,* Secretariat of Health and Well-Being

SINDIBEL	*Sindicato dos Servidores Públicos Municipais*, Municipal Public Service Servants' Union of Belo Horizonte
SINDMÉD	*Sindicato dos Médicos*, Doctors' Union
SINSAÚDE	*Sindicato da Saúde*, Health Workers' Union
SIPSSNM	*Sistema Integrado de Prestação de Serviços do Norte de Minas*, Integrated Health Service Provision System of Northern Minas Gerais
SMS	*Secretaria Municipal de Saúde*, municipal health secretariat
SMSE	*Sistema Municipal de Saúde Escola*, Municipal Health System School
SMSSS	*Secretario Muncipal de Saúde e Serviços Sociais*, Municipal Secretariat of Health and Social Services
SUDS	*Sistema Unificado e Descentralizado de Saúde*, Unified and Decentralized Health System
SUS	*Sistema Único de Saúde*, Unified Health System
TCU-RS	*Tribunal de Contas da União*, Accounts Tribunal of Rio Grande do Sul
TSE	*Tribunal Superior Eleitoral*, Supreme Electoral Court
UAMPA	*União das Associações de Moradores de Porto Alegre*, Neighborhood Association Union of Porto Alegre
UBS	*Unidade Básica de Saúde*, basic health unit
UECE	*Universidade Estadual do Ceará*, State University of Ceará
UESPAR	*Universidade Estadual da Paraná*, State University of Paraná
UFC	*Universidade Federal do Ceará*, Federal University of Ceará
UFMG	*Universidade Federal de Minas Gerias*, Federal University of Minas Gerais
UFPR	*Universidade Federal do Paraná*, Federal University of Paraná
UFRGS	*Universidade Federal do Rio Grande do Sul*, Federal University of Rio Grande do Sul

UFRJ	*Universidade Federal do Rio de Janeiro*, Federal University of Rio de Janeiro
UnB	*Universidade de Brasília*, Brasília University
UNE	*União Nacional dos Estudantes*, National Student Union
US	*Unidade de Saúde*, health unit

Movement-Driven Development

ONE

Subnational Democratization of Health

After returning to democracy and codifying a universal citizenship right to health in the mid-1980s, Brazil witnessed nothing short of a historic transformation in its public health institutions and social development outcomes. During the quarter century following the exit of its military dictatorship from national power, Brazil's largest capital cities recorded an impressive 70% reduction in infant mortality, an achievement that ranks among the most extensive improvements of any large democracy in the Global South.[1] This book argues that the transformation emerged from a locally rooted process of movement-driven development (MDD) in which Brazilian civil-society activists helped to both enshrine the country's universal right to health and reform institutions of the local state in ways that made that right more than just a grandiose, constitutional promise. To do so, these actors weakened an entrenched legacy of patronage-based health-service institutions left behind by the country's erstwhile military dictatorship and its subnational allies, who maintained a formidable presence in local government well after the regime's departure. Ultimately, such efforts rendered municipal governments more responsive to citizens, enhanced the capacities of local states to programmatically deliver basic forms of public health care, and dramatically improved social development outcomes such as infant and child mortality rates.

While this transformation echoes a growing consensus that the very notion of development entails society-wide growth in basic human capabilities,[2] it also highlights how little is known about the kinds of civil society–

state relations that can foster such holistic outcomes in democracies of the Global South. In Brazil, for instance, while marked improvements in infant and child mortality rates clearly reflect expansions in access to basic public health care and a general deepening of democratic accountability, less consensus exists about the specific ways in which elected politicians and civil-society actors have collaborated to maximize growth in such social development outcomes. Complicating matters is the fact that Brazil's 1988 codification of a constitutional right to health left municipal governments within the country's federalist system of multilevel governance with weighty responsibilities to deliver many of the basic public services on which that lofty promise relies. Among other consequences, even Brazil's largest and most important cities varied considerably in the extent of developmental progress they achieved over time. This book aims to explain how and why Brazil experienced such an extraordinary, if subnationally uneven, pattern of social development, despite a recent history of rampant infant mortality and an ignominious reputation as the worldwide champion of inequality.

The study argues that, even amid such adverse conditions, practically minded civil-society actors whom I call "pragmatist publics" have propelled Brazil's developmental strides by making subnational public health agencies more responsive to historically excluded citizens. As Brazil emerged from beneath the shadow of a twenty-one-year military dictatorship, the country's most important public health movement—the Sanitarist Movement (*Movimento Sanitário*)—established an important set of civil-society institutions that became pivotal in their continuing efforts to reform the public health state. Mobilizations by movement activists and veterans with ties to a changing public health profession—known in Brazil as *sanitaristas*—played an outsized role in codifying the new right to health, establishing a new public health system known as the Unified Health System (*Sistema Único de Saúde*, SUS), and founding the new democratic office of the SUS director on all three levels of government. While existing accounts of Brazil's social development transformation note the movement's earlier influence in establishing a right to health and the SUS,[3] they generally attribute later improvements to factors other than ongoing sanitarista control of local democratic offices that emerged alongside the SUS.[4] Yet sanitaristas in many major cities leveraged SUS directorships to advance a highly consequential state-building project that significantly expanded the capacities of municipalities to deliver basic public health services. By successfully demanding subnational SUS directorships with key managerial responsibilities for realizing Brazil's right to health—and by occupying those new offices with remarkable consistency in many cities—sanitaristas helped deepen the practical abilities of local governments to more fully enact that right over time. Ultimately, this quarter century of activism had major implications for social development outcomes throughout the country's largest cities.

More specifically, sanitaristas managed to occupy local SUS directorships to varying extents across urban Brazil, and this variation contributed to uneven degrees of subsequent institutional change and social development in the country's largest cities. Part of encompassing historical pathways of democratization in Brazil's public health sector, consistent subnational office holding by sanitaristas maximized the growth of local public health states with capacities to deliver basic public health care in a programmatic and widespread fashion. Across urban Brazil, cities generally witnessed three distinct trajectories of health democratization that differed according to how fully the local public health sector became accountable to various civil-society actors and institutions. First, through a "participatory-programmatic" trajectory of health democratization in major capitals such as Belo Horizonte, Porto Alegre, and Recife, sanitaristas consistently held key offices atop the subnational public health state, where they capitalized on inconsistently ruling right parties, supportive left-party mayors, and influential popular movements to advocate, design, and execute maximal degrees of municipal state-building for basic health care provision. This pattern led to the construction of state structures that maximized the programmatic delivery of basic public health services and generally remained open to limited oversight of the sector by everyday citizens in participatory democratic institutions such as municipal health councils (CMSs) and Participatory Budgeting (OP).

Second, through a "programmatic" trajectory of health democratization in capitals such as Curitiba and Fortaleza, sanitaristas consistently held key offices atop the subnational public health state, where they capitalized on inconsistently ruling right parties and acquiescent center-party mayors to similarly maximize service-delivery capacities in the primary health sector. Although such cities generally lacked the more deeply democratic monitoring of the sector in the cases just mentioned, office-holding sanitaristas nevertheless mobilized even centrist mayors with few ideological convictions to build roughly similar state capacities for widely and programmatically delivering basic forms of public health care. Finally, amid consistent right-party rule and a continued, dictatorship-era pattern of patronage politics, a "minimalist" trajectory of health democratization in Salvador and Rio de Janeiro saw traditional politicians obstruct sanitaristas from frequently occupying SUS directorships, effectively preventing their state-building ambitions from becoming material realities. This pattern led to a relatively incapacitated local state that lacked the ability to programmatically and widely deliver basic public health services as well as sustained participatory democratic oversight of the sector.

These three trajectories of democratization in the public health sector—participatory-programmatic, programmatic, and minimalist—also help to explain the "robust" or "nonrobust" development outcomes that major capital cities had achieved by the end of the period. The concept of a robust development outcome describes the experience of cities, whose degree of change in development between 1988 and 2014 exceeded what initial development levels at the beginning of the period would have otherwise predicted. Thus, while all cities experienced improvements in development indicators such as infant and child mortality, cities with robust development experienced unexpectedly high degrees of change over time. In all major capitals, these development trajectories reflected both sanitarista efforts to enact a constitutional right to health through local state-building and significant reactions to those efforts from other civil-society and political-society actors. And while national political actors and dynamics conditioned these local politics in nontrivial ways, the variable influence of local sanitaristas and their allies in the face of such reactions helped produce subnationally uneven local state capacities to improve human capabilities across urban Brazil. More specifically, while the outcome of robust development can be traced to both a participatory-programmatic trajectory in Porto Alegre, Belo Horizonte, and Recife and a programmatic trajectory in Curitiba and Fortaleza, the contrasting outcome of nonrobust development in Rio de Janeiro and Salvador emerged from a minimalist trajectory that more clearly echoed Brazil's nondemocratic past. Thus, subnational variations in post-1988 patterns of health democratization help account for major contrasts between the contemporary records of social development achieved throughout Brazil's largest capital cities.

1. Why Study Growth in Public Health and Social Development?

Deeper understandings of Brazil's social development transformation are critical for scholars, policy makers, and citizens interested in understanding the origins of society-wide human well-being and how civil society and democratic governments can foster it over time. Because Brazil witnessed one of the Global South's largest improvements in society-wide health outcomes during recent decades, it presents a theoretical opportunity for explaining a pattern of contemporary social progress that has been both unusual and not fully explored.[5] The project's findings thus offer insights for those interested in the human condition and how it can improve over time as well as for social scientists of inclusive social and health policies, their origins, and their ultimate effects on society-wide health. The book's analysis of subnational cases in Brazil also addresses larger questions about how societies struggling with ingrained inequality and exclusion can overcome patterns of political domination that may otherwise undermine social development and delivery of basic public services.

Few observers anticipated Brazil's impressive developmental strides, which initially drew little interest in an English-language literature on public health and health policy, welfare, and social development that has long emphasized countries of the Global North. Indeed, early analyses of the first decade following Brazil's return to democracy cast the country as a case of largely failed efforts at health care reform (Weyland 1998). Such accounts at first seemed to confirm the diagnosis of Brazil as a country suffering dire and path-dependent institutional and developmental consequences of Portuguese mercantilist colonialism.[6] In addressing years leading up to and including the three decades following Brazil's restoration of formal democracy, however, this book's argument about MDD departs from the expectations of such frameworks, which struggle to fully account for Brazil's twenty-first-century strides in social development. Although subnationally uneven colonial legacies clearly persist across the country,[7] Brazil witnessed marked progress in social development within capital cities of its northeast region such as Fortaleza and Recife, which bear particularly deep scars of colonialism. Thus, explanations are still needed for how and why basic health care provision and social development outcomes improved in such cities despite their longstanding histories of political clientelism and exclusion of most citizens from access to many public services.

Explaining such surprising outcomes also matters for humanistic reasons, because growth in society-wide well-being denotes improvement in what Amartya Sen calls the capability of all people to pursue lives they have good reasons to value (1999). Social scientists of development in the Global South have long been preoccupied with explaining economic dimensions of development using indicators such as GDP per capita that are not always or necessarily tied to society-wide improvements in human welfare. The outcomes examined in this book, however, unambiguously capture expansion in this notion of development as freedom. Declining infant and child mortality rates are clear indicators of what Sen understands to be the master capability of avoiding premature death. Further, the broadening of rights-based access to even basic forms of health care similarly captures the expanded freedom of all individuals seeking to prevent and treat illnesses that would otherwise impede their ability to live lives of their own choosing. Thus, scholars and policy makers of Brazil, Latin America, and the Global South more generally all stand to benefit from understanding the conditions under which such capabilities have improved so dramatically in recent decades. This book offers one such account that places these social development outcomes front and center and examines the conditions under which they have improved the most over time.

Assessing the subnationally uneven growth of such outcomes also sharpens our inferences about what maximizes improvements in public health and social development. Unlike much of the research on health care reform and welfare state programs in advanced industrial democracies of the Global North, work on social and health policies that target low-income populations in the Global South has not often embraced how the local level on which such policies are implemented constitutes a theoretically and analytically important unit on which to appraise their efficacy. Although states and especially municipalities play the leading role in financing and delivering primary health services in multilevel systems of democratic governance such as Brazil's, research on such interventions has tended to treat them homogenously as ones that emanate downward from the national level via wavelike processes of diffusion in which particular qualities of subnational units have little relevance.[8] Such approaches may conceal both significant local variations in public health and development outcomes as well as potential clues about what has caused such deviations. They may also miss an opportunity to forge deeper understandings of the subnational conditions under which the municipalities that hold chief responsibility for enacting a nationwide right to health can maximize the provision of public services that bring such lofty promises closer to material fruition. Knowing the diverse ways that municipalities attempt to ensure such rights to even basic forms of health care, how effective these interventions have been in improving actual health outcomes, and why and how some major capital cities have devised more effective ways of delivering such services than others is all fundamental for illuminating the politics of rights-based social policies and their human consequences. Subnational analysis is also particularly well suited to answering broader questions about government effectiveness in democratic settings and the conditions under which social movements with a nationwide presence can best advance such efforts locally. This book contributes to such pursuits.

Additionally, improved access to health care and social development in Brazil has important implications for our understanding of democratic politics and its local rhythms. The country's expansion of rights-based provision of basic public health care shows how local states have forged stronger ties of accountability to sizable majorities of the citizenry that were previously excluded from accessing such services. And beyond just these improved patterns of access to services, new public responsibilities of SUS managers arose alongside participatory democratic institutions such as municipal health councils (CMSs) that assumed comanagement authorities for the health sector and opened new spaces for citizens to express their voices and participate in health-policy-making. For any country in the Global South, much less one emerging from beneath the shadow of a decades-long military dictatorship, such transformations not only represent impressive policy accomplishments but also show that history need not become fate. Still, this remarkable trajectory of progressive social change points to key unanswered questions about their origins. What kinds of state-society configurations can maximize social development outcomes such as access to public health services and the reduction of premature death? What, if any, forms of civil-society mobilization are most likely to have concrete consequences for health-policy enactment and social development expansion?

2. *Alternative Explanations*

Existing scholarship offers several plausible, alternative explanations for Brazil's social development transformation in recent decades. Although theoretical frameworks of state-directed development, power constellations, and policy diffusion all emphasize political-society and state actors to a greater extent than does this book's explanation of MDD, such alternative explanations contribute much to the understanding of Brazilian development and cannot be dismissed out of hand. This study argues, however, that such existing accounts offer, at best, an incomplete basis for explaining changes in development and institutions throughout contemporary, urban Brazil, in part because fuller understandings of civil-society agency are needed to assess whether and how they can inform such processes.

Before individually addressing alternative explanations, two salient points about this study's theorized explanation of MDD merit emphasis here. First, the study focuses on a meso-level of generality that highlights major capital cities as especially relevant political units of analysis within the vast and heterogeneous geography, population, and society that is contemporary Brazil. Serving as important hubs within major cities that comprise approximately one-third of Brazil's more than 210 million people, these large capitals constitute a sizable and substantively relevant sample of comparable units in a country in which 86% of residents live in urban areas.⁹ As such, this approach complements both macrolevel studies that usefully cast Brazil in a cross-national light but risk homogenizing its internally heterogeneous subnational politics and society as well as microlevel studies that illuminate relevant processes within one or a few subnational cases but struggle to speak capably about Brazil as a whole. The former approach risks compromising internal validity by systematically overlooking Brazil's internally diverse record of development and institutional change, reifying the country's heterogeneous local politics, masking subnational drivers of its recent progress, and correspondingly misidentifying sources of these recent shifts. The latter approach provides compelling explanations for one or a few cities or states, but it provides an inadequate basis for generalizing about the country as a whole. By contrast, this study rejects efforts to assess the entire country based on one or a few similar cases of cities or states, and it eschews both single case-studies of cities or states that struggle to inform the understanding of countrywide dynamics and national-level studies that— especially in a country of continental size such as Brazil, with many and diverse subnational units—can suffer from "whole-nation bias" (Snyder 2001). Second, the study rejects both voluntarist and overly structural accounts that prove similarly incomplete for explaining institutional change and development in contemporary, urban Brazil. It instead seeks to reconcile historically focused arguments about the path-dependent legacies of prior eras alongside alternative theoretical perspectives and growing empirical evidence about the nontrivial roles of civil-society actors in profoundly transforming Brazilian society more recently. In doing so, the study not only rejects voluntarist approaches that risk romanticizing and exaggerating the agency of political- and civil-society actors but also aims to rethink the nature of political agency in a context for which scholars have offered path-dependent explanations emphasizing structural reproduction of institutions created during distant historical periods. Although these longer-term structural impediments figure into the analysis that follows, they will be framed within a larger context alongside more recent civil-society agents who have mediated these distant historical influences in nontrivial ways.

2.1. STATE-DIRECTED DEVELOPMENT AND ECONOMIC GROWTH

Crystallized through impressive studies by brilliant scholars such as Atul Kohli and Lant Pritchett, expectations drawn from the distinct "state-directed development" and "wealthier is healthier" paradigms similarly struggle to explain Brazil's social development improvements. Although not crafted to explain social development outcomes per se, state-directed development theories emphasize the cohesive state structures that (typically authoritarian) political leaders constructed to promote twentieth-century economic development (Kohli 2004). The technical capacities of such state structures to execute the goals of political leaders at their apex have sometimes been linked with surprising reductions in infant mortality rates (IMR) such as those facilitated by decidedly illiberal dictators like Chile's Augusto Pinochet (McGuire 2010). Nevertheless, this framework's focus on illiberal rulers as drivers of change offers little insight into Brazil's social development transformations, which instead arose from a more democratic mode of state-society relations that originated amid the departure of its dictatorship. Indeed, sanitarista visions of an equal and universal citizenship right to health were anathema to a military regime (1964–1985) that had solidified a patronage-fueled health sector that systematically excluded the vast majority of the country's population from access to basic health services. Also molded by an earlier era of generally illiberal, corporatist rule by President Getúlio Vargas (1930–1945, 1951–1954), the health sector reflected Brazil's larger, Bismarckian social-policy regime, which replicated such exclusion in most other public-service sectors. Even as Brazil returned to democracy in the 1980s, the legacies of these eras lingered in the form of traditional subnational politicians, who typically hesitated to establish new state institutions for free public provision of basic public services such as primary health care. In sum, where sanitaristas and other progressive actors managed to construct new state capacities to deliver such care as a citizenship right to health, they typically did so despite the locally ruling patronage politicians and conservative economic forces that marked Brazil's illiberal era of state-led development.

Scholars have also argued for the beneficial effects that economic growth can have on social development indicators such as IMR. As the "wealthier is healthier" hypothesis goes,[10] the improvement of average household income during the period that I examine should have improved the access of poor Brazilians to better nutrition, health care, running water, sewage, sanitation, and other established vectors of IMR reduction. Nevertheless, the unequal distribution and timing of that economic growth makes this hypothesis considerably less persuasive for the Brazilian context. Scholars have suggested that Brazil's impressive social development strides since democratization are not attributable to economic growth alone, which was tepid during and immediately before the 1985 to 2002 period in which IMR improved the most.[11] And because a consistently high IMR during Brazil's dictatorship coincided with a period of considerable economic growth, it is difficult to argue that industrialization or per capita growth in GDP can account for social development outcomes during that earlier period or the contemporary one examined in this book. Further, the statistical analysis presented in chapter 3 finds no strong, statistically significant effect of per capita income on IMR levels in Brazil's largest capitals. This raises the question of how much the benefits of economic growth extended to poorer segments of the population, which remained exposed to disproportionately high epidemiological risks that exacerbate childhood mortality. At a minimum, this study offers no evidence that urban social development is exclusively traceable to economic growth.

2.2. POLICY DIFFUSION, NETWORKS, BUREAUCRATS, AND PROFESSIONALS

The study's account of MDD describes a mechanism of institutional change that also contrasts with those articulated by policy diffusion accounts and other approaches that similarly de-emphasize the solidary underpinnings and outward civil orientations of Brazil's sanitaristas. In conventional diffusion frameworks, outcomes like those examined in this study are posited to emerge from a wavelike spread of generally homogeneous "policy models" throughout units that share certain features. For example, Natasha Borges Sugiyama (2012) cogently argues that the presence of a local sanitarista network in a given city accounts for governments' adoption of Brazil's flagship primary public-health-care program, the Family Health Program (PSF). Nevertheless, the diffusion frameworks underlying such analyses have been persuasively criticized for overlooking the reactivity, adaptation, and reinvention that typically occurs in the interplay between somewhat malleable policy templates and the heterogeneous political units that seek to enact place-specific variants of them (Chorev 2012). The application of such a framework to the Brazilian public health sector is further confounded by evidence suggesting that local-actor configurations have transformed and adapted developmentally beneficial programs like the PSF to operate differently in different municipal contexts and have supplemented them with other platforms for primary public-health-care delivery.[12] In addition to other theoretical limitations addressed in chapter 2, the framework offers little analytic leverage for explaining subnational variation across the sample of all major Brazilian capitals examined by this study because all of these cities featured sanitarista networks but only some experienced maximal degrees of institutional change and development.

To more fully account for considerable variation in local institutional change and development across a sample of major cities that exhibits no substantial variation in the mere presence of a sanitarista network, this project pursues another approach that instead examines the *conditions under which* such actors can matter for similar outcomes. Results suggest that it is not merely the presence of sanitaristas in a local context, or just their intra-institutional mobilizations within national politics, but their consistent office holding atop the subnational public health state that maximized institutional change and social development outcomes. Further, such outcomes are not attributable to any mechanistic adoption or downward dissemination of nationally formulated policies throughout the variable, subnational political contexts that constitute Brazil's highly decentralized federalist democracy. Instead, it was these actors' occupations of local state offices that maximally transformed local state institutions and constructed the otherwise missing local state capacities required to reformulate and adapt those programs to best fit local, heterogeneous circumstances.

2.3. POWER CONSTELLATIONS

The book's argument about MDD also addresses explanatory limitations of the power constellations framework, which posits that enduring experiences of democracy and nationally ruling left parties can lead to crystallization of redistributive social policy in the Global South.[13] The framework struggles to explain how in Brazil's relatively young democracy, the centrist presidential administration of President Fernando Henrique Cardoso introduced health programs such as the PSF well before national rule by more left-leaning PT members. The theory of MDD better fits Brazil's experience by highlighting how pragmatist publics helped create this program as well as a preexisting architecture of subnational democratic offices that built the local state capacities needed to maximize the program's reach and effectiveness. Indeed, the case studies in this book show how sanitaristas sometimes mobilized the support of centrist subnational executives who were otherwise uninterested in such programs. In doing so, they also created essential capacities of the local state for enacting nationwide CCT programs such as Bolsa Família (BF), which are sometimes credited as a sole product of nationally left-leaning political parties. By building local infrastructure such as basic health clinics and by meritocratically hiring the staff needed to maximally expand the PSF, these activists have also indirectly facilitated expansion of BF, which typically depends on the PSF to deliver the basic health services that its beneficiaries must access in order to meet the program's conditionalities. Thus, although left-leaning executives in national politics can and have introduced CCTs, the notion of MDD complements power constellations frameworks by showing that the ability of such programs to operate effectively has depended in part on pragmatist publics to help build the very local state capacities on which CCTs rely. Indeed, pragmatist publics have often mobilized such support of political society in the first place, both among left-leaning executives and a wider ideological spectrum of subnational executives.

3. Movement-Driven Development (MDD) and Pragmatist Publics

In answering how and why, after decades of underperformance, social development grew so much and so unevenly throughout contemporary urban Brazil, this study's MDD framework stresses how particular kinds of civil-society actors can propel the democratic state-building needed to realize ideologies of universal and equal rights. Across the country's largest capital cities, maximal gains in social development outcomes occurred when such activists more consistently occupied and leveraged new democratic offices in ways that transformed the ideology of a universal and equal citizenship right to health into material capacities of the subnational public health state to programmatically deliver basic public services. Although MDD entailed disruption of prior monopolies on local power by clientelist parties of the far right, it also featured activists who created new democratic offices atop the local public health state and wielded them to build stronger capacities for practically advancing a citizenship right to health. Epitomized by Brazil's sanitaristas and conceptualized more deeply in this book, pragmatist publics construct and wield civil-society institutions such as democratic offices to advance their solidary projects, and they adopt a self-consciously Gramscian (2000) approach to occupying trenches of the state, where they combine Deweyan (2012) approaches to public problem-solving with the use of what I call social code-switching to mobilize politicians' support for subtle material expressions of their universalistic ideologies. When local democracies exhibit these two conditions—both an infrequency of monopolistic control over the subnational executive by clientelist parties of the far right and pragmatist publics' consistent occupation of democratic offices that oversee public-service bureaucracies—they are more likely to maximize social development improvements over time.

While such dynamics of MDD thus build on a foundation of formal democracy, they revolve around pragmatist publics that not only transform universalistic ideologies into constitutional and legal responsibilities of states but also establish and control new democratic offices with direct lines of accountability for enacting those responsibilities through state-building. The framework therefore proposes that Brazil's development transformation emerged from far more than just nationwide qualities of democratization such as the restoration of competitive elections. Related, nationwide processes—especially the legal codification of a state responsibility for enacting Brazil's citizenship right to health and the tasking of a new SUS director's office with the authority for doing so (Federal Republic of Brazil 1990a, 1990b)—would all have been unlikely without sustained advocacy by Sanitarist Movement activists. Furthermore, by occupying and wielding municipal and state offices of the SUS director, sanitarista advocacy on the subnational level helped to materially advance otherwise abstract constitutional principles of equity and universality. Yet these efforts were more successful in some major cities than in others, and such unevenness had major practical consequences for access to basic forms of health care and for health outcomes more generally. Particularly consequential was how consistently activists held and leveraged the SUS directorship to expand three key state capacities: meritocratically recruited and well-trained public health workers, primary public health clinics, and tools for systematically targeting both workers and clinics to city regions whose residents faced the direst threats of premature death. Where they more consistently held such offices over time, sanitaristas generally maximized provision of primary public health care to previously excluded groups and disproportionately improved social development outcomes such as infant and child mortality rates. The historical evolution of sanitarista agency thus epitomizes how pragmatist publics can meaningfully contribute to overarching processes of democratization and social development.

MDD in urban Brazil unfolded over time through three distinct pathways of health democratization, whose locally variable incarnations had major implications for social development outcomes. In negative cases of nonrobust social development such as Salvador and Rio de Janeiro, a "minimalist" variant of health democratization was insufficient to maximize improvements in public-health-care delivery and IMR reduction because pragmatist publics failed to overcome local clientelist elites' insulation of the subnational public health state from reform pressures. In all positive cases of robust development, by contrast, pragmatist publics animated one of two "programmatic" variants of health democratization in which they more consistently wielded those offices to reform state health agencies and hold them more accountable to their public mandates and responsibilities as guarantors of a universal right to health. Ultimately, this programmatic pattern of health democratization maximized public-service-oriented statebuilding, actual delivery of primary public health care, and growth in social development over time. In positive cases such as Belo Horizonte, Porto Alegre, and Recife, this pattern coincided with a distinct "participatory" dimension of health democratization that yielded more inclusive venues in which everyday citizens could monitor the local public health state, but these cities' robust development outcomes are better explained by state-building processes that are instead traceable to the programmatic dimension of health democratization. Other positive cases of robust growth in social development such as Curitiba and Fortaleza—where subnational public health states were transformed by a programmatic dimension of health democratization despite a relative absence of the participatory dimension witnessed in Belo Horizonte, Porto Alegre, and Recife—reinforce this point by showing that even a nonparticipatory trajectory of health democratization was sufficient for maximizing social development progress across contemporary urban Brazil if office-holding sanitaristas were able to impart that path with a programmatic orientation to state-building.

Thus, beyond just mobilizing extra-institutionally to codify their universalistic ideologies into constitutions, laws, and policies, Brazil's sanitaristas exemplify how pragmatist publics also establish and occupy democratic offices accountable for enacting those commitments. After their watershed victories in codifying a constitutional right to health, for example, sanitaristas continued mobilizing for nearly three decades to transform this vision of a citizenship right to health into tangible practices of Brazil's local public health state. An underappreciated dimension of this process was how sanitaristas created and then occupied the new subnational democratic office of the SUS director in major capital cities across the country. The mere creation of the office concentrated sanitaristas' powers to expand the subnational public health state, which considerably influenced nationwide development outcomes as municipal governments became responsible for ensuring access to the most basic public health services. Sanitaristas also mounted subsequent campaigns to occupy and wield the subnational office of SUS manager across urban Brazil. Although their success in doing so varied across cities and drew on their reputations in wide-ranging professions of public health and medicine as well as their practical skills in statecraft, it also depended on a subtler but similarly decisive factor: their identities as civil-society activists and social-movement veterans. During the thirty years following Brazil's return to democracy, the way that sanitaristas embedded their universalizing, equity-focused visions of a right to health within public-service institutions of the subnational state depended on these movement lineages more than existing accounts allow for. As such, they exemplify how pragmatist publics can leverage their civil-society identities and associations to cultivate society-wide solidarities around universalizing notions of the public good. Yet a deeper conceptualization of these actors is necessary to grasp the mechanisms through which they can influence the state-society politics of public health and social development.

3.1. CIVIL SOCIETY, STATE-SOCIETY RELATIONS,
AND PRAGMATIST PUBLICS AS AGENTS OF MDD

If dynamics of MDD entailed the pursuit of a new and distinctively programmatic mode of democratic governance in Brazil's public health sector, an only partially understood transformation in civil society–state relations precipitated this shift. While this transformation involved the rise of prodemocracy activists who hastened the exit of Brazil's military dictatorship from power, the relationship of these and other civil-society activists to political society remains a topic of unresolved debate. The decades-long advocacy of sanitaristas in Brazil's state-society politics of public health, however, suggests that subnationally mobilized activists with distinctive identities and roots in civil society animated this shift in largely overlooked ways. Heightened democracy in Brazil's state-society politics of health was thus the sole product neither of the electoral incentives of political elites to accommodate civil-society demands for policy expansion nor of any agentless process of policy diffusion in which civil-society networks served as mere nodes. Rather, democratization of these politics reflected precocious and consistent (but subnationally variable) efforts by such activists to mobilize political-society actors around solidary norms of universality and equality emanating from civil society itself. In short, understanding Brazil's process of MDD requires attention to how activists mobilized political society around solidary norms of civil society, despite the distinct emphasis in existing literature on political-society actors as prime animator of this process.

Furthermore, explaining the contributions of Brazil's sanitaristas to this shift requires a different conceptualization of civil society than exemplary research on related topics can offer, and this study's notion of pragmatist public offers one such account. Studies of Brazilian local democracy often stress involvement by everyday citizens whom Avritzer (2002, 2009) calls "participatory publics" for their public decision-making roles in deliberative democratic institutions such as OP and the CMS.[14] Such actors have also been cited as the central protagonists of "encompassing embeddedness," a mode of civil society–state relations with considerable potential to generate capability-focused, twenty-first-century analogs of the developmental states that were so essential for twentieth-century economic growth.[15] This book complementarily suggests that pragmatist publics represent a distinct type of actor, who can nevertheless cultivate encompassing embeddedness through less radically inclusive and less participatory channels of democratic activism. Pragmatist publics' unique sources of agency in state-society politics flow partly from their membership in voluntary civil-society institutions and networks, as standard definitions of civil society highlight. But their efforts to remake state institutions in the image of their solidary, rights-based ideologies can have long-lasting relevance for their activism and the purposes they envision for it. Although voluntary and associative qualities of sanitarista agency were baseline prerequisites for how sanitaristas framed and implemented Brazil's constitutional right to health, this generic quality of all civil societies sheds less light on how and why these activists' multidecade span of activism endured and became as consequential as it did. Voluntary qualities of civil-society activism may well explain more about the efficacy of activism for universalistic ideologies in countries of the Global North, where enduring democratic traditions of universal and equal citizenship offer preexisting normative and legal reference points for civil-society demands to institute social policies for realizing such commitments. Brazil, however, lacked any similarly time-tested traditions when sanitaristas began demanding a universal and equal right to health, leaving them with no such beneficial legal or normative landscape to serve as a flash point. Indeed, scholars have persuasively shown that Brazilian civil societies instead confronted a hostile, preexisting political culture that prioritized rights of privileged social groups and devalued individual rights and freedoms typically associated with liberal and social democratic understandings of citizenship (Baiocchi 2006; Holston 2008). Even against such hostile backdrops, however, pragmatist publics frame demands for universal and equal rights within communicative institutions of civil society that can help sustain struggles to establish more receptive, democratic contexts over the long-term.

The concept of a pragmatist public informs how this can occur within otherwise hostile, weakly institutionalized contexts of democracy by calling attention to more than just the generic qualities they share with all civil societies. First, pragmatist publics mobilize around radically inclusive ideologies that are rooted in civil society, which Jeffrey C. Alexander usefully specifies as "a solidary sphere, in which a certain kind of universalizing community comes to be culturally defined and to some degree institutionally enforced" (2006, 31). Pragmatist publics mirror civil-society actors more generally in that their sources of influence in state-society politics flow from more than just norms, practices, and institutions of voluntary life alone. Far from the voluntary but self-referential groups (for example, bowling leagues) highlighted in the research of scholars like Robert Putnam (2000), pragmatist publics instead exhibit Tocqueville's oft-overlooked but central quality of civil society as defined "by an orientation to wider solidarity, not the act of associating per se" (Alexander 2006, 99). Throughout nearly a half century of activism straddling both authoritarian and democratic political regimes, sanitaristas have exemplified this quality in how they aimed to build society-wide solidarities around a core, universalizing ideology of all Brazilians as a community of rights-bearing citizens with equal entitlements to health and state-ensured public health services. Beyond just motivating a remarkable generation of sanitaristas to continually advocate for a right to health, the universalistic, society-wide scope of this ideology contributed an overlooked normative weight to these efforts. Further, this normative resonance was not reducible to these actors' separate technical competencies as public health experts, the social prestige of many as doctors, or their connectedness with public-health-focused policy networks of politicians and bureaucrats. As standard-bearers for solidary projects of a universalistic scope, pragmatist publics maintain publicly recognized identities that endow them with considerable normative power to animate state-society politics.

Second, pragmatist publics mirror other civil-society actors in their efforts to mold regulative institutions such as constitutions, laws, and democratic offices and to wield them to invade and infuse noncivil spheres like state agencies with such solidary norms of universality and equality. Brazil's sanitaristas exemplify this quality in how they helped draft articles of the country's Constitution and Organic Health Laws that both enshrined their own framing of a citizenship right to health and established a new public responsibility of the state to ensure that right (Federal Republic of Brazil 1988, 1990a, 1990b). As such, sanitaristas went beyond merely using communicative institutions such as their associations to propagate and advocate for a right to health in the public sphere. Leveraging these associations and the growing public opinion regarding the need for state interventions to redress deficient and unequal access to health care, they managed to further enshrine these rights and responsibilities into major regulative institutions of Brazilian civil society, none more pivotal than the country's Constitution, federal laws, and its public health system (the SUS). Less noted in existing accounts, however, is how this created another, pivotal regulative institution— the office of the SUS director (*gestor do SUS*)—atop all three (federal, state, and municipal) levels of the public health state. The way in which the SUS directorship became not just a normative authority but also a legally accountable, democratic office for enacting the country's new right to health is a more idiosyncratic quality of pragmatist publics that I return to later. Yet this effort to create a set of regulative institutions that hold sway over both state structures and economically dominant social groups in the name of civil society is itself a quality that pragmatist publics share with nearly all civil societies.

The advocacy of pragmatist publics for solidary values and norms of equality and universality, as opposed to narrower and more particularistic group interests, nevertheless differentiates them from more canonical ways of defining civil-society actors. For instance, their efforts to render state agencies accountable to regulative institutions of civil society might at first seem to resemble Gramscian (2000) wars of position since they similarly invade the state in order to reorient its structures around a distinct, counterhegemonic ideology. To be sure, pragmatist publics commonly orchestrate intra-institutional episodes of mobilization in which they seek to personally capture and wield regulative institutions such as democratic office. But even when activists describe their own efforts to do so in self-consciously Gramscian terms of counterhegemony (as Brazilian sanitaristas often characterize their advocacy for health reform), analytically reducing these struggles to wars of position overlooks how the universalistic, solidary ideologies at their core go far beyond what Gramsci could have envisioned civil-society actors advancing. In part because Gramsci understood civil society as inherently capitalist and far afield from democratic government, he remained skeptical that counterhegemonic wars of position could go beyond one particularistic social group manufacturing the consent of others for its own narrow interests. This precluded Gramsci from conceptualizing how civil society could foster an "institutionalizing solidarity of a more universalistic kind," or translate it into government control, as Alexander's concept of "civil power" (2006, 29, 110, 150) suggests is possible.

By shifting the terrain of their struggles from communicative to regulative institutions of civil society such as constitutions, law, and democratic offices—and especially by using such regulative institutions to render actual state agencies more capable of pursuing universalistic, solidary ideologies—the mobilizations of pragmatist publics qualitatively differ from the counterhegemonic actors of Gramscian theory, who instead aim to leverage their positions within noncivil spheres like class-based organizations, professions, and the state to foster their own particularistic interests. As such, the ideologically infused and universally oriented arguments that pragmatist publics make at the state-society interface of politics can themselves exert a normative weight that fundamentally differs from other sources of power such as technical expertise, the forceful manufacturing of consent, or the exertion of class power.

Third, and a quality more endemic to pragmatist publics, is a thoroughgoing pragmatism in how they leverage regulative institutions of civil society to advance their universalizing ideologies through state-building. Pragmatist publics seek to marshal civil-society institutions such as laws, constitutions, and democratic offices to iteratively construct missing state capacities, whose absence otherwise impedes the material enactment of solidary ideologies. In this respect, pragmatist publics are democrats at their core, but they are also state-builders and reformers capable of mounting cumulative struggles that endure over surprisingly long periods. Deepened by persistent deficits of state capacity in newer and more weakly institutionalized democracies of the Global South such as Brazil's, this state-building impulse exposes constraints within theories of civil society that were developed solely with longstanding democracies of the Global North in mind. Although materially enacting positive citizenship rights like a right to health typically requires considerable government intervention in nearly any democratic context, an almost defining feature of many democracies in the Global South is a persistent lack of the state capacities needed for such interventions to succeed.[16] Such bottlenecks in capacity commonly induce civil-society actors to revise how they pursue their solidary goals because, even when such goals become formally codified into constitutions and laws, their subsequent execution by state agencies can rarely be assumed. Among other effects, this fosters civil societies that exert their normative authority as advocates for legally enshrined solidary goals via state-building interventions that can bring those goals closer to material fruition.

To be sure, pragmatist publics may orchestrate such state-building efforts from atop bureaucratic agencies or professions that offer technical expertise relevant for the tasks at hand. Yet, in the eyes of both citizens and political elites, their grounding within communicative institutions such as associations ultimately bolsters their normative legitimacy as appropriate occupants of regulative institutions, especially when the regulative institutions concerned are democratic offices with legitimate authority and a public responsibility for enacting their legally enshrined solidary goals.

Pragmatist publics thus exhibit a brand of problem-solving more often thought to animate communicative institutions of civil society such as associations rather than regulative institutions such as the democratic offices that hold public responsibility for overseeing state agencies. Such problem-solving mirrors what John Dewey argued in *The Public and Its Problems* ([1927] 2012) were the efforts of publics to collectively address the practical consequences of social problems through sustained processes of communication and experimentation that treat their solutions as iterative works in progress. Yet Dewey largely envisioned such processes taking place in the realm of communicative institutions such as associations operating beyond the reach of powerful social actors and interests that he suggested would dominate the state and statecraft itself. Although they exhibit similar problem-solving orientations as Deweyan publics, pragmatist publics are distinct in their additional pursuit of such approaches through statecraft itself and the piecemeal elaboration of regulative institutions that continually facilitate ongoing iterations of state-building. Yet conceptualizing how pragmatist publics wage Gramscian wars of position to mobilize politicians who trade in the currency of political power requires supplementing Dewey's understanding of public problem-solving and Alexander's notion of civil power with an account of how these actors leverage their own locations within social hierarchies to advance universalizing ideologies.

Pragmatist publics do so through a fourth quality that I term social code-switching. As coined by communications scholars and linguistic anthropologists, the notion of code-switching describes how interlocutors alternate between and intermix multiple languages to create shared, multivalent meanings that are not fully recognizable to those fluent in only one of those languages (Auer 1998; Gardner-Chloros 2009). In describing how pragmatist publics engage politicians at the state-society interface, the notion of social code-switching revises and adapts this concept for the higher level of abstraction on which macrosociologists examine political dynamics. Through social code-switching, activists who occupy privileged social locations within class and professional structures can mobilize dominant actors in these noncivil spheres around solidary projects and ideologies that they are otherwise unlikely to support as fully, if at all. Pragmatist publics accomplish this by employing and intermixing the distinct, value-laden languages of both civil and noncivil spheres to mobilize dominant, noncivil actors around discreet projects that satisfy their interests in narrower objectives while simultaneously generating material expressions of universalistic ideologies and norms emerging from civil society. By leveraging their favored positions within class, occupational, and political-party hierarchies—and by applying their corresponding fluency in the lingua franca of such noncivil spheres—pragmatist publics appeal to the narrower interests of dominant, noncivil actors in ways that simultaneously create subtle but unmistakable material expressions of universalistic ideologies. Capitalizing on their social prestige and positions atop Brazil's professional-class structure during Brazil's dictatorship, for example, sanitaristas stealthily mobilized even authoritarian state managers to support projects that materially advanced their core ideology of a universal citizenship right to health, even though such authorities otherwise rejected that ideology as dangerous and subversive to their own grip on political power in the country. In securing political elites' support for discrete state-building projects in the public health sector, sanitaristas advocated for these projects using a narrower language of efficacy in reaching historically excluded groups, a language that cohered to these managers' interests in expanding public-service provision as a means for increasing social control over a sprawling country of continental size.

Although their privileged social positions render them more proximate to political elites whom they aim to influence, fluency in the value-laden language of such spheres equips them to frame arguments in terms that elites are more likely to view favorably, even when their proposals aim to materialize potentially subversive ideologies and norms of civil society. As such, pragmatist publics' use of code-switching expands on Baiocchi's (2006) argument that individual-oriented codes of liberty can coexist alongside nonindividualistic and illiberal codes, inciting struggles among and between civil-society and political-society actors to establish the dominance of one system over the other. Through code-switching, pragmatist publics establish more influential positions for universalistic goals and norms within state institutions in a process that Brazilian sanitaristas often compare to the installation of a Trojan horse inside the gates of the state (L. Barcelos and M. L. Jaeger, interviews, 2010; Rodrigues Neto, Gomes Temporão, and Escorel 2003). Furthermore, the code-switching efforts of pragmatist publics suggest that civil-society actors can advance values and ideologies favored in liberal codes without depending solely on deliberative or participatory democratic institutions. Indeed, pragmatist publics craft targeted arguments for political elites in ways that contradict Habermas's (1981) understanding of civil society as a realm of communicative action characterized by reason-based argumentation among actors with sincere commitments to deliberation. Through code-switching, pragmatist publics instead crystallize arguments that placate these elites' narrower goals while simultaneously advancing solidary norms and ideologies grounded in civil society. Chapter 2 expands on them in greater detail, but such qualities of pragmatist publics help account for the outsized and sustained influence of sanitaristas in democratizing access to health and improving social development across urban Brazil.

4. Mixed-Methods Research Design, Cases, and Data

By integrating statistical, fuzzy-set, and comparative-historical case-study analysis of Brazil's largest capital cities, this study offers the most comprehensive assessment to date of the country's dramatic but subnationally uneven reduction of IMR and growth in access to basic public health care between 1985 and 2014. By integrating these three analytic approaches to assess original data collected during more than two years of fieldwork in Brazil, the study both systematically tests alternative explanations of these outcomes and offers evidence to substantiate a new theory of how pragmatist publics can animate MDD processes and foster the expansion of human capabilities. First, multivariate regression analyses of a unique, cross-sectional time-series (CSTS) data set show that, even after controlling for alternative explanations, sanitarista office holding in the municipal SUS directorship was negatively associated with IMR and childhood (under five years old) mortality rates (CMR) and positively associated with rates of access to primary public health care across urban Brazil. Then, fuzzy-set analyses (FSA) deepen this finding by showing that consistent sanitarista office holding was a necessary condition within a configuration of factors that was sufficient across urban Brazil to maximize improvement in three outcomes over time: IMR reduction, growth in municipal spending on the public health and sanitation sectors, and coverage of the PSF (Brazil's flagship primary public-health-care program). The study then complements these statistical and configurational findings with a comparative-historical case-study analysis that traces these outcomes to two sanitarista-driven pathways of MDD: a participatory-programmatic variant of health democratization in Belo Horizonte and Porto Alegre and a programmatic variant in Curitiba and Fortaleza. This empirical evidence is based on original measures of office holding by pragmatist publics and of social development outcomes as well as on archival research, in-depth interviews with key informants, and participant observations of health-policy-making processes.

In part because other explanations have been proposed for Brazil's transformation in social development, chapter 3 begins the book's empirical analysis with systematic testing of alternative accounts alongside this book's theory of MDD using an original data set of annual observations between 1995 to 2014 for all eleven Brazilian capitals with more than one million residents. The first stage of analysis on this data set uses a statistical approach often applied by scholars of national and subnational social policy in Latin America (Huber and Stephens 2012, Niedzwiecki 2016): Prais-Winsten regression analyses with panel-corrected standard errors (PCSE) and autoregressive (ar1) disturbance terms. One set of regressions demonstrates that sanitarista office holding in the municipal SUS directorship was negatively associated with infant and child mortality rates in the country's largest capital cities, even after controlling for alternative explanations and controls. Additional analysis shows that sanitarista office holding had a positive net effect on both the rate of public-health-care delivery to the uninsured population and the coverage rate of the PSF. But to more fully examine this project's configurational expectations about MDD, it is necessary to draw on additional methods that explicitly model interactions between sanitarista office holding and multiple other factors that regression models somewhat unrealistically hold constant and assume to work in isolation from one another. The second stage of analysis does this using FSA models (Longest and Vaisey 2008; Ragin 2008) of the complex interactions between pragmatist publics and other factors as well as of the effects of these interactions on social development outcomes.

This mixed-methods approach aims to complement several excellent studies of social development in contemporary Brazil. These include studies examining outcomes such as health-service provision but not actual health outcomes (Borges Sugiyama 2012), the evolution of health-related development outcomes on a nationwide basis (Falleti 2010a; McGuire 2010), and large-N analyses of well-being across Brazilian municipalities whose statistical approach nevertheless struggles to assess causation (Touchton, Borges Sugiyama, and Wampler 2017). To better address questions raised in this book, this study combines statistical and fuzzy-set analysis of Brazil's eleven largest cities with a third method: comparative-historical analysis (CHA) of four city-level case studies that qualitatively examine the mechanism through which pragmatist publics contributed to robust development outcomes during three decades following Brazil's gradual return to democracy. This combination of within-case longitudinal analysis of individual cases and statistical and systematic comparative analysis of multiple cities enables a comprehensive consideration of potential factors underlying social development and allows for elaboration of new theory.

Each city-level case study employs process tracing (Bennett and Checkel 2015) of the state-building processes that led to major improvements in primary public-health-care delivery and IMR reduction as well as of instances of ineffective attempts to expand the reach of such services. By presenting detailed evidence on the local state-building processes that allowed city governments to become more capable providers of primary public health care, meticulous process tracing helps identify the causal mechanisms that precipitated robust development outcomes. It can thus also be used to assess evidence for alternative explanations of robust development outcomes by generating credible and detailed information on factors that fall short of influencing such state-building processes. By integrating this process-tracing approach to within-case analysis with systematic comparison, CHA places front and center the temporal dynamics (Mahoney and Thelen 2015) that affect local state-building for health and development. CHA allows for credible estimation of the duration of time lags between pragmatist publics' office-holding episodes and their contributions to state-building and the ways in which those lags can have consequences for IMR reduction. It also permits greater attention to how longer and more consistent episodes allow pragmatist publics to accumulate power in unforeseen ways. This book's analysis relies on original data collected from multiple sources that chapter 3 describes in greater detail.

5. Organization of the Book

The book is organized into eight chapters that articulate and reinforce its overall argument about MDD. Chapter 2 offers background on the Sanitarist Movement and applies the MDD framework to show how the movement's activists propelled a subnationally variable process of health democratization across urban Brazil. In beginning the book's empirical analysis, chapter 3 then applies the framework to statistically and comparatively demonstrate the consequences of office-holding sanitaristas for four social development outcomes: IMR, CMR, the coverage of the PSF, and rates of access to primary health care by the uninsured population. The regression analysis finds that sanitarista office holding of the SUS directorship was associated with better than average outcomes for all indicators, even after holding constant alternative explanations discussed in this chapter. In deepening this finding, comparative findings illustrate how consistent sanitarista office holding was necessary within a larger configuration of conditions for "programmatic health democratization" that I show was jointly sufficient for robust improvements in IMR. Conversely, the inconsistency or full-on absence of sanitarista office holding was necessary within a larger configuration of conditions for minimalist health democratization that was sufficient for nonrobust social development outcomes to occur.

In qualitatively deepening these findings, chapters 4 through 7 offer comparative case studies that trace robust social development outcomes in urban Brazil to two variants of health democratization: a participatory-programmatic variety in Belo Horizonte and Porto Alegre and a generic (nonparticipatory) programmatic variety in Curitiba and Fortaleza. Chapters 4 and 5 show how office-holding sanitaristas in Belo Horizonte and Porto Alegre worked alongside participatory publics and political elites from progressive and sometimes centrist parties to animate a participatory-programmatic trajectory of health democratization that helped generate robust social development outcomes. Yet the within-case analyses of both chapters suggest that it was office-holding sanitaristas who most animated the programmatic pathways that mattered for maximizing IMR reduction.

Chapters 6 and 7 provide additional case studies of how office-holding sanitaristas in Fortaleza and Curitiba advanced a programmatic trajectory of health democratization that yielded similarly robust social development, despite a relative absence of influential participatory publics. Chapter 8 applies the book's theory of MDD to a broader set of cases in the Global South and considers the implications of the book's findings beyond Brazil.

TWO

Pragmatist Publics in Urban Brazil

> Health is a right of all and a duty of the state, guaranteed by
> social and economic policies that seek the reduction of risk of
> sickness and other ailments, and universal and equal access
> to actions and services for its promotion, protection, and
> restoration.
>
> —*Brazilian Constitution of 1988, Article 196 (my translation)*

> The municipal direction of the SUS . . . manages and executes
> public health services.
>
> —*Federal Law 8,080 of 1990, Article 18 (my translation)*

Despite general agreements that progressive political elites and newly mobilized civil-society groups helped precipitate Brazil's return to democracy
and growth in social development, the civil-society actors and state-society
relations behind this historic shift have not been precisely conceptualized or systematically linked to human-capability expansion. This chapter addresses this lacuna by presenting a new theoretical framework of
movement-driven development (MDD) for explaining urban Brazil's variable degrees of improvement in access to primary public health care and
human capabilities. Although studies exploring the state-society relations
behind contemporary Brazil's improvement in public health have tended
to focus on national-level dynamics,[1] Brazil's tasking of municipalities with
the responsibility for delivering primary health care ultimately raised the
stakes of subnational health and development politics in underappreciated
ways. The framework presented in this chapter focuses on an oft-noted period of health democratization in Brazil, during which subnational and national government gradually codified and sought to enact the rights-based
and programmatic mode of delivering basic health care outlined in Brazil's

1988 Constitution (Federal Republic of Brazil 1988) and in two legal specifications of it called Organic Health Laws (Federal Republic of Brazil 1990a, 1990b). The framework holds that the period unfolded in distinct ways, even across similarly sized capital cities throughout a country of continental size with twenty-six states, over six thousand municipalities, and more than 210 million people.

The chapter differentiates between three subnationally variable experiences of the health-democratization period—what I call minimalist, programmatic, and participatory-programmatic variants—and argues that the last two pathways maximized social development transformations, while the first trajectory did not. More specifically, a participatory-programmatic variant of health democratization in Belo Horizonte and Porto Alegre and a nonparticipatory but programmatic variant in Fortaleza and Curitiba were sufficient for robust development outcomes to occur, while the minimalist variant experienced in cities like Rio de Janeiro and Salvador was sufficient for only nonrobust development outcomes by the end of the period. To contextualize this argument, the chapter first describes the dire state of public health and development in which the sanitarista pursuit of a citizenship right to health gained momentum during the early 1980s. It then conceptualizes these civil-society actors in greater detail through a discussion of their qualities as a pragmatist public. After specifying subnational variants of the health-democratization period, the chapter concludes by arguing that local state-building in the primary-care sector was a key mechanism by which office-holding sanitaristas maximized improvements over time in social development outcomes such as IMR reduction.

1. Initial Conditions of Local Politics and Social Development

As Brazil began transitioning to formal democracy in the 1980s, urban politics remained mired in a pre-democratic mode of military tutelage, with the country drawing notice for its weak social development outcomes.[2] In this initial moment, the country recorded a high, nationwide IMR of over 61 deaths per 1,000 live births that was worse than some sub-Saharan countries, such as Kenya, at the time.[3] Even as Brazil codified a constitutional right to health in 1988, the country's generally more-developed large capitals[4] recorded an IMR of over 51 deaths per 1,000 live births. Some cities, such as Manaus, recorded extreme levels as high as 80 deaths per 1,000 births, rivaling levels observed in the world's most underdeveloped countries at the time.[5] Further, this widespread infant mortality in urban Brazil could hardly be blamed on any lack of economic growth during the prior twenty years of military dictatorship, when annual economic growth rates were about five times higher than during the twenty years of democracy that followed ratification of Brazil's 1988 Constitution.[6] Rather, Brazil's surprisingly poor performance in social development as the country returned to democracy had distinctively political and social origins.

More specifically, the country's weak social development record at the dawn of re-democratization reflected damaging legacies of colonialism, slavery (which remained legal in Brazil until 1888), and more than two decades of rule by a military regime that assiduously cultivated patronage-based ties to local political leaders from the country's economic elite.[7] Indeed, one key institutional remnant of past eras throughout urban Brazil was a conservative economic and political elite in major capitals that was notorious for its personalism, antidemocratic orientation, and general disinterest in constructing programmatically oriented state institutions for improving society-wide health outcomes.[8] By the early 1980s, one result of these politics was the deepening of a Bismarckian social-service system that woefully underachieved in its delivery of basic public services, such as primary public health care, sewage, sanitation, and running water, to the vast majority of the Brazilian population.[9] Forced in 1982 to contest local power for the first time in two decades, however, many of these local political elites began to lose their holds on power in major capitals and states, and these shifts had important implications for such basic public-service sectors. Watershed electoral victories by the left-leaning Workers' Party (PT) in the mayoral races of southern capitals such as Porto Alegre in 1987 demonstrated the virtues of more democratic patterns of local governance, as its progressive administrations introduced new institutions for incorporating civil society into municipal budgeting, especially the now famous Participatory Budgeting (OP) process.

But neither the restoration of municipal elections in 1985 nor the ratification of Brazil's progressive 1988 Constitution eliminated the conservative political and economic elites who had previously dominated urban health politics during and before the dictatorship. Indeed, sanitaristas and other progressives initially encountered adverse conditions for enacting a right to health, including national and subnational resistance to reform from entrenched conservative interests. Among such opponents were private hospital and insurance interests, whom Brazil's erstwhile military dictatorship had sustained through its perpetuation of a publicly subsidized, private-sector health industry that predominantly served formal-sector workers and public employees in the country's more prosperous southern and southeastern regions (Escorel 2008). Indeed, in the Constitutional Assembly in which the right to health was framed, these actors effectively vetoed more radical *sanitarista* proposals to institute a purely state-run health system that would have altogether outlawed private-sector provision of health care and insurance (UNESCO 2005a). In alliance with such interests, conservative politicians repeatedly undermined progressive proposals to expand the democratic state's role in ensuring a universal right to health by obstructing proactive measures such as heightened public spending on basic health and sanitation provision, actual state delivery of primary public health services, and construction of the local state structures required for such interventions.[10] In short, a major institutional legacy of Brazil's prior colonial and authoritarian eras was itself a conservative elite of traditional politicians and entrenched economic interests that emerged from these eras as power brokers in the municipal politics of major capitals. And even as competitive elections on municipal and state levels generally moved local governance in more democratic directions thereafter, municipal politics emerged as a major battleground between advocates and adversaries of rights to health and democracy.

Ultimately, however, these initial conditions of local politics and social development can explain neither individual cities' subsequent paths of minimal, programmatic, or participatory-programmatic health democratization nor the robust versus nonrobust social development outcomes they achieved by the end of the period. Neither the initial restoration of free and fair elections for mayoral and gubernatorial offices nor codification of a constitutional right to health nor the mere presence of a local *sanitarista* network can explain such variations, in part because such factors did not meaningfully or systematically differ across major capitals. Indeed, the beginning of the health-democratization period saw initial, city-level IMRs that varied widely among all five positive cases that experienced robust development—Porto Alegre, Curitiba, Belo Horizonte, Recife, and Fortaleza—with the first two municipalities ranking in the best third of all major capitals (lowest IMRs or better initial development) and the last three ranking in the worst third (highest IMRs or worse initial development). And some variant of a programmatic configuration arose in all five of these positive cases, despite considerable variation in these cities' rates of progressive political representation, their initial economic development levels, and their more and less intense colonial legacies. For example, some variant of a programmatic trajectory arose and robust development occurred in major capitals with relatively lower (Curitiba and Fortaleza) and higher (Porto Alegre, Belo Horizonte, and Recife) rates of left-party office holding, in capitals with relatively lower (Recife and Fortaleza) and higher (Belo Horizonte, Porto Alegre, and Curitiba) rankings in GDP per capita during 1985, and in capitals whose encompassing territories had suffered both the most severe (Recife and Fortaleza) and least severe (Belo Horizonte, Curitiba, and Porto Alegre) legacies of Portuguese mercantilist colonialism.[11]

Even northeastern capitals such as Salvador, Fortaleza, and Recife, which were similarly notorious for clientelist politics and Brazil's highest IMRs initially, diverged from one another subsequently. Specifically, Fortaleza and Recife witnessed consistent sanitarista office holding and robust IMR reductions by the end of the period, while Salvador featured inconsistent sanitarista office holding and nonrobust IMR reductions. Conversely, the tepid performance of nonrobust developers such as Rio de Janeiro—a capital that began the period with an IMR in Brazil's highest-performing third—further reinforces the notion that relatively favorable initial conditions of infant mortality did not guarantee continued overperformance thereafter. Rio's status as a nationwide center for the Sanitarist Movement also shows that the mere presence of a dense sanitarista network at the beginning of the period hardly ensured maximal growth in social development by its end, especially if these actors remained insulated from municipal office holding. Conversely, minimalist health-democratization and nonrobust development occurred in capitals with relatively lower (Salvador) and higher (Rio de Janeiro) initial GDP per capita, in cities with comparatively lower (Salvador) and higher (Rio de Janeiro) previous rates of office holding by center-left parties, and in capitals (Salvador and Rio de Janeiro) whose encompassing regions suffered more (northeast) and less (southeast) severe colonial legacies, respectively. In sum, where democracy and social development have been concerned in contemporary urban Brazil, history has not been fate, and commonly deployed variables struggle to account for subnational variation in both.

2. *Brazil's Sanitaristas as Pragmatist Publics*

A core premise of this book is that understanding such diverse and un-explained pathways of social development across urban Brazil requires sharper conceptualizations of the civil-society actors who most animated the politics of public health and development throughout the period. Although much scholarship has chronicled the rise and advocacy of Brazil's Sanitarist Movement, existing work has not conclusively reconciled these actors with social science theories of civil-society actors and their possibilities for agency within the state-society politics of democracy and development.[12] As late as the early 2000s, sanitaristas loosely mirrored Tarrow's (2011, 9) authoritative definition of social movements as agents of "collective challenges, based on common purposes and social solidarities, in sustained interaction with elites, opponents, and authorities." Nevertheless, scholars have tended to loosely conceptualize Brazil's sanitaristas in a multiplicity of other ways, ranging from nodes within issue/policy networks (Borges Sugiyama 2012; Falleti 2010b; McGuire 2010) and actors within a larger social-movement coalition (Garay 2016) to a collective of health professionals (Harris 2017) that early commentators such as Weyland (1998) argued to have demobilized after their biggest victories of the 1980s. Beyond general agreements that sanitarista mobilizations have featured increasingly contained repertoires of contention such as policy advocacy, lobbying, and attempts to control state health institutions from the inside out, surprisingly little attention has been paid to their sources of agency in such advocacy. Yet doing so is key to understanding how more democratic patterns of access to health emerged and molded social development outcomes across urban Brazil.

This study argues that more fully understanding these actors' long-lasting political agency within Brazil's national and subnational politics of democracy and social development begins with recognizing their qualities as a pragmatist public. Sanitaristas have thrived on qualities that sociologists associate with the notion of a "public," which Emirbayer and Sheller (1999, 156) call "interstitial networks" defined by "open-ended flows of communication that enable socially distant interlocutors to bridge social network positions, formulate collective orientations, and generate a psychical 'working alliance' in pursuit of influence over issues of common concern." In this respect, Brazil's sanitaristas mirror but ultimately diverge from close cousins such as the "partisan publics" theorized in Mische's (2008) study of Brazilian youth-activist networks[13] and the "participatory publics" addressed in Avritzer's (2002, 2009) studies of civil society and participatory democracy in the country. General qualities that they share with these other actors—particularly dense social networks, flows of communication, and relations with wider groups of citizens and narrower groups of political-society elites—clearly mattered for their advocacy in public health and development politics. But such general qualities illuminate less about how sanitarista agency persisted for as long as it did and why it contributed to tangible growth in social development for as sustained a period as it did.

The more specific notion of a pragmatist public, however, further emphasizes how these actors' outward civil orientations lead them to create and wield new democratic offices through which they can engineer state machinery for tangibly enacting material expressions of their solidary ideologies. In seeking to bring previously excluded groups closer to practically realizing Brazil's universal and equal citizenship right to health for all members of society, Brazil's sanitaristas aimed to build state structures that could deliver basic health services to the vast majority of the populace that lacked access to state-provided health care. These qualities not only fueled a remarkable generation of activists who were more committed to that ideology than to any particular repertoire of contention (sanitaristas employed a wide variety of disruptive and contained repertoires). They also allowed sanitaristas to frequently and nimbly recalibrate their repertoires to fit changing political-opportunity structures that spanned both authoritarian and democratic political regimes on the national level as well as myriad varieties of municipal and state-level politics of health and development in Brazil's largest capital cities. In short, this combination of an outward public orientation, a focus on democratic office, and a deep-seeded commitment to the solidary ideology of a universal right to health enabled sanitaristas to fluidly and malleably adapt to changing political-opportunity structures in ways that made them enduring protagonists in Brazil's state-society politics of health and development.

Sanitaristas exhibit four more specific qualities of pragmatist publics that further enabled them to consistently advance their universalistic ideology of a citizenship right to health within Brazil's initial context of extreme social inequality and exclusion of access to basic health care. First, sanitaristas were committed institution builders, not just of state agencies (as existing accounts highlight) but of civil-society institutions. Essential to the longevity of their activism was how sanitaristas crafted key communicative institutions of civil society, particularly civic associations that aimed to foster society-wide solidarity around their universalizing vision of an equal, universal, democratically enshrined right to health for all Brazilians. Sanitarista activism assumed this more sophisticated form in the mid-1970s through the founding of new associations such as the Brazilian Center for Health Studies (CEBES) in 1976 and the Brazilian Public Health Association (ABRASCO) in 1979 (Escorel 2008; Paim 2007). As coming chapters address and as Belo Horizonte's experience of the Mineiro Sanitarista Party (PMS) suggests, individual cities typically featured at least some incarnation of the so-called Sanitarista Party, which was a self-conscious misnomer because its activists were civil-society activists intent on advancing their ideology of health universalism through multiple avenues into local and national politics. Such associations helped coordinate early, city-specific activism but continued to be valuable tools for the subsequent office-holding campaigns of sanitaristas well after the creation of SUS directorships across urban Brazil (J. M. Borges, M. L. Jaeger, and L. Tonón, interviews, 2010). While their specific goals changed over time and sometimes included projects of specific interest to their medical-professional and -student constituencies, these associations began propagating an ideology and political program of sanitary reform during the late 1970s and aimed to construct broader bonds of social solidarity around a new, society-wide identity of all citizens as bearers of a universal and equal right to health (Paim 2007). Over time, the repertoire of CEBES and ABRASCO has included the coordination of public discussions about the movement's core strategies and the ideology of sanitary reform, organization of widespread public mobilizations around these ideologies (including protests and demonstrations), and consolidated lobbying campaigns in national and subnational government.[14] And even after a 1980s-era episode of more disruptive mobilizations, sanitaristas remained connected to these and other movement organizations that continue to advocate for and seek to more tangibly enact Brazil's right to health.

Despite their multiple and changing purposes over time, sanitarista associations such as CEBES, ABRASCO, and city-specific branches of the Sanitarist Party exemplify how the outward orientation and universalistic ideologies of such communicative institutions can sustain the advocacy of pragmatist publics over time. Although CEBES was initially founded in 1976 by medical professionals, medical residents, students, and Brazilian Communist Party (PCB) militants to crystallize and divulge a philosophy of social medicine that could address the country's vast health inequalities, it became the primary advocate for the twin goals of restoring the country's democratic regime and codifying a universal citizenship right to health (Escorel 2008). Beginning with their underground activism during Brazil's repressive military dictatorship, CEBES organizers and other sanitaristas initially risked capture and grave danger to pursue such goals. As the repressive grip of Brazil's military regime loosened in the early 1980s, sanitarista associations increasingly pursued their goals by organizing public forums and dialogue about their proposals for a universal, democratic right to health. In 1986, for instance, activists helped organize a series of health conferences, including the Eighth National Health Conference in Brasília, which for the first time included as participants not just health professionals but users of state health services. The conference culminated in a yearlong series of regionally decentralized, open public dialogues about aspirations and proposals for the country's future postdemocratization health system. Ultimately, it generated the specific proposal to codify a universal right to health and establish a state responsibility for realizing it that sanitarista participants in Brazil's Constitutional Assembly successfully integrated into Article 196 of the country's Constitution of 1988 (Federal Republic of Brazil 1988; Escorel 2008). It was no accident that sanitarista inputs into Article 196 codified a right to health, the pursuit of which came to depend on a highly decentralized system in which municipalities assumed significant responsibilities for administering actual service provisions. Although powerful representatives of the private-sector health and insurance industries effectively vetoed proposals for an etatist system in the Constitutional Assembly, many sanitaristas favored the resulting decentralization of responsibilities for enacting the right to health because their regionally diffuse networks and associations were well positioned throughout the country's capital cities to seize control of how that right would be implemented (M. L. Jaeger, interview, 2010). As chapters 4 through 7 demonstrate, these networks played a seminal role in four major cities in implementing and institutionalizing the right to health nationwide, but this was especially so where individual sanitaristas exploited them to seize control of key offices atop the subnational public health state.

This, in turn, points to a second quality of sanitaristas as a pragmatist public: namely, how they mold regulative institutions of civil society—especially new democratic offices and Brazil's Constitution and its laws creating the public health sector—to advance their own universalistic framing of a citizenship right to health. Such institutions include Article 196 of the country's Constitution (Federal Republic of Brazil 1988), which declares an equal and universal citizenship right to health and health services; national laws such as Laws 8,080 and 8,042 that created its current public health system (the SUS); and follow-up laws of states and municipalities that specified how civil society would cogovern the health sector.[15] Often overlooked in existing accounts that focus on the agency of sanitaristas within federal health bureaucracies—as opposed to the democratic offices that control those bureaucracies—is how sanitaristas influenced these laws and subsequent SUS Basic Operating Norms (NOBs) to successfully create an architecture of new democratic offices for regulating such agencies according to public purposes. No office has been more important in this regard than the SUS directorship, which holds public responsibility for guiding how such health agencies on all three levels of government attempt to enact the country's right to health (Federal Republic of Brazil 1990a, 1990b). This brand of sanitarista agency exemplifies how civil-society actors can sometimes institute and wield democratic offices in ways that are not tantamount to a mere collapse of civil-society activists into political society elites. More specifically, for sociological theorists of civil society such as Alexander, "when the representatives of civil society, and their high-level appointees, take up the reigns of state power, they enter into an 'office,' a publicly defined role regulated by ethical and legal constraints on both corruption and self-interest. . . . When solidarity is more expansive, and the pressures of 'society' become more explicit and powerful, office becomes an outpost of civil society directly inside the state" (2006, 133–34). Subnational variation in the success of their office-holding efforts aside, sanitaristas helped establish such regulative institutions and used them to infuse noncivil spheres—especially state health bureaucracies such as the federal health ministry (MS) and state- and city-specific Health Departments (SESs and SMSs)—with the solidary norm of a universal and equal right to health. Although anathema to Brazilian political culture at the dawn of the health-democratization period, such changes gradually transformed many such agencies in the country's largest capitals, having profound consequences for human welfare in the country.

Central to these efforts was what the venerable *sanitarista* activist Dr. Eleutério Rodrigues Neto (1997) termed "the parliamentary way"— occupying high-level offices atop state agencies that they sought to reorient around sanitary reform goals.[16] Beginning in the late 1970s, *sanitaristas* initiated a campaign to occupy high-level offices atop the country's public health bureaucracy on all three levels of government (federal, state, and municipal) in Brazil. Eventually, the campaign helped to supplant old state health care institutions and establish new ones that more closely embodied the universal scope of sanitary reform ideology. For instance, these efforts hastened the extinction of Brazil's primary dictatorship-era health institution—the National Institute for Medical Assistance in Social Security (INAMPS), which was a central instrument for excluding the vast majority of the Brazilian population from access to public health care—and replaced it with a series of new programs and state institutions that gradually broadened the delivery of primary health care (Falleti 2010b; Rodrigues Neto, Gomes Temporão, and Escorel, 2003). Although existing accounts emphasize how such reforms reflected acute political pressure for change among national bureaucrats inside state agencies like the INAMPS, *sanitarista* access to such positions also reflected an ongoing restoration of civil-society regulative institutions such as voting. As active participants in the wider Direct Elections Now! movement focused on national elections and in prior efforts that helped restore competitive gubernatorial elections in 1982 and mayoral elections in 1985, *sanitaristas* were early advocates for the restoration of democratic rights and freedoms, which they had come to view as essential for codifying their goal of a right to health (Escorel 2008). And as democratically elected opposition candidates to the military won gubernatorial and mayoral office for the first time in decades, they were eager to appoint their supporters to key positions; these appointments included those of *sanitaristas* to key public health posts. *Sanitaristas* initially secured access to such positions in part because of their applied knowledge of the public health sector, their experiences as primary health care providers, their social prestige as physicians and public health researchers, and

their undeniable interest in addressing deficiencies in the country's public health system that even the generals recognized as a threat to their rule.
But their primary motivation for pursuing the parliamentary way was to
bend state institutions around universalistic civil-society norms of sanitary
reform.

Sanitarista pursuit of a right to health achieved even deeper legal grounding in 1990, when sanitaristas secured passage of two key laws—perhaps the
quintessential regulative institution of civil society as it pertains to health
in Brazil—Laws 8,080 and 8,142 (Federal Republic of Brazil 1990a, 1990b).
Most basically, the laws specified Article 196 of the Constitution by creating
the SUS and effectively establishing a new democratic office atop all three
levels of the Brazilian public health state. Law 8,080 did more than just
place municipal governments in charge of planning, organizing, and executing service delivery, as spelled out in its Article 18. As noted by Cristiani
Vieira Machado, Luciana Dias de Lima, and Tatiana Wargas de Faria Baptista, Law 8,080 also established that "more than an administrator, the SUS
manager serves as each sphere of government's 'sanitary authority,' whose
political and technical actions must be regulated by principles of Brazilian sanitary reform" (2011, 50–52, my translation). Although the national
post of health minister and the subnational positions of municipal and state
health directors predated it, Law 8,080 effectively fused those positions with
the new democratic office of SUS manager, which assumed public responsibility for formulating health policy and generally regulating the health
sector in accordance with principles of sanitary reform ideology that were
codified into the Constitution in 1988 and into law in 1990. Yet even before
founding the office of municipal SUS manager, sanitarista directors of municipal health offices had embraced normative responsibilities of sanitary
reform before Law 8,080 made them into public responsibilities of all office occupants. Thus, sanitaristas' pre-SUS-era occupations of administrative positions atop the Brazilian public health state can be more fully understood as part of a coordinated effort to remold state institutions around
the civil-society norm of a universal citizenship right to health, even before
the 1988 reestablishment of constitutional democracy. Far from incidental
or passing forays into public office holding, sanitaristas were instead self-
consciously Gramscian (2000) in strategically seeking to occupy state offices in what many viewed as a perpetual war of position to embed core ideological tenets within the practice of the democratic state (J. M. Borges and

M. L. Jaeger, interviews, 2010; Paim 2007). But unlike in Gramsci's own understanding, sanitaristas hardly pursued particularistic goals in doing so. Rather, they viewed such forays as opportunities to bring their universalistic ideology of a citizenship right to health for all Brazilians closer to material fruition.

It comes as less of a surprise, then, that in Brazil's highly decentralized federalist democracy, civil-society efforts to establish localized incarnations of such regulative institutions through the "parliamentary way" led to programs that sought to practically enact the new right to health. For instance, although sanitaristas working in the country's federal health ministry (MS) helped create the Family Health Program (PSF)—the flagship nationwide program for fulfilling the responsibility to universally deliver basic health care—municipal governments could choose whether, how extensively, and with what particular adaptations they might adopt the PSF. And because PSF adoption entailed municipalities assuming primary responsibility for the lion's share of financing, administering, and building the local state capacity required to operate the program (H. M. Magalhães, interview, 2010), the subnational regulative institution of SUS director deeply influenced the timing and extent of PSF adoption across urban Brazil, particularly amid the severe fiscal constraints of the 1990s. Curiously, however, individual sanitaristas did not always remain in SUS directorships for extended periods of time, in part because of their own desires to make discrete, piecemeal interventions into the local state-building needed for implementing programs like the PSF and then return to more traditional modes of movement advocacy, their medical practices, or their own public health research and teaching positions. Returning to conventional activism within movement organizations such as ABRASCO and CEBES and to the practice of public health care and preventative medicine were two frequent sequels to sanitarista activism within SUS directorships. Yet understanding this sanitarista orientation toward laws and especially such democratic offices begs in turn for an account of the unusual and paradoxical mixture of ideological fervor and pragmatism that many activists brought to such episodes.

Sanitaristas exemplify a third quality of as a pragmatist public in how they have adopted a distinctively pragmatist approach to creating and wielding new regulative institutions of civil society, such as the SUS manager's office, to practically enact Brazil's right to health. The fact that sanitaristas secured support for nearly a half-dozen institutional predecessors of the SUS in the decade before its inception clearly reflects oft-noted qualities of pragmatism such as an iterative and reformist approach.[17] But the calling cards of sanitarista advocacy during the quarter century following creation of the SUS also included subtler but still quintessential features of political pragmatism, such as incrementalism, a problem-driven perspective, reflexivity, and an openness to deliberation when useful for intended purposes.[18] Often overlooked in existing work is that the SUS itself is less a structure of bureaucratic state health agencies than a legal and normative latticework of civil-society institutions that sanitaristas introduced for incrementally creating such state structures. As a result, activists have had to continually defend the SUS and repeatedly leverage components of it—especially SUS directorships—to iteratively construct administrative agencies capable of enacting its otherwise amorphous legal and ideological principles. As a set of principles, laws, and operating norms mandating all three levels of Brazilian government to enact a universal right to health, the SUS is thus a quintessential regulative institution for the Global South in that enactment of its principles and prerogatives has usually defaulted back to the variable consistency and strength of civil-society efforts over time to translate such principles into the state machinery needed to more tangibly advance its core commitments. In this respect, there may well be elective affinities between civil-society regulative institutions and pragmatist publics such as Brazil's sanitaristas, who embrace the longer-term piecemeal work of defending and rendering them more capable over time.

This pragmatist approach has been especially palpable in sanitarista efforts to establish and wield the subnational democratic office of SUS manager, as coming chapters detail in particular city-level cases.[19] While sanitaristas successfully mobilized to codify Laws 8,080 and 8,142, which declared legally binding changes to the country's health system and imposed requirements for how existing state health institutions such as the federal health ministry and state and local health offices (SESs, SMSs) would be governed, this victory marked the beginning of a new stage of activism in which their pragmatism was on full display. For one, the way that sanitaristas helped craft such laws and the office of SUS manager also reflected their recognition of a master problem with Brazil's new health system. In short, sanitaristas anticipated how actual implementation of such reforms would necessarily be constrained by weak state capacities and institutional legacies of patronage imparted by preexisting health agencies such as the INAMPS that were notoriously resistant to reform and infamous for their inefficiency and exclusion of most Brazilians from health-service provisions. And if the SUS was not itself a new health care bureaucracy but a mandate to create one, many pivotal responsibilities for doing so fell to subnational governments. In particular, municipalities inherited responsibility for universalizing access to even basic health services. The fact that they received precious few federal resources for doing so only magnified the difficulty of an already monumental institution-building project to begin addressing preexisting deficits in coverage. In response, however, sanitaristas across urban Brazil set out to incrementally enact the SUS's sweeping promise of a universal and equal right to health care during a three-decade span of institutional reform in which they seized control of the SUS manager's office and its predecessors.

That formal codification of the office explicitly highlighted its normative status as a "sanitary authority" was no accident. Indeed, this reflected the view of influential sanitaristas that a central and enduring problem was likely to be an absence of the political will and ability to uproot the patronage-based, antiprogrammatic vestiges of the subnational public health state. In response, sanitarista founders of the SUS such as Sergio Arouca and Eleutério Rodrigues Neto sought to craft the office of SUS manager as a permanent space atop the public health state in which activists could confront this overarching problem over the long term. Crystallization of the office as a sanitary authority encoded SUS directorships in a way that systematically favored future sanitarista occupation and control of the office. Founding the office as a sanitary authority simultaneously yielded SUS directorships with a bias toward authorities versed in the ongoing problems faced by public health systems and individuals whose own biographies symbolized commitment to tenets of sanitary reform ideology—especially the democratic value of a universal and equal right to health—that undergirded the SUS. In both the Brazilian public sphere and at the state-society interface of public health politics, no actors symbolized this combination of expertise and fidelity to this solidary norm of universalism more than sanitarista activists themselves.

But even this overt and skillful piece of statecraft on the part of sanitaristas could do little more than thrust future SUS managers into the vexing and often contextually specific problems of subnational health reform. To be sure, different city governments faced the same problem of bridging the yawning gap left between Brazil's right to health and the enduring weakness of local state capacity to achieve even minor material expressions of it. But as borne out in greater detail by coming chapters, localized manifestations of this master challenge abounded, making the reflexivity of sanitarista occupants an essential tool for navigating this difficult landscape in ways that ultimately produced more capable state administrative agencies. Learning from failed efforts to build such capacity, sanitaristas often improvised reforms and expansions of SMSs and SESs in ways that reflected grounded learning about the ways these agencies had failed to address vexing public problems such as rampant infant mortality. Local state-building improvisations of sanitaristas were especially essential for cities to expand the federally initiated but locally run Family Health Program (PSF), the country's flagship primary health program. Across the cities explored in this study, the sanitaristas who occupied the SUS directorship and embraced the continual institution-building processes the office demanded often spoke of the hard-won lessons accumulated from failed attempts to implement it. Sanitaristas were notably reflexive in learning from failed attempts to build essential capacities to implement the PSF, particularly when it came to the hiring of qualified health professionals, the construction and renovation of primary health clinics, and the use of technical tools for allocating those resources.

Another dimension of sanitarista pragmatism has been activists' enduring openness to the inputs of democratic deliberation in general, especially Brazil's deliberative health councils. Alongside other vociferous advocates for Brazil's return to democracy, sanitaristas successfully demanded that creation of the SUS include an elaborate institutional architecture of deliberative health councils nationwide. Mandated to exist on federal, state, and municipal levels, health councils reserve half of their seats for civil-society actors and possess formal co-governing authorities in the health sector, including the right to veto budgets and review state expenditures in the sector annually (Avritzer 2009; Wampler 2015). While sanitaristas have typically focused more intently on populating SUS directorships historically, they have also generally supported health councils' more open-ended democratic deliberations about state-building and policy formulation in the sector. In remaining open to the inputs of other activists and citizen participants in these bodies and in civil-society institutions more generally, sanitaristas thus differ sharply from other categories of actors such as professionals and technocrats, who more often seek to unilaterally wield their technical expertise, training, knowledge, and professional experience to pursue narrower objectives with comparatively little input from nonexperts. They have thus remained committed democrats from an early moment and have generally viewed such deliberations as opportunities to broaden the basis of social support for solidary ideologies such as universal rights to health. Sanitarista office holders of the SUS directorship have, however, typically been more consistently and meaningfully engaged with power brokers in political society than with the participatory publics who animate health councils, as coming chapters show.

Sanitaristas also epitomize a fourth defining quality of pragmatist publics in how they have subtly deployed what I call social code-switching to reframe state-building proposals for the public health sector. These proposals advanced their own core ideological concerns with equality and universality but in ways that resonated surprisingly with subnational political elites who did not typically share such concerns otherwise. Social code-switching refers to the way that activists sometimes leverage both their privileged positions atop class, occupational, and political-party hierarchies and their corresponding fluency in the lingua franca of such noncivil spheres to formulate appeals to the noncivil actors that dominate these spheres in a language that appeals to their narrower interests. Often doctors from the high-prestige medical profession, sanitaristas have done so by cloaking projects that advance the ideology of health universalism in the narrower languages of programmatic effectiveness and sometimes even social control in which Brazilian political elites during the dictatorship were fluent. This skillful approach was detectable even before sanitaristas crafted Article 196 of the Constitution and the Organic Health Laws, which codified solidary principles of universal and equal access to health care into law and established active advancement of those principles (via tangible state delivery of public services) as a requirement of office holding for local elected officials and SUS directors. Even before the restoration of democracy, well-known sanitaristas such as Arouca and Rodrigues Neto first gained entrée into rarified discussions about health-sector reform among the country's military rulers in large part because of their social status as representatives of the high-status medical profession. Here, sanitaristas adeptly exploited their positions near the top of a pre-democracy-era social hierarchy that Baiocchi (2006) has shown was structured by a corporate code of discourse that valued qualities such as social connectedness among elites and related privileges of the well-connected while devaluing individual citizenship rights. During incipient, pre-democratic moments, including the creation of institutional forerunners of the SUS, sanitaristas sought to reorganize the public health state to better foster principles of equality, universality, and individual citizenship rights to health. Clearly, such liberal principles rejected the Bismarckian foundations of Brazil's pre-democratic health state, which remained structured by a corporate code that defined access to public health care as a privilege of well-connected, high-status individuals. Yet they framed discrete state-building projects in a way that exploited a mistaken belief among such political elites that projects to expand access to health would help maintain the order and control of such elites. If sanitaristas were able to first frame the issue of public health for political elites in such a way only because their social prestige as medical professionals granted them a measure of proximity to such elites in the first place, they succeeded in gleaning elite support for this universalistic framing in part by emphasizing the value of such a system for advancing narrower and more parochial interests of the era's political elites in maintaining a highly unequal social order.

The pre-democratic public health system in which sanitaristas first exhibited this code-switching approach featured a mainstream of private-sector health providers and insurers and a medical profession dominated by actors who generally embraced (and profited from) a patronage-fueled, fee-for-service model of privately administered services that overwhelmingly benefited patients from high-status class, race, and gender strata. Initially a small and heterodox undercurrent in the profession, sanitaristas drew their solidary ideology of a universal right to health care from a competing liberal code around which they sought to refashion the country's medical profession, its public health system, and, more generally, its political regime. Commonly overlooked, however, is how sanitaristas—motivated by the chance to materially advance such otherwise nebulous, universalistic principles through health-sector reform—periodically cloaked their reform proposals in the languages of efficiency and benefits for the existing political order, even the military's thoroughly antidemocratic order. Thus, sanitarista code-switching has involved leveraging their favored positions near the top of a social order defined by the corporate code to (somewhat surreptitiously, at first) orchestrate broader social support for health institutions that reflected a nearly diametrically opposed set of values—especially an individual right to health—taken directly from the country's competing liberal code. In what amounted to a Trojan horse approach to political reform in the dying days of the dictatorship, sanitaristas first won support from generals for what they mistakenly regarded as benign proposals for public-health-care expansion in the poorer northeastern region of the country. As a member of the elite medical profession, Rodrigues Neto secured a position within an early-1980s, dictatorship-era health bureaucracy through which he garnered the military's support to introduce a health program known as the Integrated Health Actions (AIS) program. Observers generally agree with Rodrigues Neto's own assessment that the intervention meaningfully contributed to subsequent institutional reforms and eventual adoption of the SUS (Escorel 2008; Falleti 2010b; Rodrigues Neto, Gomes Temporão, and Escorel 2003). Less noted is how these interventions benefited from a social code-switching approach in which sanitaristas skillfully framed state-building proposals for political elites in their narrower lingua franca of securing and maintaining political power while conspiring among themselves and broader groups of civil-society activists to reorient the public health state around a broader and more universalistic set of commitments. In essence, sanitaristas smuggled the ideological germ of a universal health system into a carefully articulated but unassuming proposal for rural health care expansion that soon garnered an unexpected level of support for a universal health system among northeastern state governors and mayors that few in the military seem to have anticipated.

If sanitaristas initiated this code-switching approach when mobilizing to help reestablish democracy and codify the country's new citizenship right to health, they also artfully honed it during three subsequent decades of efforts to enact that right through subnational politics. After Brazil's return to democracy, some subnational executives became otherwise unlikely advocates for creation of the SUS and expansion of its primary health programs, not because of any deep-seeded ideological commitments to a universal and equal right to health but because of how sanitaristas successfully articulated the promise of the new system's expanded public-service delivery as instrumentally beneficial for electoral success. If their pre-democratic code-switching efforts couched state-building proposals in the language of maintaining social order, their newer efforts appealed to the electoral calculations of political-society elites. Indeed, doing so became a central preoccupation for individual office-holding sanitaristas in SMS directorships in the early 1980s amid the return of competitive local elections. Yet even in this newly competitive landscape of subnational electoral politics, sanitaristas adopted the same code-switching approach to make their proposals for pursuing health universalism legible and appealing to incumbents and challengers from a wide variety of political ideologies (not just to left-leaning parties), all of whom were primarily interested in the new currency of accessing state power: winning elections. In particular, office-holding sanitaristas have often couched their proposals for building the municipal state capacities needed to expand the PSF in the instrumental language of electoral benefits, despite describing their own primary motivations for doing so as grounded in a fidelity to sanitary reform principles of universality and equity in access to health (L. Barcelos, J. M. Borges, M. L. Jaeger, and L. Tonón, interviews, 2010). Examined in more depth by the case studies in chapters 4 through 7, these social code-switching abilities of sanitaristas are an oft-overlooked dimension of their advocacy that complemented an ideological fervor for a universal right to health, a remarkable ability to construct new regulative institutions of civil society in the image of that principle, and a pragmatist embrace of incrementalism, problem solving, reflexivity, and deliberation.

3. Democratization of Health across Urban Brazil

This study argues that contemporary Brazil witnessed a period of movement-driven development (MDD) in which civil-society efforts to democratize access to health profoundly transformed both the national and especially subnational public health states. Stretching from the 1970s into the early 2010s, the period was defined by the struggles of sanitaristas to both legally codify core tenets of its sanitary reform ideology and reorient the practice of Brazil's democratizing state around these principles. While sanitarista mobilizations between the late 1970s and early 1990s led to the codification of Brazil's right to health, a subtler but extended period of mobilization during the nearly quarter century that followed saw efforts to enact that right through subnational state-building. The variable success of locally active sanitaristas in doing so across urban Brazil had far-reaching but subnationally variable consequences for institutional reform and development. But precisely because sanitaristas maintained social networks in all major capitals explored in this study, the mere local presence of their networks cannot explain such variations. Rather, accounting for these subnationally variable records of institutional change and development requires both a careful accounting of the extent to which sanitaristas asserted themselves in the local politics of public-health-related state-building throughout the period.

3.I. DEFINING THE HEALTH-DEMOCRATIZATION PERIOD

The study defines Brazil's health-democratization period as a contemporary sequence in which (1) civil-society actors who embraced sanitary reform as an ideology came to exert considerable influence in the state-society politics of health and development, and (2) these actors advanced a political project for constitutionally codifying a citizenship right to health and revising state institutions to enact that right. During this period, actors from Brazil's Sanitarist Movement helped to both propagate an ideology of universal citizenship rights to health and mobilize political elites around their political project for enacting that right through national and subnational state-building. Whereas discussions of the period commonly underscore the movement's success in drafting and securing approval for Article 196 of the Constitution, less attention has been paid to the subnational state-building dimensions of this political project. Thus, the definition of the period formulated here emphasizes how the movement propagated and subnationally advanced a Brazil-specific formulation of "sanitary reform"—a core movement ideology that framed universal access to basic health care and sanitation as a democratic right of all citizens.[20] It also highlights the palpable but locally variable state transformations set in motion by a political project that sanitaristas undertook to mobilize national and subnational politicians around tangible state transformations for realizing that ideology.

Three key tenets were especially notable within this formulation of sanitary reform: (1) the social norm of political activism as a defining quality of the medical profession, (2) the eventual embrace of a social democratic liberalism as the most feasible political system for enacting a right to health, and (3) an anticorporate critique of capitalist threats to democratizing health. A first notable component of sanitary reform as an ideology was its normative claim that the medical profession be made a terrain of political struggle to enact a right to health. In particular, the movement's "social medicine" doctrine heterodoxically framed the medical profession as demanding political activism by practitioners to correct society-wide health inequalities. The prominent place that the doctrine took within Brazilian sanitary reform owed much to social ties between seminal Brazilian and other Latin American public health activists. For example, the scholarship and political advocacy of Juan César García, an Argentine physician and public health activist, proved enormously influential in helping institute one of Brazil's first social-medicine master's programs at the State University of Rio de Janeiro in 1972 (Escorel 2008, 411; Galeano, Trotta, and Spinelli 2011). The Brazilian formulation of social medicine not only spelled out a Marxist-inspired historical-structural critique of disease as caused by unequal socioeconomic structures and ruling-class power but also framed the medical profession as a realm of inherently political—as opposed to simply epidemiological, clinical, or other forms of technical—practice and action. As noted by Sanitarist Movement scholar-activists such as Sarah Escorel (2008, 397) and Jairnilson Silva Paim (2007), this heterodox vision of the medical practice crystallized within the academic work of venerable sanitaristas, especially Sergio Arouca's *O Dilema Preventista: Contribuição para a Compreensão e Crítica da Medicina Preventiva* (2003). Distinct from alternative formulations such as "public health" and "preventive medicine" that lacked a structural Marxist diagnosis of health inequalities, the ideas of social medicine formulated by these early activists helped politicize a remarkable generation of health professionals and helped generate a new activist-oriented identity of sanitaristas throughout urban Brazil.

Second, while various antiauthoritarian ideologies suffused the intellectual currents of sanitaristas after Brazil's military seized power in 1964, it was ultimately a progressive and social democratic liberalism that undergirded sanitary reform's prescribed actions and beliefs regarding the most feasible political arrangements for realizing a right to health. Particularly as the country's military regime became increasingly brutal and repressive, sanitary reform rejected positivist notions of individuals as pieces within a necessarily hierarchical society that required an illiberal state willing to rigidly impose order. In this sense, the early health-focused activism of sanitaristas such as Sergio Arouca flowed from their other activism within underground political parties such as the Brazilian Communist Party (PCB), which opposed the dictatorship and was forced underground by it. Sanitary reform's increasing embrace of proposals for a democratic state predicated on liberal rights and freedoms constituted a marked shift from the contrasting views of early-twentieth-century public health advocates in Brazil and beyond, who had at the time generally mirrored their counterparts in Iberia and throughout South America in tolerating supposedly "enlightened" republican dictatorships and other illiberal regimes that promoted exclusive definitions of citizenship. Indeed, dominant tenets within the formulation of sanitary reform that emerged during the 1970s increasingly emphasized liberal democratic principles such as universal rights to free speech and associational freedoms as the most promising platform from which a more encompassing citizenship right to health could be effectively pursued.[21] Additionally, Brazilian sanitary reform increasingly emphasized local political autonomy and envisioned the subnational state as a guarantor of such rights and freedoms in the face of historically ingrained, regional political elites that otherwise dominated local politics.

Third, late-twentieth-century sanitary reform in Brazil was also notable for its anticorporate orientation. As militants with pedigrees in communist organizing and other related political spheres, sanitaristas leveraged health-specific critiques of large capitalist organizations such as the private health insurance and hospital industries that dominated service provision during the military dictatorship. They not only opposed such private-sector interests because of the military dictatorship's patronage-based support of these actors but also more generally exposed their deleterious influences on society-wide health-service provision and health status. Sanitary reform especially critiqued the patronage nexus between the dictatorship and the private health industry for cultivating a private-sector health industry that almost uniformly excluded poor populations in both urban and rural areas. These critiques highlighted problematic realities such as the fact that the industry delivered mostly high-cost health services to middle and upper classes within health care facilities located in wealthier neighborhoods of major southern and southeastern cities (Lobato and Burlandy 2000) as well as the fact that the percentage of all hospital beds in private-sector facilities climbed from only 14% in 1960 to 73% by 1976 (McGuire 2010, 161). To be sure, sanitaristas lost a decisive political battle when these conservative interests defeated their proposal for proposed language in the Constitution that would have eliminated all private-sector provision of public services. Nevertheless, the ideological stance against large private-health-sector interests remained a consistent and consequential theme in the movement's discourse well into the twenty-first century.

In addition to the presence of sanitaristas who embraced these core ideological principles of sanitary reform, these actors' subnational pursuit of a shared political project for enacting these tenets constitutes a second defining feature of the health-democratization period. In all the capitals examined below, the period witnessed dramatic improvements in the capacities of subnational states to deliver disease-preventing basic public services such as primary health care, running water, sewage, and sanitation. As state capitals, these cities shared a similarly central position within the country's evolving federalist system of multilevel governance and benefited from roughly similar increases in national-level support for these sectors. Yet the health-democratization period was also defined by considerable subnational variation in the extent to which the political project of sanitary reform came to material fruition in terms of tangible state structures for enacting a universal right to health. And in general, pursuit of sanitary reform in national politics had important local precursors in most of the cities examined in this study. To be sure, one largely unquestioned result of sanitarista influence in nationwide reform processes was an explosion in nationwide provision of basic services such as primary public health care, running water, and sewerage on a scale that few had previously imagined (McGuire 2010; Falleti 2010a). And if localized differences across major cities have remained a fact of life, the subnational pattern of that variation shifted palpably with many erstwhile underperformers becoming urban Brazil's leaders and vice versa. Thus, in examining the full period of these changes—and by investigating connections between national-level and local-level health politics—this definition of the health-democratization period differs from other accounts, including those arguing that the constitutional codification of a right to health was an unexplainable critical juncture that launched subnationally uniform, path-dependent changes in motion throughout urban Brazil (Arretche 2004). Furthermore, conceptualizing the period as extending into the present day expands on Falleti's (2010b) analysis of intrainstitutional health reform on the national level by accounting for several subsequent decades after creation of the SUS in which unexplained, subnational variations in institutional change and development transformations left a profound mark on the human condition across urban Brazil.

3.2. TYPES OF HEALTH DEMOCRATIZATION

Beyond these shared qualities, however, the health-democratization period unfolded in three distinct ways, and this study provides an account of the causes and consequences of these differences. For purposes of highlighting the developmental consequences of this period throughout urban Brazil, the most important distinctions concern the extent to which democratic reforms of political opportunity structures occurred within the country's largest capitals and the way these shifts permeated the local public health state. Focusing on seven salient dimensions of this variation reveals that three types of health democratization characterized urban Brazil during the period: minimalist, programmatic, and participatory-programmatic variants.

First, health democratization in all major Brazilian capitals was defined by a restoration of formal democratic procedures, freedoms, and rights. Political leeway and momentum to establish a universal citizenship right to health fundamentally depended on—but were not reducible to—these underlying shifts in the country's political opportunity structure. Brazil's democratization was predicated on decisive shifts such as the restoration of basic voting rights, the freedom to associate and organize political parties, and formal freedoms for the press and media. Thanks in part to formidable pressure from the nationwide Direct Elections Now! (*Diretas Já*) movement, Brazil's military regime gradually reintroduced opposition-party organization in 1980 and voting rights in direct elections, first for state governors in 1982, then for municipal mayors in 1985, and, finally, for president in 1989.[22] Existing accounts show how these major shifts unsettled an ingrained pattern of decentralized despotism in which regional oligarchs dominated the country's subnational state structures through a fusion of coercive, legal, and economic power that persisted well into the 1980s (Baiocchi, Heller, and Silva 2011, 40; Hagopian 2007). These disruptions aided sanitaristas' pursuit of a right to health by fundamentally weakening these historical adversaries of programmatic approaches to delivering public goods. Indeed, generic features of local democratization, especially the newly competitive electoral landscape in urban Brazil, generally undermined these decentralized despots, whose hold on power depended on a system of selective, patronage-based distribution of services that fundamentally rejected the sanitarista ambition to adopt rule-bound, democratically accountable, and programmatic procedures for universally delivering public health services.

Second, health democratization in all major Brazilian capitals reflected both the formal codification of a universal citizenship right to health in federal laws and the Constitution as well as local governments' embrace of a new mandate and public responsibility to enact that right. Alongside the specification of a larger set of positive rights in the country's 1988 Citizens Constitution, the new right to health set in motion a series of institutional transformations, which would prove to be especially consequential for efforts to alter the country's public health state during subsequent decades. Due in large part to the influence of venerable sanitaristas such as Dr. Sergio Arouca in drafting the document during Brazil's Constitutional Assembly, Article 196 came to declare health as a right of all citizens and a duty of the state to enact through social and economic policies that ensure universal and equal access to an array of health services (Federal Republic of Brazil 1988). Nevertheless, the formal right to health care for all Brazilians did not automatically translate into a lived reality for every citizen in any of the capitals examined in this study. The process of bringing this right to fruition was a different matter, and reflected still other dimensions of institutional change during Brazil's health-democratization period.

Third, decentralization reforms throughout urban Brazil accompanied the restoration of formal democracy in ways that ultimately favored sanitarista ambitions by enabling subnational configurations of political actors to pursue local institutional change. In particular, political, fiscal, and administrative decentralization jointly transformed the balance between national and local authority in ways that generally empowered municipalities vis-à-vis national- and state-level authorities (Falleti 2010b, 151). The ratification of the 1988 Brazilian Constitution gave municipalities unusually sweeping political autonomy not only by designating them as "state-members" with roughly similar status as states but also by authorizing them to promulgate so-called organic laws that functioned like municipal constitutions and have been used by local political actors to hold municipalities responsible for local needs (Baiocchi, Heller, and Silva 2011, 46). In addition to creating a free and universal health system (the SUS) that replaced the system installed by the military, these reforms created new political opportunity structures in state- and municipal-level politics that sanitaristas skillfully exploited in their efforts to establish and enact a democratic right to health. Additionally, fiscal-decentralization measures promulgated through a piecemeal series of constitutional amendments, laws, regulations, a federal pact, and NOBs of the SUS created new funding streams for health that considerably improved the resources on hand for local political actors to programmatically enact a right to health.[23] Finally, although administrative decentralization created unfunded mandates for subnational states and generated considerable ambiguity regarding which levels of government would ultimately be held accountable for provision of certain public services, these reforms empowered municipalities to provide basic health care services and gradually created a patchwork of financing mechanisms that left them far more empowered than at the advent of democratization.

Fourth, Brazil's health democratization was characterized by the subnationally variable extent to which local political actors disrupted the monopoly on municipal power that right-leaning parties, notorious for the antidemocratic and antiprogrammatic management of social-policy sectors such as the health sector, had maintained in many capitals. Although nationwide democratization generally eliminated prior patterns of decentralized despotism throughout urban Brazil, the political-party vestiges of traditional politicians remained far more resilient in some large capitals than in others. The newly competitive electoral environment and opportunities for social-movement political influence introduced by formal democratization and decentralization in Belo Horizonte, Porto Alegre, Recife, Curitiba, and Fortaleza significantly disrupted similar monopolies on local power that predated the health-democratization period. Although elected politicians from the country's most important, programmatic, left-leaning political party, the Workers' Party (PT), were especially forceful in unseating traditional politicians in some of these capitals, centrist-party actors played surprisingly similar roles at times. The shared record of left and centrist parties in dislodging traditional politicians from power underscores the record of nationwide democratization processes in empowering reformers from a broad ideological spectrum, not merely those constrained to the left-leaning PT.

By contrast, in Rio de Janeiro and Salvador, generic processes of formal democratization and democratic decentralization failed to disrupt the monopoly on local state power traditionally held by conservative regional elites working through patronage-oriented political parties. In Salvador, these transformations failed to disrupt political domination by the Carlista group of Antônio Carlos Magalhães (ACM), who rose to prominence as an appointed mayor and state governor under Brazil's military government and subsequently concentrated political power for much of the first two decades following democratization. By monopolizing the executive in Salvador's encompassing state of Bahia during a nearly uninterrupted period between 1982 and 2007—and by holding a majority of Salvador's municipal executives and state and federal legislative seats during this period—the infamously clientelist rule of various Carlistas thoroughly stunted the city's public health state through highly discretionary distribution of patronage and low prioritization of social spending.[24] Similar dynamics prevailed in the capital of Rio de Janeiro, where the dominance of infamously clientelist mayors such as César Maia and Luis Paulo Conde compounded the antidemocratic impulses of governors that consistently obstructed political autonomy for the capital and severely weakened its capacities for programmatic public-service provision.

Fifth, another subnationally variable quality of health democratization was unevenness in the reach of Brazil's flagship antipoverty program, Bolsa Família (BF). Although the conditional cash transfer (CCT) program is federally run, means tested, and the largest in the world as of the mid-2010s, its reach has varied considerably within urban Brazil. Indeed, the analysis in chapter 3 suggests that some major Brazilian capitals experienced far superior coverage and targeting of the program than did others. The program's ability to actually reach eligible recipients in five capitals—Belo Horizonte, Porto Alegre, Recife, Curitiba, and Fortaleza—considerably exceeded that of other capitals, such as Rio de Janeiro and Salvador. Specifically, the former group of cities witnessed higher rates of actual enrollment in the program among families that were eligible for its benefits as well as greater proportions of the overall population that ultimately received benefits through Bolsa Família. Although existing literature often presumes that the program's accessibility to eligible recipients has been largely constant across urban Brazil because of its status as a nationwide program that is administered by the federal Social Development Ministry (MDS), the unevenness documented in this book instead raises questions about the extent to which uneven local state capacities in the primary health sector may affect the uneven reach of BF. Because CCTs such as BF require recipients to demonstrate that they've received regular medical attention before they can receive cash transfers, the program's subnationally variable reach may well reflect the reach and effectiveness of arguably more fundamental social-policy sectors like the primary public health sector emphasized in this book. Such unanswered questions aside, the uneven reach of BF speaks to the depth of health democratization across urban Brazil if only because the program has likely induced uneven proportions of eligible recipients to access primary public health care and receive transfers that, depending on the city in question, could be spent on primary health care. At a minimum, the universalism at the core of the health-democratization period achieved a deeper expression, to the extent that conditions in cities allowed for greater reach of BF.

Sixth, Brazil's largest capitals varied considerably in the extent to which subnational state-building constructed new capacities for primary health care delivery. In five cities—Belo Horizonte, Porto Alegre, Recife, Curitiba, and Fortaleza—programmatically oriented actors such as sanitaristas maximized the expansion of these institutions. During the period, a variety of social and political actors critiqued the weak or nonexistent public health states that Brazil's largest capital cities had inherited from the prior period of military authoritarianism. Such structures lacked bureaucratization, professional staffs, and the power and resources to programmatically and equitably deliver basic public services such as primary health care to citizens. To the extent that local public health states existed at all in capitals, they tended to be weakly institutionalized, clientelist vectors between the military regime and private hospitals or clinics. In part because local representatives within Brazil's prior national health bureaucracy (INAMPS) channeled the flow of national resources directly into private health care facilities in a discretionary manner that largely circumvented municipalities, subnational health bureaucracies tended to remain underdeveloped prior to the period.[25] Compared to those of earlier periods, the new state structures that progressive political and social actors demanded and in some cases helped build were much larger, more centralized, and more bureaucratically institutionalized. As such, such structures accumulated greater capacities to penetrate cities through more programmatic modalities of basic service provision that reached poorer citizens living in neighborhoods with considerably higher health risks. By contrast, such state-building in the primary-care sectors of Rio de Janeiro and Salvador was less extensive.

Finally, Belo Horizonte, Porto Alegre, and Recife differed from all other capitals in the considerable extent to which tangible participatory democratic monitoring arose in the public-service sectors that most affect social development outcomes, and especially the public health sector. Here, it is particularly illuminating to assess the consistency with which Brazil's two most central institutions of participatory democracy—Participatory Budgeting (OP) and the Municipal Health Council (CMS) in each capital—operated in practice throughout the period. In these three cases, sanitaristas allied with participatory publics to institute and maintain these

TABLE 2.1
Types of health democratization in urban Brazil

	Minimalist (Rio de Janeiro, Salvador)	Programmatic (Curitiba, Fortaleza)	Participatory-programmatic (Belo Horizonte, Porto Alegre, Recife)
Return of formal democracy creates more competitive local elections	Yes	Yes	Yes
Local governments assume legal mandate to enact a universal and equal citizenship right to health	Yes	Yes	Yes
Municipalities assume the lead responsibility for primary health care	Yes	Yes	Yes
Nonright parties disrupt monopoly on local power by right parties	No	Yes	Yes
Bolsa Família achieves maximal coverage and targeting locally	No	Yes	Yes
Local governments consistently expand capacities of the public health state for primary service delivery	No	Yes	Yes
Participatory democratic institutions are capable monitors of health sector	No	No	Yes

mechanisms for citizen input into budgeting and monitoring of the relevant sectors in a consistent fashion. In this way, such capitals experienced a far more sustained and robust institutionalization of participatory democracy. Specifically, in all three of these cases, both OP and the CMS operated in a substantive (rather than purely cosmetic) way during well over half the period. As a result, the institutionalization of OP and the CMS in these three cities translated into heightened participatory-democratic monitoring of the public health sector as well as of other health-relevant sectors such as the sewage, running water, and sanitation sectors.[26] In such cases, health democratization achieved its fullest expression in all of urban Brazil. By contrast, similar demands for participatory-democratic oversights of key sectors in Curitiba, Fortaleza, Rio de Janeiro, and Salvador gained little or no sustained political traction, as evidenced by these capitals' only infrequent and superficial or nonexistent experiences of OP and CMS.

In sum, patterns of cross-case variation along these parameters suggest that urban Brazil witnessed not one but three different types of health democratization (see table 2.1). Next, I turn to the consequences of this variation.

4. Consequences of Health Democratization

The fact that nearly all major capitals had traveled at least some ways toward assembling minimally effective municipal public health states testifies to how nationwide democratization processes helped disrupt prior institutional legacies of Brazil's colonial and authoritarian eras. Compared to the mid-1980s, for example, all major Brazilian capitals had markedly increased spending and actual delivery of basic health and sanitation services and had reduced IMR by the end of the period.[27] Yet subnational variation in the health-democratization period had important consequences for both the type of local public health institutions that had emerged and the degree of institutional change and social development progress that had occurred in major capitals by the end of the period. First, the period generated key transformations of the local public health state with some major capitals, such as Belo Horizonte, Porto Alegre and Recife, emerging with "deliberative healthy states," while "healthy states" arose in Curitiba and Fortaleza, and "incapacitated states" emerged in Salvador and Rio de Janeiro. Second, these institutional transformations precipitated robust social development outcomes in cities with some version of a healthy state (Belo Horizonte, Porto Alegre, Recife, Curitiba, and Fortaleza), while those with incapacitated states (Salvador and Rio de Janeiro) experienced only non-robust development.

The MDD processes observable during the health-democratization period correspondingly entailed three subnational trajectories. First, through a participatory-programmatic path in Belo Horizonte, Porto Alegre, and Recife, office-holding sanitaristas not only maximized growth in municipal spending on basic health and sanitation provision, actual state delivery of primary public health services, and construction of the local state structures required for such interventions but also facilitated the rise of participatory-democratic institutions that became more active monitors (if not equal cogoverning partners) of the public health sector. Second, Curitiba and Fortaleza witnessed programmatic configurations that propelled moderate state-building and maximized the duration and depth of expansions of the municipal public health state's service-delivery arms but not its participatory institutions for monitoring this sector. This process maximized growth in municipal spending on basic health and sanitation provision, actual state delivery of primary public health services, and construction of the local state structures required for such interventions, but it did not institu-

TABLE 2.2

Consequences of health democratization in urban Brazil

	Type of health democratization trajectory		
	Minimalist (Rio de Janeiro, Salvador)	Programmatic (Curitiba, Fortaleza)	Participatory-programmatic (Belo Horizonte, Porto Alegre, Recife)
Extent of democratic state-building in primary health sector	Minimal	Moderate	Maximal
Institutional legacy	Incapacitated state	Healthy state	Deliberative healthy state
Social development legacy	Nonrobust development	Robust development	Robust development

tionalize democratic processes for sustained civil-society monitoring or co-governance of the health sector. Nevertheless, all five of these cases constructed some variant of a health-developmental or healthy state during the period. Far outperforming baseline levels of improvement across urban Brazil, the healthy states of Curitiba and Fortaleza and the deliberative healthy states of Belo Horizonte, Porto Alegre, and Recife lifted average spending on health and sanitation above the 255 reais per capita threshold, expanded average primary public-health-care coverage rates throughout the period beyond 30% of the population, and raised this rate above the 40% mark by 2012. Furthermore, the two variants of a healthy state in these five cities helped reduce IMR by more than what their initial conditions would have predicted.

Third, Rio de Janeiro and Salvador contrastingly saw clientelist configurations allow for only minimal degrees of state-building that featured, at best, brief and isolated moments of expansion in the public health state's service-delivery arms and its participatory-democratic institutions for monitoring the sector. In stark contrast to the maximal and moderate state-building processes that yielded some variant of a healthy state in the five positive cases just discussed, this led to only minimal growth in municipal spending on basic health and sanitation, in actual state delivery of primary public health services, in construction of the local state structures required for such interventions, and in capacities for participatory-democratic oversight of the sector. The "incapacitated states" that emerged as a result performed strikingly far below average, with expenditures hovering around

130 reais per capita, while both the period average and ending level of primary health coverage lingered below the 5% threshold. Ultimately, IMR reductions underperformed relative to initial conditions.

Table 2.2 summarizes this argument regarding the consequences of these variable paths of health democratization for the country's overall dynamics and outcomes of MDD. Given their many other similarities as cities in Brazil—their geographic proximity; their shared policy-making authorities within a highly decentralized federalist democracy; and Brazil's damaging legacy of slavery, Portuguese colonialism, and military authoritarianism—the presence of these contrasting institutional and development outcomes within the same country are striking. For instance, the political transformation undergone by capitals like Recife and Fortaleza remains nothing short of remarkable when one considers their encompassing region's history as a slave-trading hub within a country that received more African slaves than any other in world history. Far from representing a final distribution of social development, however, such outcomes instead represent consequences of the quarter-century health-democratization period at a moment in the mid-2010s in which few could dispute its clear denouement, if not outright collapse. Further, the study does not dismiss out of hand the possibility that other factors, including colonial legacies, power constellations, nationally administered social policies, policy diffusion, and women's political representation, could have contributed to such social development outcomes. Rather, the statistical and configurational analysis presented next will systematically examine predictions of this study's MDD framework alongside such alternative explanations.

THREE

Sanitaristas and Infant Mortality Reduction

This chapter begins the book's empirical analysis of how sanitaristas affected state-building and social development outcomes across urban Brazil's largest cities during the health-democratization period. The regression analyses that follow first demonstrate that, even after holding canonical alternative explanations constant, sanitarista office holding in the SMS directorship was negatively associated with child and infant mortality rates (CMR & IMR) and positively associated with rates of access to primary public health care across urban Brazil between 1995 and 2014. Then, configurational fuzzy-set analyses (FSA) show that consistent sanitarista office holding was a necessary condition for maximizing IMR reduction and growth over time in both municipal spending on the public health and sanitation sectors as well as on the reach of the PSF (Brazil's flagship primary public-health-care program) within major capitals. Thus, the chapter situates the coming comparative-historical analyses of individual capitals by first illustrating an overall relationship in recent decades between pragmatist publics—a central, hypothesized driver of local state-building according to this book's theory of MDD—and social development outcomes across Brazil's largest capitals.

More specifically, the chapter first demonstrates subnational variation in four outcomes annually: IMR, CMR, PSF coverage, and the ratio of primary public-health-care provision to the uninsured population. It also documents cross-case variation in sanitarista office holding in the SMS directorship and a host of variables capturing alternative explanations. Then, Prais-Winsten regression analyses using panel-corrected standard errors and autoregressive disturbance terms show that sanitarista occupation of the SMS was negatively associated with IMR and CMR across urban Brazil, even after controlling for alternative explanations such as ruling political-party ideology, women's political representation, coverage by Brazil's conditional cash transfer program (*Bolsa Família*), influential participatory publics, and other factors. Next, FSA results complement these findings by showing that consistent sanitarista office holding was a necessary condition within all combinations of factors that were sufficient for achieving robust development outcomes, while inconsistent sanitarista office holding was a necessary condition within all such configurations that were sufficient for nonrobust development. FSA results also show that office-holding sanitaristas were part of the only configuration that was consistent with maximal local spending on health and sanitation and with maximal coverage of municipally delivered primary public health care via the Family Health Program (PSF). After section 1 introduces the data, measures, and results from regression analysis, section 2 moves to an extended discussion of the FSA findings. This is followed by section 3's concluding discussion of the insights, complementarities, and limitations of these findings.

1. Statistical Data and Regression Analysis

Despite their limitations, the statistical methods of multivariate regression analysis used here complement and reinforce the comparative-historical case studies of coming chapters in several ways. Particularly when addressing a country of continental size such as Brazil, studies aiming to offer general insights about nationwide dynamics benefit from the broad scope that multivariate regression analyses like the ones that follow can offer. The approach also permits testing of several theories of social development alongside one another and of the study's central argument about sanitarista office holding throughout all of Brazil's largest capital cities. Particularly as a growing number of scholars seek to explain Brazil's social development transformation, these methods also allow for the study's findings to be replicated more broadly. As an initial step toward assessing the drivers of this transformation, the statistical analyses below employ cross-sectional time-series (CSTS) data that are especially useful in illustrating associations—though not causal relationships—between sanitarista office holding and social development throughout urban Brazil.

These data include annual data points for all eleven major Brazilian capital city municipalities, defined here as those capitals that averaged greater than one million residents during the 1995 to 2014 period. These include São Paulo, Rio de Janeiro, Salvador, Fortaleza, Belo Horizonte, Manaus, Curitiba, Recife, Belém, Porto Alegre, and Goiânia. The study omits Brasília from consideration because its status as the national capital entails different governing practices that undermine its comparability to these cities. For methodological and theoretical purposes, capital city municipalities are an especially appropriate unit of analysis to examine because they faced significant pressures from federal and state government to assume responsibility for the primary public health sector after 1994. Serving as important public-service provision hubs within major cities that contain approximately one-third of Brazil's more than 210 million people, these large capitals constitute a substantively relevant sample of comparable units within a country in which 86% of residents live in urban areas. I statistically analyze the period after 1994 because data for all alternative explanations and relevant controls do not become available in a nationally comparable form until then. Use of lagged independent variables resulted in analysis of 198 city-years, including 18 years of observations for all eleven major capital cities.

I.I. DEPENDENT VARIABLES: MEASURING SOCIAL DEVELOPMENT

I analyze four indicators of social development annually at the municipal level. First, the *logged infant mortality rate (uimr)* applies the log function to the ratio of all infant (under one year old) deaths per 1,000 infants aged one year and younger. As highlighted earlier, such measures of premature death constitute a generally agreed upon measure of social development in the Global South and beyond. Echoing Sen's capability approach, scholars, policy makers, and international institutions such as the World Bank and United Nations have for decades named reductions in infant mortality as a key indicator of developmental progress.[1] As is common practice in studies of child health, taking the logarithmic function of the variable improves the normality of its distribution. Second, as a robustness check, the regression analysis that follows also operationalizes the *logged under-5 mortality rate (u5mr)* as the logged ratio of deaths among children five years old and younger per 1,000 children aged five years and younger. As with the infant mortality measure above, lower values of this variable also indicate a higher level of social development. Both operationalizations represent a common-place measure of social development in the Global South similar or identical to those used in cross-national analyses and other subnational analyses of Brazil.[2]

These first two indicators demonstrate that major Brazilian capitals varied from one another in their *absolute* levels of social development during recent decades. Further, these absolute levels of infant and child mortality—and their variability from city to city—declined considerably during later years in the sequence examined. Whereas in 1995 unlogged *u1mr* averaged 32.33 deaths per 1,000 infants with a standard deviation of 9.72, this indicator declined to 15.21 deaths per 1,000 with a standard deviation of only 2.82 by 2012. Similarly, whereas in 1995 the average under-five-year mortality rate was 7.19 deaths per 1,000 with a standard deviation of 2.13, the mean had declined to 3.52 with a standard deviation of .63 by 2012. The convergence in infant mortality rates observable at the end of the period owes much to large improvements achieved in the regions of the country that bear Brazil's most adverse institutional legacies of colonialism. Indeed, cities in Brazil's heavily colonized northeast region such as Fortaleza and Recife witnessed the largest declines in IMR between 1988 and 2014 (52.91 deaths per 1,000 and 53.06 deaths per 1,000, respectively). By contrast, southern- and southeastern-region cities such as Porto Alegre and Rio de Janeiro experienced the most modest declines during that period (18.84 deaths per 1,000 and 21.60 deaths per 1,000, respectively). Thus, absolute levels of social development in urban Brazil have grown across the board but particularly in capitals within the country's historically poorest and most heavily colonized regions.

Additionally, the particular subnational pattern of these declines yielded major, surprising changes over time in *relative* levels of development among major capitals. Indeed, major differences in the rankings of these cities relative to one another during earlier (for example, in 1988) versus later moments (for example, in 2014) constitute a surprise vis-à-vis existing theory. Specifically, such differences defy the continuity in contemporary outcomes that theories of colonialism and postcolonial development would predict. Mahoney's comparative-historical analysis of regional development in Brazil shows that the country's regions generally maintained their positions relative to one another throughout most of the twentieth century (2010, 242–52). Yet during the late-twentieth and early-twenty-first centuries, the position of the country's largest capitals relative to one another shifted away from this relatively stable hierarchy in development levels. Indeed, a fundamental reordering in relative levels of social development in major capitals occurred after 1988.

For instance, no major capital had maintained its 1988 IMR ranking among major Brazilian capitals by 2012. The correlation between these cities' infant mortality rankings in 1995 and their rankings in 2012 was only .32. This correlation is even weaker (.21) when comparing 2012 rankings to rankings in 1988, when colonial legacies were even more firmly entrenched. This reordering especially reflects major changes in the relative position of northeastern cities such as Fortaleza and Recife, which climbed from ninth and tenth place in 1988 to third and sixth place by 2012, respectively. Yet these improvements in relative development were not simply confined to the northeast region; indeed, some of the worst-performing southeastern cities in 1988, such as Belo Horizonte, climbed from eighth to fourth place by 2012 and to third by 2014. Thus, the particular subnational pattern of contemporary change in social development throughout urban Brazil requires explanations that—while attentive to longstanding legacies of colonialism—can speak to other, more recent drivers of change.

Two additional dependent variables measure primary public-health-care provision. Using the federal health ministry's estimate, the *PSF coverage rate* captures the proportion of the municipal population reached by the PSF.[3] PSF coverage varied widely across cities in all years, including 2013, when, for instance, Belo Horizonte achieved over 73% coverage while Salvador recorded only 23%. The *primary-care rate* measures how some cities deliver such services through non-PSF platforms and feature higher numbers of users who are effectively priced out of the market for private health care. It captures the proportion of all primary public health services (PSF and non-PSF) delivered to the estimated population of uninsured residents.

1.2. SANITARISTA OFFICE HOLDING AND OTHER INDEPENDENT VARIABLES

Two measures assess sanitarista office holding. *Sanitarista municipal health secretary* is a dichotomous variable coded equal to one if the municipal SUS directorship was occupied by a sanitarista for at least half the year. *Sanitarista state health secretary* is a dichotomous variable equal to one if a sanitarista directed the State Health Department (SES) in the capital's encompassing state for at least half the year. Using a variety of archival records;

TABLE 3.I.
Data sources used for scoring of sanitarista office-holding variables

Type	Description
Archival records	Periodicals and newsletters of two key movement organizations: CEBES's *Health in Debate* (*Saúde em Debate*) journal (http://www.saudeemdebate.org.br/); and *ABRASCO Bulletin* (*Boletim da ABRASCO*; http://www.abrasco.org.br/site/)
	Newsletters and other archives of three organizations founded by sanitaristas: the National Council of Health Secretaries (CONASS; http://www.conass.org.br/); the National Health Council (CNS; http://conselho.saude.gov.br/); and the National Council of Municipal Health Secretaries (CONASEMS; http://www.conasems.org.br/)
	Newspaper articles from Brazil's national newspaper of record, *Folha de São Paulo* (http://www.folha.uol.com.br/), and five other Brazilian newspapers: *Estado de Minas* (http://www.em.com.br/), *Diário de Pernambuco* (http://www.diariodepernambuco.com.br/), *O Globo* (http://oglobo.globo.com/), *Correio do Povo* (http://www.correiodopovo.com.br/), and *A Tarde* (http://atarde.uol.com.br/)
	Minutes of Municipal Health Council (CMS) meetings held between 1992 and 2012 in multiple capitals
	Searchable online database of medical specializations for physicians as recorded and reported by the Federal Medicine Council (CFM; www.cfm.org.br)
	Searchable online database of the curriculum vitae for Brazilian public health scholars maintained by the federal Brazilian research funder, the National Council of Scientific and Technological Development (CNPq; http://lattes.cnpq.br/, last accessed July 2015)
Participant observations	Participant observations of Municipal Health Council (SMS) meetings in multiple capitals between 2008 and 2010
In-depth interviews	Interviews with nationally prominent sanitaristas published as UNESCO (2005a, 2005b)
	Original, semistructured interviews with sanitaristas and other key informants in multiple Brazilian capitals between 2008 and 2010

NOTE: All online sources last accessed in August 2015 unless otherwise noted.

publicly available, online data sources; and self-reporting through in-depth interviews wherever possible (table 3.1), I coded the occupants of these two offices as sanitaristas when their backgrounds and experience indicated clear involvement with Sanitarist Movement organizations or political projects. Descriptive analyses of all city-years (see table 3.2) exhibit surprisingly high levels of office holding by sanitaristas on both the municipal (37%) and state levels (30%). I expected to find that municipal office holding by sanitaristas was negatively associated with childhood mortality rates and positively associated with primary public health delivery.

TABLE 3.2

Descriptive statistics and sources for PCSE model variables

Variable	Mean	St. dev.	Min.	Max.	N
Social development outcomes[a]					
Logged infant mortality rate—$(ln)u1mr$	2.81	.33	2.10	3.85	198
Logged under-5 mortality rate—$(ln)u5mr$	1.34	.33	.66	2.42	198
PSF coverage rate	21.92	19.34	0	76.69	198
Primary-care rate	5.76	4.06	.16	18.06	198
Sanitarista office holding[b]					
Sanitarista municipal health (SMS) director	.37	.49	0	1	198
Sanitarista state health (SES) director	.30	.46	0	1	198
Ruling party ideology[c]					
Ideology of mayor's party	5.83	1.49	3.10	7.98	198
Ideology of governor's party	5.61	1.07	3.10	7.98	198
Women's political representation[d]					
Female mayor	.10	.30	0	1	198
Female municipal health secretary	.12	.32	0	1	198
Female governor	.07	.25	0	1	198
Female state health secretary	.07	.25	0	1	198
Participatory democratic institutions[e]					
Participatory Budgeting	.43	.50	0	1	198
Federal social-policy delivery[f]					
Bolsa Família coverage index	49.97	53.72	0	172.60	198
Local state spending[g]					
(ln) Per capita municipal health and sanitation expenditure	5.28	.97	2.20	7.17	198
Controls					
(ln) GDP/capita[g]	9.10	.38	8.47	9.80	198
(ln) Birth rate[h]	2.84	.21	2.51	3.44	198
(ln) Maternal illiteracy rate[i]	1.33	.65	−.72	2.66	198

NOTE: All statistics are calculated for the years that each variable was analyzed in regressions. Mortality rates are calculated for 1997-2014; *PSF coverage rate* and *primary-care rate* are calculated for 1996–2013. Statistics for other variables are for 1995-2012. All websites were last accessed in March 2016 unless otherwise mentioned.

[a] For mortality rate variables, data on deaths are drawn from civil registry, and population estimates for each age group are from Brazil's Geographic and Statistics Institute (IBGE). *PSF coverage rate* is the MS's calculation of the proportion of the municipal population reached by the PSF. *Primary-care rate* equals the ratio of primary health services (http://www2.datasus.gov.br/) to the Supplementary Health Agency's (ANS) survey estimate of un-insured population (http://www.ans.gov.br/).

[b] See table 3.1 for detailed description of data sources.

[c] To identify mayors, governors, and their parties, I use data from Brazil's Supreme Electoral Court (TSE) web-site (http://www.tse.jus.br/eleicoes/eleicoes-anteriores/) as well as archival sources (see table 3.1) to track party-switching between elections. For party coding, I use the survey-based ratings produced by Power and Zucco (2009) and linear interpolations and projections for nonsurvey years. Although these rankings use a 10-point scale on which 1 = furthest left and 10 = furthest right, I reverse the scale's direction to ease interpretation.

[d] Data on officeholder identity drawn from TSE (http://www.tse.jus.br/eleicoes/eleicoes-anteriores/).

[e] This variable was coded from archival sources and city government websites for all capitals. See table 3.1.

[f] The index sums together two distinct variables that passed scalability tests and are highly correlated with one another. The first component is the targeting rate, which is the ratio of the total number of families enrolled to the number of families who met federal-state eligibility criteria in a given year. The second component is the popula-tional coverage rate, which is the ratio of the total estimated number of individual beneficiaries to the total resident population. Data were downloaded from MDS's website (http://www.mds.gov.br/bolsafamilia) and from http://aplicacoes.mds.gov.br/sagi/FerramentasSAGI_menu/internet.php.

[g] Data in Year 2000 constant reais are from Research and Analysis Institute (IPEA; http://www.ipeadata.gov.br/).

[h] Data are from the health ministry website (http://www2.datasus.gov.br/).

[i] Data are from representative samples of IBGE's 1991, 2000, and 2010 censuses (Minnesota Population Cen-ter [2013], *Integrated Public Use Microdata Series, International: Version 6.2* [Minneapolis: University of Minnesota], https://www.ipums.org/, last accessed May 2014). Linear interpolations are used for other years.

A first set of independent variables assesses predictions from power constellation theory that left-party executives generally advance social development, whereas right-party executives undermine it. To measure party ideology, I adapted Power and Zucco's (2009) survey-based scoring of Brazilian party ideologies such that higher numbers indicate more left-leaning parties and lower numbers indicate more right-leaning parties. By enabling empirically based estimates of party ideology using continuous variables, these data permit a more cautious approach to estimating party effects and avert the severe multicollinearity resulting from inclusion of separate dummy variables for right- and left-party rule. *Ideology of mayor's party* is a continuous variable measuring the party-ideology score for mayors during each city-year, whereas *ideology of governor's party* is a continuous variable measuring the party ideology of governors in each municipality's encompassing, state-level government. While the party-ideology variable was strongly correlated with sanitarista office holding, the association was weak (municipal level: $r = .41$, $p < .05$; state level: $r = -.27$, $p < .05$). Further, sanitarista office holding was not solely traceable to PT rule of the executive: 36% of city-years with sanitarista SMS directors featured non-PT mayors, whereas 81% of city-years with sanitarista SES directors featured non-PT governors. Although existing theories predict that above-average values on both variables (more left-leaning executives) should be associated with stronger development outcomes, I treat this as an empirical question.

To assess women's political representation, *female mayor* and *female governor* are dichotomous variables coded one if the executive during each year was female. Because existing literature suggests that developmental effects of women's electoral representation are most likely to arise when women reach a critical mass of at least 20% of all seats in a national legislature (Swiss, Fallon, and Burgos 2012), lower rates of female representation in both the mayorship (10%) and governorship (7%) make such effects somewhat unlikely in the Brazilian context (rates of women's legislative representation are also low). *Female municipal health secretary* and *female state health secretary* are dichotomous variables coded one if women occupied directorships atop the SMS and the SES, a more plausible effect of women's political representation in Brazil. Additionally, *Participatory Budgeting (OP)* dichotomously measures the presence or absence of this process (Baiocchi, Heller, and Silva 2011), which helps assess the influence of participatory publics in formulating the capital improvement budgets of cities. Following Touchton and Wampler (2014) and Gonçalves (2013), *Bolsa Família (BF) coverage* measures the targeting and coverage of Brazil's CCT. *Per capita health and sanitation expenditure* captures municipal government spending in logged, inflation-adjusted, Year 2000 Brazilian *reais*. Controls include *(ln)GDP per capita,* a continuous measure of economic development using logged, inflation-adjusted (Year 2000) Brazilian reais; *(ln)birth rate*, a logged continuous variable calculated from federal birth registry statistics; and *(ln)maternal illiteracy rate*, a logged continuous measure.

1.3. RESULTS OF REGRESSION ANALYSIS

The multivariate regression models below test the sanitarista office-holding hypothesis alongside controls and alternative explanations, using Prais-Winsten models with panel-corrected standard errors (PW-PCSE), a first-order autocorrelation correction *(ar1)*, and lagged independent variables. Models of primary health care delivery (table 3.4) employ a one-year lag of all independent variables, reflecting qualitative findings that sanitarista office holding typically required a year to affect the rollout of new on-the-ground capacities for service provision. Mortality regressions (table 3.3) employ a two-year lag to recognize that sanitarista office holding required another year for such capacity-building efforts to affect actual health outcomes.

By analyzing predictors of infant and child mortality across cities and over time, these models represent a commonly adopted approach in political sociology, economic sociology, and political economy to correcting violations of assumed error independence and constant variance (Brady, Beckfield, and Seeleib-Kaiser 2005; Bandelj 2009; Kristal 2010; Vasi and King 2012). If left uncorrected, such violations can lead to biased and misleading significant tests (Frees 2004). Beck and Katz's (1995) technique of PCSE with an *ar1* term represents a generally agreed-upon approach to adjusting for contemporaneous and serial error correlation and heteroscedasticity, particularly for temporally dominated data sets (Beck 2001; Plümper, Troeger, and Manow 2005) like mine (eleven cities, eighteen years). Panel-specific *ar1* is used to model nontrivial, cross-city variations in the degree of within-panel autocorrelation.

A first set of results (table 3.3) demonstrates that sanitarista office holding of the municipal SUS directorship was negatively associated with childhood mortality rates, even after controlling for canonical explanations. Models 1 and 2 show that municipal office holding by sanitaristas had

TABLE 3.3
Predictors of (logged) infant and child mortality rates, 1995–2014

	PW-PCSE		PW-PCSE	
	(1) $(ln)u1mr$	(2) $(ln)u5mr$	(3) $(ln)u1mr$	(4) $(ln)u5mr$
Sanitarista office holding				
Sanitarista municipal health director	−.081***	−.074***	−.077***	−.067**
	(.022)	(.020)	(.024)	(.022)
Sanitarista state health director	−.087**	−.086**	−.010**	−.096**
	(.032)	(.029)	(.033)	(.032)
Ruling party ideology				
Ideology of mayor's party			−.009	−.007
			(.010)	(.010)
Ideology of governor's party			.012	.016
			(.012)	(.011)
Women's political representation				
Female mayor			−.073	−.079*
			(.038)	(.034)
Female municipal health secretary			−.043	−.027
			(.028)	(.026)
Female governor			−.016	−.014
			(.038)	(.037)
Female state health secretary			−.071*	−.038
			(.034)	(.031)
Participatory democratic institutions				
Participatory Budgeting			.033	.026
			(.034)	(.031)
Federal conditional cash transfers				
Bolsa Família Coverage			−.000	−.000
			(.001)	(.000)
Local state spending				
(ln) Per capita municipal health and sanitation expenditure			−.083**	−.071**
			(.029)	(.026)
Controls				
(ln) GDP/cap	.008	.026	−.007	.016
	(.057)	(.055)	(.060)	(.060)
(ln) Birth rate	.686***	.763***	.537***	.614***
	(.168)	(.156)	(.147)	(.141)
(ln) Maternal illiteracy rate	.253***	.233***	.161**	.169**
	(.056)	(.054)	(.057)	(.056)
Constant	.511	−1.301*	1.637*	−.370
	(.665)	(.640)	(.702)	(.689)
R^2	.945	.854	.951	.873
N	198	198	198	198

NOTE: All results are from Prais-Winsten regression with panel-corrected standard errors (reported in parentheses) and a panel-specific ar1 term. All independent variables are lagged by two years.

*$p < .05$; **$p < .01$; ***$p < .001$ (two-tailed tests)

strongly negative and highly significant effects on logged under-one-year and under-five-year mortality rates after controlling for economic development, birth rates, and maternal illiteracy rates. With an r^2 of .95 and .85, respectively, these models explain an overwhelming amount of variation in both outcomes. Given likely unobserved sources of heterogeneity, however, the qualitative case studies that follow complementarily illustrate the subnational state-building mechanisms by which sanitarista office holding mattered for both outcomes.

Models 3 and 4 in table 3.3 show that sanitarista office holding continues to be a strongly negative and highly significant predictor of both infant and child mortality, even after considering controls and alternative explanations such as ruling-party ideology, women's political representation, participatory-democratic institutions, the reach of CCTs, and municipal health and sanitation expenditures. Model 3 suggests that with 99.9% confidence, municipal-level office holding by sanitaristas was negatively associated with infant mortality, even after controlling for such explanations and demographic predictors. As a robustness check, model 4 suggests with 99% confidence that, on average and with all else equal, municipal office holding by sanitaristas was also negatively associated with under-five-year mortality rates. Although ruling left-party ideology, participatory-democratic institutions, and federal conditional cash transfers all fall short of statistical significance, municipal spending on health and sanitation—a key channel through which such factors can matter for mortality—is associated with both outcomes at the lower 99% level. Both models offer only weaker support (at only $p < .05$) for the arguments that women's political representation in the state-level health department was associated with lower infant mortality rates (model 3) and that women's political representation in the mayorship was associated with lower under-five-year mortality rates (model 4). Ultimately, the separate effects of spending and women's representation do not nullify those of sanitarista office holding, inviting further qualitative examination of its underlying mechanisms.

Models 3 and 4 fail to support the commonplace expectation that ruling-party ideology, influential participatory publics, and economic development are associated with social development. After scoring party ideology using data on self-reported differences between left and right parties, the party ideologies of neither mayors nor governors are significantly associated with mortality in these models. Neither the state- nor the municipal-level measures of women's electoral representation as mayors or governors is significant at the highest levels of statistical significance. Still, few substantively meaningful conclusions can be inferred from this result because both variables exhibit office-holding rates that fall well short of critical mass thresholds outlined in existing literature. Finally, the presence of influential participatory publics, as indicated by the presence of a Participatory Budgeting process, is not a statistically significant predictor of development in these tests.

Additional models (see table 3.4) further suggest the relevance of sanitarista office holding for development by showing that sanitarista occupation of the municipal health directorship was positively and significantly associated with both measures of primary public health delivery. Model 1 suggests with 95% confidence that municipal-level office holding by sanitaristas was, on average, associated with a 2.66 percentage-point increase in the PSF coverage rate, even after controlling for ruling-party ideology, women's political representation, participatory democracy, CCT coverage, municipal health and sanitation expenditures, and per capita GDP. Interestingly, sanitarista office holding positively affected PSF coverage, even when considering separate, significant effects of per capita municipal health and sanitation spending. This suggests that sanitarista office holding affects development via channels other than just sheer public health spending. Model 1 also suggests that means-tested CCTs such as Bolsa Família, which require children in recipient households to undergo regular medical exams, may have helped expand provision—or may have reflected expanded provision—of primary public health services.

Model 2 in table 3.4 further supports the argument that sanitarista office holding on the municipal level mattered for the primary-care rate as well. With 99% confidence and all else equal, sanitarista office holding of the SMS directorship was on average associated with an increase of 1.11 in the primary-care rate, even after controlling for the separate influence of per capita GDP. The model again suggests that women's office holding in the directorship of the state health department was also positively and significantly associated with this outcome, further suggesting that the identity of cabinet-level officeholders mattered for primary public health care. In sum, the models suggest that sanitarista office holding mattered for policy implementation and social development, net of longstanding explanations and controls.

TABLE 3.4
Predictors of primary public health care delivery, 1995–2013

	PW-PCSE	
	(1) PSF coverage rate	(2) Primary-care rate
Sanitarista office holding		
Sanitarista municipal health director	2.655*	1.108**
	(1.280)	(.356)
Sanitarista state health director	−1.180	−.405
	(1.748)	(.492)
Ruling party ideology		
Ideology of mayor's party	.362	−.264
	(.573)	(.166)
Ideology of governor's party	.005	.284
	(.685)	(.210)
Women's political representation		
Female mayor	1.933	−.596
	(2.136)	(.462)
Female municipal health secretary	−.433	.490
	(1.656)	(.394)
Female governor	−2.638	.135
	(1.968)	(.557)
Female state health secretary	2.158	.856**
	(1.704)	(.325)
Participatory democratic institutions		
Participatory Budgeting	2.407	.212
	(1.714)	(.506)
Federal conditional cash transfers		
Bolsa Família coverage	.0679*	.005
	(.033)	(.006)
Local state spending		
(*ln*) Per capita municipal health and sanitation expenditure	6.924***	.625
	(1.471)	(.340)
Controls		
(*ln*) GDP/cap	.152	4.284***
	(2.492)	(1.202)
Constant	−24.310	−35.506***
	(23.767)	(10.576)
R^2	.389	.286
N	198	198

NOTE: All results are from Prais-Winsten regressions with panel-corrected standard errors (reported in parentheses) and a panel-specific *art* term. All independent variables are lagged by one year.
*p < .05; **p < .01; ***p < .001 (two-tailed tests)

Nevertheless, the statistical models mentioned earlier have several limitations and rely on numerous assumptions, some of which are more tenuously upheld than others. First, such analyses assume that key independent variables are not correlated with factors that are related to the dependent variable but are excluded from the model. Although few research designs can eliminate this possibility, the high r-squared values in all mortality models (.86 and above) demonstrate that the variables in the model explain over 85% of the variation in each of the outcomes examined, suggesting that such potential for omitted variable bias is not a major issue.

Second, the assumption that the independent variables were not correlated with one another was only tenuously upheld, with some variables more closely related to one another than is ideal for such an analysis. For instance, the configurational and qualitative analyses that follow illustrate that sanitarista office holding likely contributed to municipal-development interventions, such as PSF coverage and municipal spending on health and sanitation. Still, the statistical significance and negative association between social development and each one of these three independent variables persisted after deducting the others from models. The FSA models below, however, explicitly recognized that conditions of development overlap with one another, something that contrastingly limits the inferences possible from the aforementioned statistical models.

Indeed, the configurational and case study analyses that follow aim to address these and additional limitations of the statistical findings. For one, such statistical models assume that, when included, interaction terms can adequately assess all interaction effects among independent variables. But the theory of MDD suggests that office-holding pragmatist publics work alongside multiple factors to foster social development outcomes. In this sense, the fuzzy-set methods employed later offer a more realistic modeling of sanitarista office holding and development because they allow for the likelihood that two or more conditions of development may overlap with one another. A second and related constraint in the aforementioned regression analyses is that they offer few insights into the causal mechanisms connecting sanitarista office holding with social development. Indeed, the study makes no claim that these analyses themselves demonstrate causation. Rather, to illustrate causal mechanisms at work, subsequent chapters offer within-case analyses of the local state-building processes through which office-holding pragmatist publics fostered gradual institutional changes for social development on subnational levels throughout urban Brazil. Third, although focusing somewhat narrowly on major capital cities helps maximize the unit homogeneity of the cases examined, differences between the populations of the cities compared were sometimes considerable, a factor considered more overtly in the configurational and case study analyses to come. Finally, while the aforementioned statistical analyses somewhat tenuously assumed independence of the cases examined, the configurational and comparative-case-study analyses better accommodate the possibility that the experiences of cities examined in the analysis affected one another in nontrivial ways.

2. *Fuzzy-Set Analysis (FSA)*

The theory of MDD articulated in preceding chapters predicts that consistent local office holding by sanitaristas maximized expansion of the public health state, which in turn yielded robust development outcomes by broadening access to primary health care across urban Brazil. Although the theory posits that office-holding sanitaristas animated this process, it suggests that they did so alongside a host of other conditions that together comprise a programmatic configuration. Examining the theory's predictions about the configurations of conditions that aligned with sanitarista office holding to maximize health-related state-building and social development outcomes is a task classically suited to systematic comparative analysis. In what follows, I assess these multiple, overlapping conditions using fuzzy-set analyses (FSA) of all eleven Brazilian capitals that averaged greater than one million residents during the 1995 to 2014 period. Thus, I examine the same cities examined in the regression analyses mentioned earlier. Because FSA eschews the "net effects thinking" of such regression analyses for a configurational logic of causation (Vaisey 2007; Ragin 2008), it is especially useful for assessing whether and how such conditions overlap with one another in particular cases of interest. Ultimately, the results of these analysis suggest that two subtypes of programmatic configurations—a participatory-programmatic variant in Belo Horizonte, Porto Alegre, and Recife and a more generic programmatic variant in Curitiba and Fortaleza—yielded robust development outcomes in these capitals, whereas clientelist configurations produced nonrobust development outcomes in Rio de Janeiro and Salvador.

As argued in Ragin (2008, 6–10), set-theoretic claims such as the ones that follow differ in crucial ways from the measures of association used in the multivariate regression analyses mentioned earlier. First, FSA models set-theoretic relationships between causal and outcome sets, as opposed to correlational connections between independent and dependent variables.

The measures of association used in the aforementioned statistical analysis—both correlations and regression coefficients—assumed that a key independent variable of interest such as sanitarista office holding was symmetrically related to infant mortality rates at all levels of consistency over time in different cities. Set-theoretic analysis, by contrast, excels at assessing asymmetry in the relationship between a theorized causal condition such as sanitarista office holding and an outcome such as robust development at different levels of each. In other words, instead of examining the net effect of a unit increase above the average, cross-case level of an independent variable, FSA assesses the relevance of a causal condition for an outcome in individual cases that exhibit both high and low degrees of membership in that set. Here, for example, set-theoretic analysis allows for a theoretically defined level of frequency in office holding by pragmatist publics rather than an average across the cases, to be defined as the threshold above which robust development is nearly always present. Conversely, it allows for that threshold to be defined as the one below which nonrobust patterns of development are nearly always present. Further, FSA allows analysts to define multiple such conditions of an outcome of interest.

Second, FSA's examination of whether configurations of multiple conditions were necessary and/or sufficient for an outcome to occur fundamentally differs from the statistical models mentioned earlier, which instead assumed that all independent variables operated independently from one another. In set-theoretic analyses, such combinations can instead be usefully thought of as exemplifying a "causal" recipe, or specific combination of causally relevant ingredients linked to an outcome (Ragin 2008, 9). FSA operationalizes this approach by assessing the degree to which each of several cases is a member in a causal recipe composed of several intersecting conditions. Later, I test degrees of membership that cities with robust development outcomes had in recipes composed of six conditions, something not possible using the aforementioned statistical methods.

Finally, whereas the statistical models mentioned earlier examined the net effects of independent variables, the fuzzy-set analysis that follows instead embraces a set-theoretic approach to causal complexity that integrates systematic, counterfactual analysis. Although case study researchers often aim to shore up their causal arguments by specifying plausible counterfactual cases, set-theoretic analyses do so in an especially systematic fashion using truth tables. Here, a counterfactual case can be understood as a combination of causal conditions that does not exist empirically. In the set-theoretic analyses conducted as follows, Boolean truth tables are used to systematically examine the outcomes that would have been likely to occur if such counterfactual cases did, in fact, exist. Using systematic comparisons of counterfactuals and the full array of cases with actually existing configurations of causal factors, the analyses that follow assess the consistency with which a given configuration was sufficient for an outcome to occur.

2.1. DEFINING OUTCOME AND CAUSAL SETS

To develop such a configurational analysis, however, it is first necessary to explicitly define both outcome and causal sets by drawing on the theoretical discussions of social development and sanitarista office holding from preceding chapters. To facilitate FSA, I first define fuzzy sets that specify the degree of each capital's membership in a specified causal condition. This approach contrasts with a common alternative approach of defining "crisp sets," which instead specify case membership in a causal condition using one of only two possible scores: a 1 denoting full membership in a given set or a 0 representing full nonmembership in the set. Because they include eighteen years of annual observations that have been triangulated by fieldwork findings and additional qualitative research, my data allow for finer-grained distinctions to be drawn regarding each case's degree of membership in a given set throughout the period examined. To define these fuzzy sets and perform FSA, I use tools that Ragin pioneered and Longest and Vaisey refined and routinized in their "fuzzy" package for Stata 13.1 (Ragin 2008; Longest & Vaisey 2008).

I specify a first outcome, *robust developmental trajectory* (Y_1), which captures the set of cities that achieved degrees of infant mortality reduction exceeding what initial development conditions predicted. I define this set in three steps. First, I calculate the annual infant mortality rate (IMR), defined here as the ratio of all infant (under one year old) deaths per 1,000 infants. Then I divided each city's 1995 to 2012 reduction in IMR by the amount of expected reduction estimated by the predicted value from a bivariate, cross-sectional regression ($R^2 = .92$; $n = 11$; $p < .000$) in which the dependent variable was the eighteen-year change in IMR and the independent variable was IMR during 1995, the initial year of the sequence. Substantively, this ratio is meaningful because it recognizes cities' widely variable initial conditions and defines development in terms of the degree of overperformance (or underperformance) that is unexplained by well-known demographic and historical correlates of IMR during an initial moment.[4] Finally, I standardized this ratio and then calibrated the fuzzy-set scores that this produced using case-based knowledge.[5] The resulting fuzzy-set scores range from 0 to 1, with scores greater than 0.50 indicating membership in the set and scores below this threshold signifying nonmembership in the set. This approach of capturing the extent of each city's membership or nonmembership in the set is especially useful because it permits systematic assessment of how such degrees of membership or nonmembership in this and other outcome sets are related to configurations of membership or nonmembership in causal sets.

Table 3.5 presents the resulting fuzzy-set scores for Y_1 as well as for three other outcome sets and all causal sets examined using FSA. These initial results suggest that five positive cases are members in the set of capitals with *robust developmental trajectories* (Y_1): Curitiba, Porto Alegre, Fortaleza, Belo Horizonte, and Recife. Interestingly, half of the six cases that score greater than or equal to the 0.5 threshold for membership in Y_1 (Recife, Fortaleza, and Manaus) are capitals in Brazil's northern and northeastern regions, which suffered the most severe, path-dependent effects of Portuguese colonialism. Scores for Y_1 capture membership in the set of *robust* developmental trajectories—that is, the achievement of developmental progress not merely attributable to initial conditions of infant mortality, which were disproportionately higher in cities with deeper colonial legacies. As such, these northeastern cities' membership in Y_1 indicates a record of development despite intense colonial legacies.

A second outcome, *nonrobust developmental trajectories* (Y_2), refers to the set of cities that experienced development during the same period but not at levels exceeding those predicted by initial conditions. Thus, Y_2 is simply the negation of Y_1 and therefore describes the experiences of São Paulo, Goiânia, Rio de Janeiro, Belém, and Salvador. Two additional outcome sets—Y_3 and Y_4—assess membership in two different categories of institutional change over time. *Maximal spending expansion* (Y_3) operationalizes the set of cities that experienced above-average expansions in per capita municipal spending on health and sanitation. It does so by standardizing the amount that per capita municipal expenditure on public health and sanitation increased from 1995 to 2012. *Maximal health-service expansion* (Y_4) captures the set of cities that experienced above-average expansion in primary public

TABLE 3.5
Fuzzy-set scores for outcome and causal sets

Capital	Y_1	Y_2	Y_3	Y_4	S	B	L	R	P	W
Curitiba	1.00	0.00	0.70	0.60	1.00	0.70	0.00	0.41	0.00	0.00
Porto Alegre	0.90	0.10	1.00	0.30	0.58	0.51	0.83	0.00	1.00	1.00
Fortaleza	0.80	0.20	0.40	0.40	0.58	0.60	0.47	0.00	0.59	0.00
Belo Horizonte	0.70	0.30	0.90	1.00	0.84	1.00	0.83	0.00	1.00	0.00
Recife	0.60	0.40	0.30	0.90	1.00	0.90	1.00	0.29	0.71	0.00
Manaus	0.50	0.50	0.00	0.20	0.21	0.80	0.00	0.53	0.00	0.67
São Paulo	0.40	0.60	0.50	0.50	0.21	0.00	0.29	0.88	0.24	0.00
Goiânia	0.30	0.70	0.80	0.80	0.74	0.20	0.65	0.00	0.41	0.67
Rio de Janeiro	0.20	0.80	0.60	0.70	0.00	0.10	0.00	1.00	0.00	0.47
Belém	0.10	0.90	0.20	0.10	0.22	0.40	0.21	0.65	0.82	0.87
Salvador	0.00	1.00	0.10	0.00	0.42	0.30	0.42	0.76	0.41	0.00

health coverage by standardizing coverage rates of the municipally administered Family Health Program (PSF).

To examine configurations of conditions that led to these outcomes across cases, the same standardization procedure was used to score all cases along six hypothesized causal conditions suggested by dominant explanatory frameworks of development, the regression findings mentioned earlier, and the hypothesized expectations about the consequences of pragmatist publics. As with the outcome set, each causal set is the result of standardizing eighteen-year means of these variables. In line with the expectation that such a factor should matter the most when it endures over time, each set can be understood as the frequency of a given condition over the period of cross-sectionally variable decline in IMR. First, *consistent sanitarista office holding (S)* captures the set of cities in which Sanitarist Movement activists consistently held the municipal health department directorship. It standardizes the *sanitarista municipal health secretary* variable used in the aforementioned regression analysis. Six cities exhibit scores on *S* that exceed the 0.50 threshold for membership in the set: Belo Horizonte, Curitiba, Recife, Porto Alegre, Fortaleza, and Goiânia.

Four additional sets capture the combined implications of the encompassing embeddedness model of development. *Federal social-policy implementation (B)* defines the set of cities with effectively implemented federal antipoverty policies by standardizing the Bolsa Família index used earlier, thereby capturing variation in the populational coverage and targeting of the program. *Left-party mayor (L)* defines the set of cities in which politicians from the Workers' Party (PT)—Brazil's most important, programmatic left party—consistently held the mayorship. *Right-party mayor (R)* captures the set of cities in which politicians from parties with right- and center-right ideologies consistently held the elected office of mayor. It does so by standardizing period averages for mayoral rule by parties that Zucco and Power (2009) establish as right-leaning parties. Both *L* and *R* provide a clearer and more substantively meaningful interpretation than is possible by instead "fuzzifying" the party ideology variable used in the earlier regressions, which leads to substantively meaningless sets. Both *L* and *R* reflect agreements among experts (Mainwaring 1999; Power and Zucco 2009) regarding the ideologies of Brazilian political parties relative to one another. *Influential participatory publics (P)* assesses membership in the set of cities in which popular movements succeeded in institutionalizing public control over policy making through a consistent Participatory Budgeting process that incorporated citizen preferences into the municipal budget.

A final causal set, *women's political representation (W)*, assesses membership in the set of cities in which women occupied the state-level health secretary position at an adapted "critical mass" threshold. It does so by standardizing the *female state health secretary* variable, generating a 10% crossover point for membership in the set, meaning that cases in which women occupied the SES director position during more than 10% of years examined receive a fuzzy-set score for *W* that is greater than 0.50. Although Fallon, Swiss, and Viterna (2012) and Swiss, Fallon, and Burgos (2012) propose a 20% threshold in their cross-national analysis of women's representation in national legislatures, scoring *W* using this more admissive threshold is a sensible approach because it recognizes that although women's representation in the subnational Brazilian executive lags behind what these authors cross-nationally document for national legislatures, meaningful variation around this lower threshold may still matter in large cities of federalist systems that decentralize considerable authority to key offices of the subnational executive, as in Brazil.

2.2. FSA OF CONFIGURATIONAL CONSISTENCY WITH DEVELOPMENT AND STATE-BUILDING OUTCOMES

Rather than statistically analyzing the individual relationship between outcomes and each of these factors, the fuzzy-set "consistency" analyses that follow instead test propositions about the logical sufficiency of particular causal configurations for the occurrence of outcomes in specified cases. Unlike in other applications of fuzzy-set analysis to the analysis of development outcomes (Mahoney 2010), no single causal set was, by itself, sufficient for any of the spending, service provision, or robust development outcomes to occur in the cities examined. As such, the following tests instead examine combinations of these conditions (or their absence) that were jointly sufficient for these outcomes to occur. In particular, they examine all eleven cases to identify configurations of the aforementioned causal sets that were sufficient for four outcomes to occur: robust development, nonrobust development, maximal spending on public health and sanitation by municipalities, and maximal expansion in the reach of primary public-health-care provision.

In doing so, these FSA tests examine predictions from cross-fertilizing my expectations about the developmental effects of consistent sanitarista office holding with other predictions from the standard encompassing embeddedness model about the likely contributions of federal antipoverty policy, women's political representation, subnational left-party rule, and the existence of participatory-democratic institutions often favored by participatory publics. Doing so yields an expected configuration of conditions for social development that roughly conforms to the participatory-programmatic configuration of causes described earlier. In FSA, this prediction translates into the concrete expectation that a configuration of $S*B*L*r*P*W$ should be consistent for the occurrence of robust social development outcomes. (In FSA, an asterisk [*] indicates the logical operator "and," whereas uppercase letters indicate the presence of the condition, and lowercase letters indicate its absence.) In English, this expectation reads as follows: robust development trajectories are likely to emerge from the combination of consistent office holding by pragmatist publics (S), optimal implementation of federal antipoverty programs (B), sustained left-party mayoral rule (L), sustained absence of sustained right-party rule (r), influential participatory publics (P), and women's political representation at an adapted critical mass threshold (W).

Importantly, this elaboration of the encompassing embeddedness framework posits that sustained office holding by pragmatist publics is an essential feature within all configurations of conditions that are jointly sufficient for maximizing social development outcomes. The fuzzy-set analyses to come use the following equation to test this expectation by examin-

ing the consistency between all possible combinations of these causal conditions (x_i)—including the $S*B*L*r*P*W$ configuration—and each of the
four outcomes (y_i) sets I specified earlier:

$$I_{XY} = \frac{\Sigma \min (x_i, y_i)}{\Sigma x_i}$$

The resulting consistency scores for a given configuration can range between zero and one with higher numbers indicating greater consistency between a configuration and an outcome set. Ultimately, this test systematically examines the evidence that a given causal configuration is sufficient
for an outcome to occur with a stated level of consistency in the cases examined. Next, I examine all eleven cases to identify which, if any, configurations were jointly sufficient for four outcome sets: Y_1, Y_2, Y_3, and Y_4.

2.3. FSA OF ROBUST VERSUS NONROBUST
DEVELOPMENT OUTCOMES IN ALL CASES

First, I examine the consistency of all possible causal configurations with
the first outcome set of robust developmental trajectories (Y_1) in all eleven
of Brazil's major capital cities. Stata's "fuzzy" commands produced these
results by calculating consistency scores for the inclusion of all possible
configurations of conditions with this outcome set, or its "*y*-consistency"
(Longest and Vaisey 2008). Defining six causal sets means that there are
2^6, or 64, theoretically possible configurations that could be consistent with
Y_1 (or with any other outcome set used in such a test). Only eight combinations, however, are consistent with the outcome of a robust developmental trajectory more than 80% of the time when using a Wald test of the
difference with a 95% confidence interval. Among them is the hypothesized $S*B*L*r*P*w$ configuration, whose *y*-consistency value, or c_y, of .89 is
greater than the null hypothesis of .80 (denoted c_y of .89 > set value of .80;
$p <$ .023).

To narrow down these eight configurations to those supported by the
most compelling evidence, I follow Vaisey (2007) in additionally examining whether the data are more supportive of calling a given configuration
a sufficient condition for the presence of robust developmental trajectories
(Y_1) or a sufficient condition for its absence $(1 - Y_1)$, here understood as a
nonrobust developmental trajectory equivalent to Y_2. If the difference between a given configuration's consistency score with the set of cities exhib-

iting a robust developmental trajectory (its c_y) and its consistency with the set of cities exhibiting a nonrobust developmental trajectory (its c_n) is not statistically significant (again using a Wald test with $p < .05$), then the configuration fails this n-consistency test, suggesting a more ambiguous relationship to the outcome. Only one of the eight y-consistent configurations also passes an n-consistency test: again, the $S*B*L*r*P*w$ configuration (c_y of .89 > c_n of .53; $p < .002$). Thus, when analyzing all positive and negative cases, the $S*B*L*r*P*w$ configuration is the only one whose consistency with the outcome (.887) was both significantly higher than Ragin's (2008) suggested benchmark of .80 (using a 97% confidence interval) *and* more consistent with the set of cities exhibiting robust developmental trajectories (Y_1) than it was with the set of cities exhibiting nonrobust developmental trajectories ($1 - Y_1$). Substantively, this means that the combination of six factors that characterizes the participatory-programmatic configuration— frequent office holding by pragmatist publics (S), optimal implementation of federal antipoverty programs (B), sustained left-party mayoral rule (L), the absence of sustained right-party rule (r), frequent influence by participatory publics (P), and women's political representation below a critical mass threshold (w)—were jointly sufficient for robust developmental trajectories to occur. Crucially, the inclusion of S in this configuration suggests that sustained office holding by pragmatist publics combines with other, longer-theorized factors to foster robust trajectories of social development.

Next, I again use consistency tests to examine which configurations of conditions are consistent with a second outcome: the set of capitals with nonrobust developmental trajectories (Y_2). Substantively, this outcome refers to the set of cities that experienced IMR reduction (all cities in the sample did during the eighteen years examined) but not robust trajectories that eclipse what initial conditions predicted. Again, using Wald tests ($p < .05$), only two configurations are consistent with nonrobust developmental trajectories more than 80% of the time. Among them is the hypothesized $s*b*l*R*p*w$ configuration, whose y-consistency value is greater than the set value (c_y of .95 > .80; $p < .004$). To again narrow down results to those supported by the most compelling evidence, the results of additional n-consistency tests identify five configurations that are more consistent with nonrobust developmental trajectories than they are with robust developmental trajectories. But only one of these two configurations—$s*b*l*R*p*w$—passes both n-consistency and y-consistency tests (c_y

of .95 $> c_n$ of .42; $p <$ .01) when using Wald tests with 95% confidence. Taken together, these results suggest that the $s*b*l*R*p*w$ configuration is the only one whose consistency with the outcome of nonrobust development was both significantly higher than the benchmark of .80 (using a 99% confidence interval) *and* more consistent with the set of cities exhibiting nonrobust developmental trajectories (Y_2) than it was with the set of cities exhibiting robust developmental trajectories ($1 - Y_2$). Substantively, this means that the combination of six factors—infrequent office holding by pragmatist publics (s), suboptimal implementation of federal antipoverty programs (b), absence of sustained rule by left-party mayors (l), sustained right-party rule (R), infrequent influence of participatory publics (p), and women's political representation below a critical mass threshold (w)—were jointly sufficient for nonrobust developmental trajectories to occur. Notably, the absence of frequent office holding by pragmatist publics (s) was a necessary condition within this configuration, which was the only one that was sufficient for the occurrence of nonrobust development across all cases.

2.4. FSA OF DEVELOPMENT IN POSITIVE CASES,
NEGATIVE CASES, AND INDIVIDUAL CASES

Additional consistency tests of just positive cases point to the developmental importance of frequent office holding by pragmatist public actors such as Brazil's sanitaristas. These tests suggest a more parsimonious set of causal factors that yielded robust development in positive cases only, and those that were sufficient for nonrobust development in just the negative cases. First, results from a simplified FSA of just the positive cases of robust development (Belo Horizonte, Porto Alegre, Curitiba, Recife, and Fortaleza) reveals that these capitals shared only one, reduced-form configuration: $S*B*r$. Results from the y-consistency test find that this $S*B*r$ configuration is the only one whose consistency with the outcome of robust developmental trajectories was significantly higher than the benchmark of .80 ($c_y =$ .925 $>$ .80; $p <$ .039).[6] In other words, the only configuration of conditions that all five positive cases of robust development shared was sustained office holding by sanitaristas (S), infrequent mayoral rule by right parties (r), and optimal implementation of Bolsa Família (B).

Results from another y-consistency test of just the five negative cases (Salvador, Rio de Janeiro, Belém, São Paulo, and Goiânia) shows that no single reduced-form configuration was shared by these cities,[7] unlike the prior consistency analysis of just positive cases. Nevertheless, four of these five negative cases—Salvador, Rio de Janeiro, São Paulo, and Belém—shared a reduced-form combination ($s*b*l*R$) that was highly consistent ($c_y = .929 > .80; p < .011$) with the outcome of nonrobust development.[8] In other words, these negative cases of nonrobust development all featured infrequent sanitarista office holding (s), suboptimal implementation of Bolsa Família (b), infrequent rule by left-party mayors (l), and frequent rule by right-party mayors (R).

Using yet another variety of FSA known as a "best-fit" test (Longest and Vaisey 2008), it is possible to further scrutinize the aforementioned findings by identifying a single causal configuration that best characterizes each of the five positive cases of robust development individually rather than an as a collective. In FSA, any given case can only receive a consistency score greater than .50 for exactly one configuration, making it possible to identify this best-fit combination of conditions that most accurately describes each case's relationship to the outcome. Comparing each positive case's best-fit configuration to each of the others reveals that these five cities differ on only two causal conditions: first in consistent rule by left-party mayors (L) versus inconsistent rule by left-party mayors (l) and second in infrequent influence by participatory publics (p) versus their frequent influence (P). Specifically, Belo Horizonte, Recife, and Porto Alegre all respectively post their highest score for the participatory-programmatic pathway represented by the $S*B*L*r*P*w$ configuration. By contrast, Curitiba and Fortaleza record their highest consistency score for two different configurations: $S*B*l*r*p*w$ and $S*B*l*r*P*w$, respectively. These two deviations between the best-fit configuration for Belo Horizonte, Recife, and Porto Alegre and the best-fit configurations for Curitiba and Fortaleza further reinforce the earlier finding that three conditions within all programmatic configurations—whether the generic or participatory variety—constituted the central-most causes of robust development: sustained office holding by sanitaristas (S), optimal implementation of Bolsa Família (B), and infrequent mayoral rule by right parties (r). By contrast, two other conditions that constitute the core of the participatory-programmatic configuration—namely, rule by left-party mayors (L) and influential participatory publics (P)—were present only in Belo Horizonte, Recife, and Porto Alegre, while Curitiba and Fortaleza featured inconsistently ruling left-party mayors (l) and no shared pattern in participatory publics' influence or lack thereof.

In sum, these elaborated FSA results suggest that three core features of programmatic configurations—sustained office holding by pragmatist publics (*S*), optimal implementation of federal antipoverty policy (*B*), and infrequent mayoral rule by right parties (*r*)—have jointly constituted deeper-level causes of robust development in Brazil's largest capitals. Next, I turn to additional analyses, which triangulate and deepen this basic insight with additional findings about the patterns of public-health-sector expansion through which both programmatic and participatory-programmatic configurations fostered social development outcomes.

2.5. FSA OF PRIMARY HEALTH-SERVICE AND SPENDING OUTCOMES

Additional consistency analyses suggest that a key mechanism by which programmatic configurations fostered robust development was the realization of two central sanitarista goals: the maximization of health spending and primary health care delivery through the PSF. The first of these intermediate outcomes—maximal growth in municipal development spending in the health and sanitation sectors (Y_3)—denotes a comparatively sophisticated municipal public health state, a core mechanism by which sanitaristas aimed to foster social development locally. Analyzing the *y*-consistency and *n*-consistency of all configurations with this outcome reveals that the $S*b*L*r*P*W$ configuration is the only one whose consistency with the outcome of maximal spending growth (Y_3) was both significantly higher than the benchmark of .80 ($c_y = .99 > .80$; $p < .000$) *and* more consistent with maximal spending (Y_3) than it was with nonmaximal spending growth $(1 - Y_3)(c_y$ of .99 $> c_n$ of .37; $p < .02$) at the 95% confidence threshold. Thus, the results once again confirm that frequent sanitarista office holding (*S*) was an essential condition within the only configuration of causal factors that was sufficient for an important development outcome: this time, the outcome of maximal growth in municipal development spending on public health and sanitation.

Finally, I assess configurations that are consistent with the outcome Y_4, the set of cities that maximized coverage of Brazil's flagship primary health care program, the PSF. These analyses reveal that the $S*B*L*r*P*w$ configuration is the only one whose consistency with the outcome of maximal health-service growth (Y_4) was both significantly higher than the benchmark of .80 ($c_y = .96$, $p < .001$) *and* more consistent with maximal health-service growth (Y_4) than it was with nonmaximal service growth $(1 - Y_4)$ (c_y of .96 $> c_n$ of .39; $p < .05$) with 95% confidence. Here, too, frequent office holding by pragmatist publics (*S*) was necessary within the only configuration that was sufficient for maximal expansions in municipal delivery of primary health care.

2.6. SYNTHESIS OF FSA FINDINGS

The aforementioned analyses of maximal IMR reduction in all cases and in positive and negative cases separately ultimately complement the last analyses of health spending and service-provision outcomes in substantiating three components of the study's core analytic argument. First, they reinforce the claim that both participatory-programmatic democratization of health in Belo Horizonte, Porto Alegre, and Recife and programmatic health democratization in Curitiba and Fortaleza were sufficient for robust development outcomes in these capitals, while minimalist health democratization in Rio de Janeiro and Salvador was sufficient to produce nonrobust development outcomes. The reduced-form analyses are consistent with the argument that further-reaching, programmatic modes of health democratization achieved in positive cases of robust development ultimately complemented and emerged from more generic qualities of democratization throughout urban Brazil. Specifically, they underscore that the presence of three conditions (S^*B^*r) in all positive cases of robust development overlapped with two background conditions that were constant throughout all major capitals following Brazil's redemocratization: namely, the replacement of decentralized despotism with formal democratic procedures and the considerable municipal autonomy yielded by political, fiscal, and administrative decentralization. This combination of formal democracy, robust decentralization, municipal-level sanitarista office holding, infrequent right-party mayoral rule, and maximal reach of Bolsa Família constitute the most foundational, generic qualities of programmatic health democratization. And because this configuration of five conditions was shared by all positive cases of robust development—and not by any negative cases— the FSA findings reinforce the claim that a generic variant of programmatic health democratization was sufficient for the occurrence of robust development in the cases analyzed.

Second, the FSA results also suggest that major capitals in urban Brazil witnessed not one but two varieties of programmatic health democratization: a participatory and a nonparticipatory variant. Simply stated, participatory-programmatic democratization of health involved all of the five qualities of programmatic health democratization plus a sixth: consistently influential participatory publics. This becomes apparent when comparing the particular causal configuration for which different positive cases received their highest consistency score. In FSA, any given case can only receive a consistency score greater than .50 for exactly one configuration, making it possible to identify this best-fit combination of conditions that most accurately describes each case. Comparing elaborated versions of these best-fit configurations for just the positive cases reveals that these five capitals differ on only two causals conditions: consistent left-party mayoral rule (*L*) versus inconsistent rule by left-party mayors (*l*), and influential participatory publics (*P*) versus noninfluential participatory publics (*p*). Specifically, Belo Horizonte, Recife, and Porto Alegre all register their highest elaborated consistency score for the configuration $S*B*L*r*P*w$, whereas Curitiba and Fortaleza record their highest elaborated consistency score for two different configurations: $S*B*l*r*p*w$ and $S*B*l*r*P*w$, respectively. The two deviations between the best-fit configuration for Belo Horizonte, Recife, and Porto Alegre and the best-fit configurations for Curitiba and Fortaleza suggest that the former group experienced a participatory-programmatic mode of health democratization, while the latter group experienced only a generic mode of programmatic health democratization that lacked consistently ruling left-party mayors.

The within-case qualitative analysis in coming chapters reinforces the additional inference from FSA that, although Belo Horizonte and Recife exhibit all baseline conditions for a participatory-programmatic mode of health democratization, Porto Alegre's combination epitomizes perhaps its purest representation. To be sure, Belo Horizonte and Recife clearly exemplify all the core features of participatory-programmatic health democratization, observable in the fact that both capitals shared the best-fit configuration of $S*B*L*r*P*w$. In Belo Horizonte, amid a routine absence of right-party mayors (*r*) and strong cooperation from influential participatory publics in Participatory Budgeting (*P*), frequent office holding of the Municipal Health Office by sanitaristas (*S*) such as Dr. José Maria Borges, Dr. Cezar Rodrigues Campos, and Dr. Helvécio Miranda Magalhães Jr. mobilized formidable support for their public-health-focused state-building programs from mayors in left parties (*L*) such as the PT (Patrus Ananias from 1993 to 1996, Fernando Pimentel from 2002 to 2008) as well as from center-left-party mayors such as the Brazilian Social Democratic Party, or

PSDB (Pimenta da Veiga and Eduardo Azeredo from 1989 to 1992), and the Brazilian Socialist Party (Dr. Célio de Castro from 1997 to 2000). Additionally, the PT-led municipal government of Fernando Pimentel in Belo Horizonte undertook one of urban Brazil's most effective rollouts of Bolsa Família (B). In Recife, similar configurational patterns arose amid a similar dearth of right-leaning mayors and an effective cessation of decentralized despotism in the local state. Recife's robust developmental transformation undoubtedly owes much to post-2000 factors, such as the public health goals of PT mayors João Paulo Lima e Silva and João da Costa Bezerra Filho between 2001 and 2012, participatory publics that successfully institutionalized Participatory Budgeting, and a well-targeted rollout of Bolsa Família that ranks among urban Brazil's most successful and far-reaching expansions of the program. Sometimes overlooked in existing accounts, however, is the considerable political support for state-building programs in the municipal public health sector that office-holding sanitaristas (S) such as Dr. Humberto Sérgio Costa Lima, Tereza de Jesus Azevedo Couto, and others garnered from these actors while directing the Municipal Health Office (SMS).

In Porto Alegre, these baseline conditions for a participatory-programmatic mode of health democratization were present along with an additional condition: women's representation at a critical mass threshold. Porto Alegre's best-fit configuration of $S*B*L*r*P*W$ echoes the fact that its municipal politics of public health were heavily influenced by the relative infrequency of right-party mayors (r), consistently ruling left-party mayors (L), maximal coverage and targeting of Bolsa Família (B), and its famously influential participatory publics for participatory-democratic inputs into municipally organized, public goods provision through Participatory Budgeting (P). Yet, the FSA analysis of Porto Alegre also draws attention to other, more commonly overlooked drivers of its robust social development trajectory, especially consistent occupation of the capital's SMS office by sanitaristas (S) such as Maria Luiza Jaeger, Dr. Lucio Barcelos, and Dr. Henrique Fontana. In addition, Porto Alegre featured comparatively frequent occupation of the SMS and the state-level health office (SES) by politically influential women (W), especially by the venerable sanitarista Maria Luiza Jaeger. Thus, Porto Alegre's best-fit configuration of $S*B*L*r*P*W$ mirrored the $S*B*L*r*P*w$ configuration of Belo Horizonte and Recife in all other respects except in the presence of this one additional condition. Thus, Porto

Alegre not only joins Belo Horizonte and Recife in exhibiting all core features of the participatory-programmatic trajectory of health democratization outlined in previous chapters but also demonstrates the additional condition of women's political representation in the SES at an adapted critical mass threshold.

Third and perhaps most importantly, the FSA results intimate that it may well have been more important for a city's configuration to contain a programmatic dimension than a participatory one, since both variants of a programmatic configuration (participatory or nonparticipatory) were sufficient for robust development. The two positive cases of robust development that shared a generic programmatic configuration—Curitiba and Fortaleza—shared three and only three conditions with the other positive cases that exhibited a participatory-programmatic one (Belo Horizonte, Recife, and Porto Alegre): consistent sanitarista office holding (S), maximization of Bolsa Família's reach (B), and a relative infrequency of right-party mayors (r). Notably absent within this reduced-form, $S*B*r$ configuration was the presence or absence of consistently ruling left-party mayors (L or l) as well as the presence or absence of consistently influential participatory publics (P or p). Ultimately, this suggests that the most important driver of robust development was the combination of frequent office holding by pragmatist publics, maximal reach of a federal CCT (B), and the absence of right-party executives (r). Neither consistently ruling left-party mayors (L or l) nor consistently influential participatory publics (P or p) had as much bearing on this outcome. In this regard, the distinction between the two variants of programmatic health democratizations is perhaps of greater relevance for students of democratization than it is for those seeking explanations of Brazil's development transformation. Bracketing for a moment their considerable virtues for the deepening of democracy in capitals that experienced participatory-programmatic democratization, the reduced-form, configurational analyses of all positive cases showed that neither ruling left parties nor influential participatory publics were necessary for robust development. This basic finding reinforces the project's core argument about the greater importance for robust development of frequent office holding by pragmatist publics.

Observing the elaborated, best-fit configurations in the remaining positive cases of Curitiba and Fortaleza bears out this inference in greater detail, particularly when noting the ways in which these configurations deviate from those that comprise the participatory-programmatic variant of health democratization described earlier for Porto Alegre, Belo Horizonte, and Recife. When analyzed alongside all other cases, Curitiba and Fortaleza scored above the .50 consistency threshold for neither the $S*B*L*r*P*w$ configuration that best characterized Belo Horizonte and Recife nor the $S*B*L*r*P*W$ configuration that best characterized Porto Alegre. Rather, each exhibited its own distinctive best-fit configuration: Curitiba with $S*B*l*r*p*w$ and Fortaleza with $S*B*l*r*P*w$.[9] Two important differences between the best-fit configurations of these two positive cases and those of the other three positive cases reinforce the notion that Curitiba and Fortaleza have experienced a nonparticipatory variant of programmatic health democratization. For one, both capitals featured only inconsistently ruling left parties (p), as opposed to the consistently ruling left parties (P) that characterized the other three positive cases. This suggests that consistently ruling left parties were not necessary for a robust development outcome to occur. Additionally, the fact that the positive case of Curitiba experienced a near absence of influential participatory publics (p) suggests that the presence of such actors was also unnecessary for robust development to occur.

Although coming within-case analyses reinforce the point in greater detail, these FSA results support the argument that whereas Fortaleza exhibits all baseline conditions for a nonparticipatory mode of programmatic health democratization, Curitiba's combination epitomizes perhaps its purest expression. Curitiba's best-fit configuration of $S*B*l*r*p*w$ points to the fact that the PT, Brazil's most progressive nationwide political party during the period, never captured mayoral office in the capital (l), while participatory publics never successfully demanded the introduction of Participatory Budgeting (p), and women never held the position of SES director. But in addition to a general infrequency of right-party mayors (r) and the considerable reach of Bolsa Família (B), the capital is unsurpassed in its record of sanitarista office holding, with a long line of sanitaristas such as Dr. Armando Marinho Bardou Raggio, Dr. Luciano Ducci, Michele Caputo Neto, and others consistently occupying the SMS position (S) in a nearly uninterrupted fashion that predates even the eighteen-year period examined by FSA. This pattern suggests that, although there may be a cross-case tendency for left-party mayors to more frequently appoint sanitaristas to the position than non-left-party mayors do, office-holding sanitaristas have not solely relied on sitting PT mayors for their access to powerful positions atop the local public health state. Indeed, the case of Curitiba demonstrates that—unlike influential participatory publics—office-holding pragmatist publics can exert political influence even amid a nearly complete absence of left-party rule. In Fortaleza, too, one finds another example of the (nonparticipatory) ideal type of programmatic health democratization epitomized by Curitiba. Somewhat counterintuitively for a less economically prosperous capital located on the other side of Brazil in its northeast region, Fortaleza's local state-society politics have oddly mirrored these qualities of Curitiba, with a few minor exceptions that were especially pronounced in the Bolsa Família era. Although not to the same extent, Fortaleza featured a pattern of consistent office holding by sanitaristas (S) such as Dr. Luiz Odorico Monteiro de Andrade, who occupied the SMS position, as well as a similarly extensive and well-targeted rollout of Bolsa Família (B) and a notable infrequency of right-party mayors (r). As is addressed by the coming case study analysis, Fortaleza's post-2005 period differed from Curitiba's in the extended mayoral rule of the PT's Luzianne de Oliveira Lins and the sustained experience of Participatory Budgeting (P) that she and participatory publics helped to introduce. Nevertheless, by clearly indicating the necessity of consistent sanitarista office holding (S) within the combination of factors that was sufficient for robust development in Curitiba, even these condensed FSA findings support the coming argument that many of the most important institutional changes to Curitiba's local public health state occurred with sanitaristas consistently occupying the directorship of the Municipal Health Office (SMS).

2.7. RECONCILING NEGATIVE CASES WITH
FSA FINDINGS: THE CASE OF SALVADOR

Although coming chapters focus their analysis on positive cases, the negative case of Salvador perhaps best epitomizes the $s*b*l*R*p*w$ combination that the just-mentioned FSA analysis found to be sufficient for nonrobust development outcomes to occur. Although a similarly sized capital in neighboring Bahia state, Salvador recorded a much weaker postdemocratization record of primary health care provision and infant mortality reduction than did Belo Horizonte. Despite beginning the period with a nearly identical infant mortality rate, Salvador managed to reduce its 2013 rate to only 18.39, a level nearly twice as high as Belo Horizonte's. Among the major reasons for this contrasting outcome in an otherwise similar capital was the inconsistent office-holding record of sanitaristas in Salvador's SMS and in Bahia's SES. Aggravated by sustained right-party control of the subnational executive, the relative infrequency of sanitarista office holding delayed and weakened the construction of municipal state capacities required for fostering public health. Despite continually mobilizing for such reforms in the public sphere, Salvador's otherwise cohesive sanitarista organizations remained largely insulated from municipal state-building levers. By 2013, the capital's infant mortality rate remained higher than that of any other major Brazilian capital.

As in Belo Horizonte, sanitaristas in Salvador (Brazil's third-largest capital) mobilized extensively in the public sphere to codify and enact core tenets of sanitary reform ideology after the late 1970s (M. L. Jaeger, interview, 2010). The city's movement began organizing within the Department of Preventive Medicine (DMP) of the Federal University of Bahia (UFBA) during Brazil's dictatorship and later helped form its Public Health Institute (*Instituto de Saúde Coletiva*, ISC), which became an important coordinating center for sanitaristas (Paim 2008). Among Salvador's many influential activists were nationally recognized sanitaristas such as Dr. Jairnilson Paim, Dr. Jorge Solla, Dr. Luis Fernandes de Souza, and Dr. Luiz Pinheiro. During the late 1980s, Pinheiro and Paim helped author the official State Health Plan for the 1988 to 1991 period, which established epidemiological criteria for allocating Bahia's public resources for disease prevention and mortality reduction (Alves 2012). Yet this proved to be a brief moment of efficacy during an overarching period in which otherwise robust demand making in the public sphere by Salvador's sanitaristas precipitated comparatively fewer tangible state interventions to improve public health.

In contrast to Belo Horizonte, Salvador's sanitaristas enjoyed little office-holding success, partly due to a pattern of sustained rule by right-leaning mayors who quashed programmatic social-policy proposals of any kind, including the health-focused state-building project of sanitaristas. One clear source of this antiprogrammatic bent was the well-documented coalition between a string of Salvador mayors and Bahia's longtime regional hegemon Antônio Carlos Magalhães (ACM). ACM's "Carlista" political machine and clientelist network effectively dominated the city's politics for approximately a quarter century stretching from ACM's installation into power by Brazil's erstwhile dictatorship to as late as 2007 (Dantas Neto 2006a). Carlista mayors opposed primary public health reforms, and even the more centrist mayors who attempted to defy control by Carlistas, including Lídice da Mata (1993–1996) and Fernando José Guimarães Rocha (1989–1992), generally lacked the autonomy to do so in practice. Two brief exceptions to the overall rule of sanitarista exclusion from control of the SMS were the directorships of Solla in 2005–2006 and Dr. Eduardo Mota from 1993–1996. Yet the mayors who appointed them generally lacked political autonomy from the Carlista machine and the overall pattern remained one in which Salvador's sanitaristas found their office-holding strategy obstructed at nearly every turn (Alves 2012). Ultimately, sanitaristas managed to occupy the city's SUS directorship during only a third of the eighteen years between the 1995 to 2012 period.

This infrequent pattern of sanitarista office holding in Salvador all but ensured that primary-health-oriented state-building proposals demanded by sanitaristas in the public sphere rarely became political priorities, much less material realities, of mayors. Insulated from these reformist pressures, Salvador's mayors consistently delayed, ignored, or otherwise thwarted sanitarista proposals for building local capacities to expand primary care. Among the intermediate consequences of this dynamic were delays in municipalization of an already sparse network of public health facilities in the capital, weak subsequent expansions of that network, scant provision of primary public health care through the PSF, low per capita spending on health and sanitation, and a general dearth of professionally trained primary health workers. Even as the federal health ministry (MS) began offering municipalities financial incentives to introduce the PSF in 1996, the Carlista mayor Antonio Imbassahy refused to adopt the program, instead opting to pursue a neoliberal-oriented, World Bank–funded platform for outsourcing primary health care delivery to private nonprofits known as health organizations (OSs). Imbassahy's nonsanitarista health director, Aldely Rocha Silva, also became subject to a number of federal corruption investigations for public procurement fraud and misuse of federal transfers (Alves 2012).

Salvador's more recent divergence from this ingrained pattern of obstructing sanitarista office holding has ameliorated but not erased decades of neglect in the city's health sector. With ACM's weakening hegemony and the 2006 election of the center-left mayor João Henrique de Barradas Carneiro (PDT), sanitaristas captured the SUS directorship and initiated a small and exceptionally delayed state-building project in the sector. In particular, Luis Eugênio Portela, a sanitarista-appointed SMS director even before Carneiro's election, leveraged the office to formalize a partnership with UFBA in which the ISC contributed technical health-planning expertise and assisted the SMS in drafting its Municipal Health Plan, a mandatory five-year blueprint for health-sector interventions. Benefiting from connections to sanitaristas in the federal MS, Portela also negotiated full management status in 2006, which placed Salvador's health facilities under municipal control for the first time (Nunes Rocha, Cerqueira, and Fontes Teixeira 2010), over a decade after Belo Horizonte did so. But by 2012, Salvador's primary health sector still bore deep scars from nearly two decades of right-party rule and exclusion of sanitaristas from control of its SMS. When compared to other major Brazilian capitals, Salvador's per capita spending on health and sanitation of 383 *reais* ranked second to last, its 104 PSF teams ranked third to last, its 13% PSF populational coverage rate ranked last, and its primary appointment rate of just over 3 tied for last. Indeed, Salvador's record encapsulates how late and inconsistent sanitarista office holding contributed to relatively weak IMR decline by stunting state-building for primary public health provision.

3. Conclusion

Taken together, these statistical and configurational analyses jointly supported predictions of the study's movement-driven development (MDD) theory that consistent office holding by pragmatist publics not only advanced programmatically rooted democratization processes in the primary health sector but also maximized public-service provision and social development across urban Brazil. The analysis offered two distinct and mostly complementary kinds of empirical support. First, the statistical models suggested that sanitarista office holding on the municipal level was, on average, negatively associated with infant and child mortality rates and positively associated with primary public-health-service delivery and coverage, net of several other theoretically relevant factors and controls. But while the regression analysis reinforced the study's core prediction, it somewhat unrealistically assumed that office-holding pragmatist publics mattered independently of other factors. This effectively ignored likely interactions between such office-holding episodes and multiple other conditions, whose joint effect on social development is difficult to assess with statistical models.[10]

In response, the chapter offered an FSA of such relationships that complemented these limitations of the statistical analysis by offering a truer-to-life model of this causal complexity. It found that no single condition (including routine sanitarista office holding) was individually sufficient for robust (or nonrobust) social development outcomes, perhaps underscoring the truism that statistical associations from regression analyses do not necessarily or by themselves constitute evidence of a causal relationship. Specifically, the FSA models suggested that although neither consistent nor inconsistent office holding by pragmatist publics was individually sufficient for robust or nonrobust development, consistent office holding was necessary within the only two configurations that were sufficient for robust developmental trajectories. Conversely, inconsistent office holding by pragmatist publics was a necessary component of the only combination that was sufficient for nonrobust developmental trajectories, as the brief discussion of Salvador showed. Further, consistent office holding by pragmatist publics was necessary within the only configuration of conditions that was sufficient for two additional outcomes to occur: maximal local spending on health and sanitation and maximal coverage of municipally delivered primary public health care.

But if these regression analyses identified *associations* between sanitarista office holding and social development and the FSA findings suggested complex interactions between a broader set of *conditions* for robust development, neither fully illuminated the *mechanisms* by which office-holding sanitaristas propelled such historic shifts. The next four chapters aim to do so by complementing these cross-case inferences with more detailed comparative-historical analyses of individual cities, highlighting the municipal state-building processes by which office-holding sanitaristas expanded primary public-health-care delivery and social development outcomes. I specifically focus on two types of cases most relevant for reinforcing the theory of MDD: participatory-programmatic trajectories of health democratization in Belo Horizonte and Porto Alegre and the programmatic trajectories of Curitiba and Fortaleza. Next, I turn to the first of these cases, Belo Horizonte.

FOUR

Belo Horizonte

> Some of us [in the Mineiro Sanitarista Party] entered into the
> fray of [political party] politics more than others but from
> the point of view of health, we always shared the convictions
> to democratize health and construct a new model that could
> deliver health care for all in a democratic, inclusive, and
> equitable manner.
>
> —*Dr. José Maria Borges, sanitarista director of Belo Horizonte's*
> *SMS (1984–1992)*

Belo Horizonte, the capital of Minas Gerais state, is Brazil's sixth-largest
município, with about 2.5 million residents living in the geographic core
of the country's third-largest metropolitan area. The city's encompassing
state has long been one of Brazil's most important political centers alongside its prosperous southeastern- and southern-region neighbors, São Paulo,
Rio de Janeiro, and Rio Grande do Sul. At the beginning of the health-
democratization period, however, social development outcomes in Belo
Horizonte more closely resembled those in Salvador, the capital of Bahia
state and a northeastern-region neighbor with which Minas Gerais shares a
border. In 1988, for example, Belo Horizonte's IMR of 57.57 was higher than
Salvador's (55.24) and ranked among urban Brazil's worst, with only Recife (67.07) and Manaus (80.67) recording higher levels. By the early 2000s,
however, Belo Horizonte had undergone a remarkable transformation to
become one of urban Brazil's top performers in such social development
outcomes, a status it maintained into the mid-2010s.

This chapter traces Belo Horizonte's robust development outcomes to
a participatory-programmatic trajectory of health democratization that
locally rooted sanitaristas animated throughout nearly four decades surrounding Brazil's return to formal democracy. In certain processual re-

spects, this pathway was more intricate than the generic programmatic trajectories witnessed in Curitiba and Fortaleza in that Belo Horizonte's participatory-democratic institutions became more active monitors of the health sector. In particular, the city's participatory publics established and transformed the city's Municipal Health Council (CMS) and its Participatory Budgeting (OP) process into civic arenas in which citizen-participants monitored health-sector state-building more consistently than occurred in Curitiba or Fortaleza. But as concerns actual expansion in the primary health sector and other state-building processes that are most essential for IMR reduction, such institutions rarely lived up to their billing as power-sharing bodies. Indeed, this chapter's within-case analysis of Belo Horizonte's participatory-programmatic trajectory shows that sanitarista officeholders in the city's SMS directorship and mayorship propelled construction of the municipal public health state's service-delivery arms in far more influential, sustained, and consequential ways.

The apogee of sanitarista office holding in Belo Horizonte featured two consecutive mayoral victories by Dr. Célio de Castro (PSB, 1997–2001), arguably the city's most consequential sanitarista. Among its other effects, Castro's mayorship made sanitary reform ideologies of universal and equal access to health into political priorities of the city's highest democratic office to a degree rarely seen in urban Brazil. Yet sanitarista exertion of such civil power suffused the cabinet-level offices of the SMS directorship too and differed largely in degree but not in kind from the influence that Castro exerted from within the mayor's office. The consistency with which Belo Horizonte sanitaristas occupied the office of SMS director in the period was possible because of these civil-society actors' localized communicative and regulative institutions, including the so-called Mineiro Sanitarista Party discussed later in this chapter. Further, democratic office holding by sanitaristas mattered for IMR reduction because it afforded them the power needed to sustain a precocious and prolonged period of state-building in the primary health sector. The city's sanitarista directors of the SMS included Dr. José Maria Borges (1984–1992), Dr. Cezar Rodrigues Campos (1993–1996), and Dr. Helvécio Miranda Magalhães Jr. (2003–2008). All told, sanitaristas held Belo Horizonte's office of SMS director for over three-quarters of the twenty-five years between 1988 and 2012 and during all four years between 1984 and 1987. The office-holding tenures of such sanitaristas account for nearly all of the largest and most significant expansions in Belo Horizonte's formidable network of primary health clinics and municipal primary-care professionals; these tenures also account for major redistributions of existing health professionals to clinics in city regions facing higher epidemiological risks of premature mortality. Thus, the municipally focused state-building efforts of office-holding sanitaristas were a defining feature of participatory-programmatic health democratization and a central mediator of the period's effect on Belo Horizonte's robust development outcomes. Next, I examine the context of the civil and political society into which the city's sanitaristas emerged.

1. Initial Conditions of Civil and Political Society in Belo Horizonte

Minas Gerais is well-known in Brazil's modern politics for producing some of its most iconic statesmen, including President Juscelino Kubitschek (1956–1961) and Tancredo Neves, who died in 1985 before he could be inaugurated as the country's first (indirectly) elected president after the military's 1964 seizure of power (Skidmore 2010). Although his presidency is perhaps most closely associated with the construction of Brasília as the country's new capital, Kubitschek first began earning a reputation as a social and economic reformer when he was mayor of Belo Horizonte between 1940 and 1945. But beyond producing such individual politicians, the state is also well-known for constituting part of Brazil's long-enduring "coffee with milk" governing alliance of political and economic elites from the dairy- and cattle-producing plantations of Minas Gerais and Rio Grande do Sul and from the coffee plantations of São Paulo. Indeed, traditional families of a few coronels rooted in Minas Gerais's dairy-producing regions continued to dictate the state's politics well into the military dictatorship through patronage-fueled, oligopolistic alliances (Hagopian 1997). Like most other capitals in this study, Belo Horizonte's pre-SUS-era politics were largely animated by conservative, political-society elites, often from traditional families.

In comparative perspective, however, Belo Horizonte's politics began wriggling free from the unfettered influence of the state's coronels earlier and in a fuller way than occurred in other capitals such as Salvador, Recife, and Fortaleza. In contrast to these other capitals, this shift reflected a stronger impetus among segments of Minas Gerais's political elites who sought to promote economic development, although such efforts were initially modest. Certain segments of the subnational political elite in Minas Gerais had been pursuing industrialization since the First Brazilian Republic, although such efforts conflicted with the state's larger context of political domination by rural, dairy-producing elites, whose use of labor-repressive agriculture otherwise yielded little in the way of appetites for economic or political reform. But such countering impulses to foster economic growth gathered increasing force in Belo Horizonte during early stages of the dictatorship, as governors of Minas Gerais began coordinating with the military regime to more aggressively foster industrialization (Wirth 1977). Such efforts contributed significantly to Belo Horizonte becoming Brazil's most important economic center outside of São Paulo even before the end of the dictatorship (Eakin 2016; Wampler 2015).

Such patterns of industrialization in Minas Gerais considerably expanded middle and working classes, who organized into two major groups in Belo Horizonte that became increasingly vocal in demanding a return to democracy. As early as the 1960s, formal-sector workers and emerging professional classes were organizing increasingly powerful labor unions and associations of teachers, bankers, and journalists in the capital as well as civil-society associations focused on human rights, the environment, and health (Keck 1992). Progressive grassroots Catholic activists in the liberation theology tradition complemented such organized leftist groups in forming the city's nascent PT organization and demanding restoration of democracy (Avritzer 2009, 52). But as in other urban centers, the 1964 seizure of power by the military drove these civil-society and union groups underground—and health activists were no exception. A second group associated with the military's only approved opposition party, the Brazilian Democratic Movement (MDB), was equally important, in part because its more visible public profile helped it to lead large-scale mobilizations demanding direct elections for president through the nationwide *Diretas Já* campaign (Avritzer 2009).

It was within these various mobilizing currents that students, medical residents, and faculty on university campuses in Belo Horizonte began organizing themselves into initially clandestine groups of Sanitarist Movement activists. In the fifteen years prior to the MDB's successful pressuring of federal legislators to elect Neves president, Belo Horizonte's campus of the Federal University of Minas Gerais (UFMG) became an important hotbed for student activists, who helped create the Brazil-wide National

Student Union (UNE) and its local precursors in the capital. Some *hori-zontino* (resident of Belo Horizonte) sanitaristas began their activism in the student movement but became increasingly involved with sanitarista campaigns over time. For instance, Dr. Lídia Tonón, an early sanitarista organizer in the capital, was initially UFMG's student-body president and later a cofounder of the UNE's local chapter. But UFMG's medical school—particularly its Department of Preventative Medicine (DMP), which roughly mirrored those on other federal university campuses in the capitals examined in this study—became a hub for student activists simultaneously mobilizing for a right to health. The DMP on UFMG's campus produced many of the sanitaristas who thereafter went on to occupy key democratic offices atop the public health state in the capital, including Borges and Castro (J. M. Borges, P. C. Perreira, and L. Tonón, interviews, 2010).

As early as 1970, the DMP within UFMG had become an important center for budding sanitaristas, who began mobilizing against the dictatorship under the cover of the group's initial function as a body tasked with redesigning medical school pedagogy to incorporate training for primary health workers. The military regime allowed for the creation of DMPs as it began searching for low-cost ways of extending basic forms of health care to rural regions, where it hoped to shore up support during the 1970s. Yet the regime underestimated how their allowance of a DMP with UFMG and in the federal universities of other major capitals, such as Rio de Janeiro, would inadvertently incubate fervent opponents of the dictatorship. Although operating with less-direct ties to the CEBES than was the case for the DMPs of Curitiba and Rio de Janeiro, Belo Horizonte's DMP also convened weekly meetings throughout the 1970s that were roughly similar to the CEBES-inspired Community Health Studies Weeks (SESACS) forums in these other capitals. Among the group's earliest participants were not just activists of the organized left but also MDB activists such as José Maria Borges, who later became one of Belo Horizonte's longest serving directors of the SMS (1984–1992). Also connected to Belo Horizonte's DMP were other influential sanitaristas and MDB activists such as Dr. José Saraiva Felipe, the future SES director in Minas Gerais (1991–1993), who in 2005 became federal health minister in President Lula da Silva's cabinet (L. Tonón, interview, 2010).

Despite the fact that two leftist factions circulated within Belo Horizonte's DMP, the group was united around the goal of expanding public access to primary health care on a statewide and nationwide basis. Participants in Belo Horizonte's DMP organized in diverse activist networks, including those of communist, Mandela-inspired, and Trotskyite groups of socialist democrats that animated then clandestine protoparties such as the Communist Party of Brazil (PC do B), the Brazilian Socialist Party (PSB), and, later, the city's PT organization. But one group, the democratic socialist tendency in which Tonón organized, generally favored more radically participatory modes of health-policy-making for incorporating larger segments of the citizenry. The second faction was a more centrist group of PC do B activists, such as Borges, as well as MBD activists such as Saraiva and his UFMG professor, Francisco "Chicão" de Assis Machado. This group shared prioritization of the creation of new and more programmatic models for delivering integrated health services but were also heavily involved in union campaigns. Crucially, however, "there were various participants in the nucleus of the group, who were not from the party of Zé Maria [José Maria Borges], Saraiva, or sometimes from any party, but we all shared points of convergence in the need for a proposal for expanding primary health care" (L. Tonón, interview, 2010). Further, the fact that such diverse currents of the left all convened within Belo Horizonte's medical school was somewhat unique across urban Brazil, where such tendencies sometimes splintered into more factionalized infighting. Compared to otherwise similar cities such as Porto Alegre, Belo Horizonte featured a noticeably weaker divide between the two segments.

Amid the relative blurring of such divides within the sanitaristas of Belo Horizonte's DMP, participants began designing an agenda-setting primary-health-care model in the município of Montes Claros in northern Minas Gerais. Dr. José Saraiva Felipe, in particular, joined other *mineiro* (residents of Minas Gerais) sanitaristas such as Machado, who coordinated what became known as the Montes Claros Project, or PMC (Escorel 2008). During the early 1970s, these actors persuaded the director of Minas Gerais's SES, Fernando Megre Veloso, to begin sending trained health care workers into the state's less developed northern region through a program called the Integrated Health Service Provision System of Northern Minas (*SIPSSNM*). Machado helped found a research institute in Montes Claros called the Training and Research Institute for the Development of Rural Sanitarist Care (*IPEDASAR*) that assisted in the design and study of the service-provision model developed there. The Montes Claros Project contributed an early programmatic model that yet another group of sanitaristas in a federal research agency called the Institute of Economic and Social Planning (IPEA) eventually adopted and revised into the forerunner of an important nationwide program called the Internalization of Health and Sanitarist Actions (PIASS) program in 1976. It also widened intra-Brazil networks of sanitaristas in a manner that the growing PIASS program extended upon, ultimately leading to the 1982 creation of CONASS, the National Council of Health Secretaries (Escorel 2008; Falleti 2010b).

I.I. EARLY SANITARISTA CONSTRUCTION OF CIVIL-SOCIETY INSTITUTIONS:
THE "MINEIRO SANITARISTA PARTY"

But in Belo Horizonte, these actors helped launch more than just a process of national-level institutional change, although such dynamics demonstrated the subnational rather than federal origins of major nationwide reforms in the Brazilian health sector. Sanitarista veterans of Belo Horizonte's DMP also established key local communicative institutions of the movement such as the so-called Mineiro Sanitarista Party (PMS). It was not incidental that horizontino sanitaristas such as Machado, Borges, and Saraiva referred to this loosely organized association of statewide activists as a party, although its title was technically a misnomer, since the group was never an official political party. Its members would later permeate an unusually broad set of union and party organizations, especially three key labor unions and five major left and center-left political parties that influenced debates about state expansion in the public health sector after the return of electoral democracy. These parties included the Workers' Party (PT), the Brazilian Socialist Party (PSB), the Communist Party of Brazil (PC do B), the Brazilian Social Democratic Party (PSDB), and the Brazilian Democratic Movement Party (PMDB). As a result, sanitaristas in Belo Horizonte faced few fatal threats to their agenda of improving public health through the expansion of relatively low-cost primary-care provision in city peripheries facing high epidemiological risks of infant mortality. For similar reasons stemming from their involvement in the founding of the Doctors Union of Minas Gerais (SINDMÉD-MG), the Health Workers Union of Minas Gerais (SINSAÚDE-MG), and the Municipal Public Servants Union of Belo Horizonte (SINDIBEL-BH), sanitaristas also faced few serious setbacks at the hands of these actors.

The question of how the Mineiro Sanitarista Party (PMS) achieved such deep penetration into Belo Horizonte's most powerful parties and unions speaks to the considerable ability of the PMS to widely propagate the ideology of sanitary reform locally. The PMS echoes Alexander's observation that civil-society associations sometimes aim to "regulate political power, then, not only by putting their representatives into the state, but by making efforts to control them when they are there" (2006, 133). The PMS sought to play both roles and focused its efforts on controlling the nonbureaucratic top of the subnational public health state in the capital. Borges and Saraiva particularly epitomized the association's efforts to capture powerful offices atop the capital's subnational public health state in the hopes of building its tangible material capacities to execute the movement's core ideologies of universal, equal access to health. Yet sanitarista motivations for pursuing office were based on something other than an appetite for sheer political power. And their successful campaigns in this regard had a greater effect than that of just establishing Belo Horizonte's sanitaristas as credible public problem solvers in the eyes of reformist political elites throughout the state and the capital.

Indeed, the motivations of sanitaristas in the PMS revolved around a carefully cultivated, deep-seeded fidelity to the universalizing ideology of establishing a citizenship right to health for all citizens, as Borges's account in the epigraph illustrates. PMS activists aimed to infuse such universalizing principles of citizenship into the practice of a local state apparatus that had rarely served as anything more than a tool for political-society elites to cultivate particularistic relationships of patronage with their subjects. Crucially, the currency of success for this project was not reducible merely to the exercise of simple political power. Rather, influential actors in seminal communicative institutions such as Belo Horizonte's PMS gained access to protodemocratic offices atop the capital's public health state in part by relying on normative tools more endemic to civil society itself. More specifically, such office-holding sanitaristas began exerting civil power to achieve their state-building goals. Sanitaristas were able to bend impersonal state institutions around the principles of universal and equal access to health crystallized in sanitary reform ideology in part because their own activist trajectories and professional careers as caregivers personified a kind of fidelity to such goals among political-society elites and civil-society activists and among broader publics. In this regard, sanitarista motivations and sources of power in capturing and wielding democratic offices diverged in fundamental ways from the sort of rational calculation of interest maximization famously described by Lipset and colleagues in *Union Democracy* (1956). For Lipset, party members who capture a democratic office may well seek to keep it by observing democratic norms of responsibility and accountability to laws. But their prime reason for doing so is predominantly a by-product of the rational, self-interested motivation to maintain holds on power in a politically competitive environment. In short, such political societies typically fear that breaches of norms of the office will cost them their jobs at the hands of ambitious competitors in other parties, who seek to oust and replace them in the office.

The accounts of Belo Horizonte's sanitaristas suggest that civil power was instead a key currency underlying the efficacy of sanitarista mobilizations to capture and wield offices for purposes of institutionalizing sanitary reform. In part, this is detectable in concerted efforts by movement leaders to inculcate an ethic of public service and a fidelity to Sanitarist Movement ideologies of rights-based, universal, and equal access to health. Illustrative of these efforts is a moralizing piece written by the venerable Fortalezan sanitarista Dr. Armando Raggio in an article published in the nationwide journal of the National Council of Health Secretaries (CONASS), didactically prescribing principles that all SUS officers should uphold:

> You are firable *ad nutum*. You can be dismissed at any moment for diverging from or failing to comply with the established program of the government, and even when your job becomes the object of interest for a different political party supporter of the government. . . . To stay in the position, cling to the public commitments that underlie it and don't relinquish it, even when pressured. Above all, stay true to the mission of serving society, even if puts your position at risk. Never depend on the position" (Raggio 2016).

By cultivating a sense of what Raggio (2016) calls the "honorable mission" of occupying SUS directorships responsible for enacting core tenets of sanitary reform, mineiro sanitaristas have long sought to cultivate a morality of service in this and other democratic offices (J. M. Borges, L. Tonón, and P. C. Perreira, interviews, 2010). These efforts have certainly been nascent in Brazil, where democratic office is a far more recent phenomenon than in democracies of the Global North with longer-standing traditions. But such attempts not only echo Alexander's (2006, 137, 141) arguments that "the meaning of office obligations also is crucial" to the exercise of civil power but also suggest that many sanitaristas themselves view office as "the most immediate hands-on institution for controlling the instrumental force of political power."

In this sense, early sanitarista mobilizations in Belo Horizonte can be read as efforts to exert civil power, a form of "solidarity translated into government control" by establishing civil-society regulative institutions as "gatekeepers of political power" (Alexander 2006, 110). Here, it is especially notable how Borges and other sanitaristas describe such civil-society ideologies as superseding a range of left and center-left parties in which they were sometimes members, whereas others belonged to no parties at all (J. M. Borges, L. Tonón, and P. C. Perreira, interviews, 2010). Such accounts further reinforce the view that efficacious sanitarista pursuits of democratic office were not merely by-products of these actors' simultaneous membership in political parties. Rather, sanitarista political agency in Belo Horizonte was partially underwritten by what Raggio described as the sense of moral purpose at the root of these activists' efforts to bend state practices around the universalizing civil-society ideology of sanitary reform.

The analysis that follows further suggests that the ability of Belo Horizonte's sanitaristas to capture SMS directorships and expand primary-care provision depended in part on efforts to wield civil power through office holding. Mayors and governors in Belo Horizonte quickly recognized the practical benefits that appointing sanitaristas to SMS directorships could yield for contending with pressing public problems such as rampant childhood mortality. This played no small role in their consistent appointment of sanitaristas to the SMS directorship in coming decades and their devolution of increasing degrees of state-building power to them thereafter. But sanitaristas aimed to render the subnational public health state more accountable to emergent regulative institutions of democratic office while in them, all in ways that leveraged their own activist histories in the Sanitarist Movement as normative justification for becoming occupants of positions such as the municipal SUS directorship. In this sense, it is most meaningful to speak of the programmatic pathways of health democratization that such actors forged, not as products of political parties or as state actors per se but as the fruits of civil-society actors, who infused the ideology of health as a universal and equal citizenship right into parties, states, and especially democratic offices at the "nonbureaucratic top" of the subnational public health state. Crucially, however, this process was more intensively localized across urban Brazil than has commonly been recognized, which contrib-

uted to unevenness across major capitals that had important human consequences. And although Belo Horizonte exemplifies an especially consistent
period of *sanitarista* office holding that built on the strength of civil-society
communicative institutions such as the PMS, its relevance for development
outcomes shaped and reflected a broader context of democratization in the
city that I turn to next.

2. Participatory-Programmatic Democratization of Health in Belo Horizonte

Belo Horizonte's participatory-programmatic trajectory entailed seven core
dimensions, including the three baseline qualities that characterized generic processes of health democratization throughout urban Brazil. First,
Belo Horizonte embraced the nationwide return of free and fair local elections for the subnational executive through universal suffrage in the early
1980s. Increasingly competitive elections for the subnational executive were
relevant in the health sector for many reasons, not least because they helped
to begin reorienting the state's notoriously clientelist political culture
around more programmatic public policies.[1] And while the capital shared a
history of *coronelismo* more similar to northeastern cities than its southeastern neighbors, competitive elections began replacing traditional political
elites in the subnational executive with ones who proved generally more receptive to civil-society actors, including sanitaristas. Second, although Belo
Horizonte's responses to decentralization differed from other capitals, the
city mirrored the rest of urban Brazil in that local government assumed increasing political, fiscal, and administrative control of the primary health
sector throughout the period. Third, although the constitutional declaration of a right to health became the law of the land in the late 1980s, an especially relevant corollary to this was the infusion of Belo Horizonte's SMS
directorship with new public responsibilities of the SUS manager that ultimately favored continuing occupation of the post by sanitaristas.

Fourth, Belo Horizonte's electoral politics featured a relative absence of
the right-leaning, unabashedly clientelist and traditional mayors that previously exercised power in the capital. The city shared this trait with Porto
Alegre, Curitiba, Fortaleza, and Recife. In particular, Belo Horizonte's
health-democratization period witnessed nothing like the continuation
of monopolistic local rule by patronage-oriented, regional hegemons such

as Antônio Carlos Magalhães, who dominated subnational politics in the neighboring state of Bahia well into the mid-2000s. Unlike in Salvador, the more competitive, nationwide playing field for local rule in Belo Horizonte fundamentally disrupted similar, previous patterns of subnational rule by conservative, traditional politicians. Although not unique in this respect, the PT mayors Patrus Ananias (1993–1996) and Fernando Pimentel (2002–2008) emphasized social justice and expanded popular participation in governance more than any of the mayors who succeeded or followed them did (Wampler 2015). In narrow terms of efforts to expand primary public-health-care delivery, PT mayors resembled mayors from other left and left-center parties, such as the PSB of mayor Dr. Célio de Castro (1997–2002) and Marcio Lacerda (2009–2016), as well as more centrist parties, such as the Brazilian Social Democratic Party (PSDB) of Pimenta da Veiga (1989–1990) and Eduardo Azeredo (1990–1992). Despite other differences, all these mayors refrained from walling off decisions about the local state's interventions in public-service sectors from civil-society consultation and allowed for at least minimal civil-society influence, unlike the experience of Belo Horizonte and other capitals like Salvador before the early 1980s. Indeed, an extended sequence of mayors from both left and center political parties generally remained open to civil-society actors such as sanitaristas who presented workable solutions to trenchant public problems, including widespread infant mortality in the city as late as the early 1990s.

A fifth dimension of its participatory-programmatic trajectory was that Belo Horizonte maximized the reach of Brazil's most important federal antipoverty program, Bolsa Família (BF), after 2003. Indeed, the city was among urban Brazil's top performers in the BF's targeting rate—the proportion of eligible families who actually received transfers through the program. With an average targeting rate of 93.57% between 2004 and 2016, Belo Horizonte outranked all other cities in the study except for Porto Alegre (96.78%), another case of participatory-programmatic health democratization and robust development. And while the proportion of enrolled families to total families in the city during the period was only about 50%, this lower coverage rate likely reflects how the capital's higher average standard of living diminished the number of eligible families in Belo Horizonte vis-à-vis poorer northeastern cities such as Fortaleza and Recife. Indeed, when more aptly compared to other capitals in the southern and southeastern regions with roughly similar levels of economic prosperity, Belo Horizonte was again outpaced only by Porto Alegre (61.58%), whereas it eclipsed Curitiba (47.75%), Rio de Janeiro (48.32), and São Paulo (40.86%). Thus, in no other economically comparable major capital did Bolsa Família reach higher proportions of all families than in Belo Horizonte. Although it is beyond the scope of this study to systematically analyze why Belo Horizonte had such success in serving eligible families, the program's considerable significance for a large proportion of residents likely improved rates of access to basic forms of health care, if only because of BF's condition that program recipients attend regular medical checkups.

A sixth feature of the path that Belo Horizonte shared with Curitiba, Fortaleza, Porto Alegre, and Recife was relatively early and sustained institutional expansion of the subnational public health state's service-delivery arms, particularly when compared to Salvador and Rio de Janeiro. For instance, Belo Horizonte had developed infrastructure by 2016 for delivering primary public health care through the PSF that was unsurpassed by any other major capital. In terms of primary public-health-care facilities per capita, it ranked among urban Brazil's top performers, with 161 primary-care-focused health units (US) serving well over one million exclusive SUS users. Between 2005 and 2012, each PSF team on average served fewer than 2,513 exclusive SUS users, a record that was unmatched by any city in this study. By the end of 2016, the federal health ministry estimated that Belo Horizonte's 575 PSF teams reached approximately 1.98 million residents, or 82.8% of the city's population. Section 3 of this chapter shows how office-holding sanitaristas played an outsized role in helping construct such formidable service-provision capacities.

Finally, a defining feature of Belo Horizonte's pathway was how civil-society actors quite apart from the city's sanitaristas established and expanded a distinct set of participatory-democratic institutions for influencing the municipal public-infrastructure budget and monitoring the public health sector. Existing literature particularly chronicles the empowered forms of citizen involvement in Belo Horizonte's Municipal Health Council (CMS) and the Participatory Budgeting (OP) process introduced by the city's PT mayor Patrus Ananias (1992–1996) in 1993 (Avritzer 2009; Wampler 2015). Indeed, whereas OP has been altogether absent in Rio de Janeiro, Salvador, Curitiba, and Fortaleza until much more recently, Belo Horizonte mirrors Recife and especially Porto Alegre in the presence of a long-standing OP process. Although Belo Horizonte's CMS councillors have almost always lacked the power required to exert the body's formal authority to "cogovern" the health sector alongside the SMS, it shares this feature with all major capitals in Brazil. But what sets Belo Horizonte's CMS apart from every other capital except Porto Alegre is how actively its CMS councillors monitor the public health sector. Belo Horizonte's participatory publics, who have allied with but are conceptually distinct from the city's sanitaristas, clearly harnessed both institutions in a way that deepened the democratization of health and civic life to degrees rarely witnessed in urban Brazil.

Yet the powers of CMS councillors and OP participants to direct municipal state-building in the public health sector are simply not tantamount to those of SMS directors, and Belo Horizonte offers an especially persuasive example of this. Even in their moments of greatest agency, Belo Horizonte's CMS councillors, who are widely considered some of the most empowered and influential in all of urban Brazil, fall far short of exerting their cogovernance authorities. For example, although they have the authority and potential to veto proposed interventions of the SMS, such as the construction of a new hospital or clinic, its councillors have never exercised this veto. In part, this reflects the fact that councillors typically do not perceive the exercise of vetoes as being in the interests of the larger public that such projects would serve.[2]

Whereas Belo Horizonte's CMS and OP have consistently dialogued with the city's SMS, mayors and office-holding sanitaristas atop the city's SMS have increasingly wielded the comparatively cohesive powers of their offices to pursue state-building with little substantive direction from the city's participatory publics. Indeed, the sanitarista mayor Dr. Célio de Castro (1997–2002) concentrated and centralized power for health-policy planning within an encompassing "super-secretariat" for social policy that other sanitaristas such as Dr. Helvécio Miranda Magalhães Jr. subsequently came to control—in his case, for three years (2009–2011) following his six years as SMS director (2003–2008). And although the earlier health-focused state-building plans that emerged from the super-secretariat and the SMS have sometimes reflected inputs of the CMS, the CMS has never permanently halted major state-building plans of which it disapproved, even if they have triggered discussions between the CMS and SMS (Wampler 2015). Perhaps more importantly, the CMS and the OP exert little to no actual power in decisions to hire municipal health workers, arguably the single most important state capacity in the primary public health sector—and one in which Belo Horizonte has particularly excelled vis-à-vis other major capitals. Ultimately, this helps explain why participatory dimensions of Belo Horizonte's path of health democratization have been less important than its programmatic dimensions for social development outcomes, even if the city witnessed a clear deepening of civil society deliberation about public health planning. Next, I turn to the factors that more clearly expanded Belo Horizonte's capacity in the primary public-health-care sector.

3. Sanitarista Office-Holding and the Expansion of Belo Horizonte's Public Health State

As with most other cases in this study, Belo Horizonte achieved the lion's share of IMR reductions well before the advent of national-level factors such as the consolidation of Bolsa Família and the PT presidencies of Lula and Rousseff. Furthermore, the capital's biggest improvements occurred during an approximately eighteen-year period from 1985 to 2002 in which the centrist PSDB and PMDB parties and the center-left PSB party together held the city's mayorship over three times as often (thirteen years) as the left-leaning PT did (four years). Furthermore, scholars have noted how the Participatory Budgeting process at work in Belo Horizonte during these years devolved participants the decision-making authority for only about half of the overall resources that Porto Alegre's participants directed, while a technocratic formula devised partly by the city's sanitaristas effectively directed the other half. This raises the question of how Belo Horizonte achieved so much progress in such a short period of time amid the relative weakness—and often the outright absence—of factors commonly thought to cause such reductions in Brazil. This section argues that consistent office holding by the city's sanitaristas in democratic and protodemocratic offices atop the public health state forged sustained capacity-building processes that go a long way toward explaining Belo Horizonte's robust social development outcomes by the mid-2010s.

3.1. SANITARISTA-DRIVEN PRIMARY-CARE EXPERIMENTS AND MORTALITY REDUCTION, 1983–1992

In Belo Horizonte, sanitaristas began propelling early expansions of the municipal public health state shortly after the restoration of state-level elections for governor in 1982 and for mayor in 1985. When Tancredo Neves (then of the PMDB) became the first directly elected governor of Minas Gerais since the 1964 military seizure of power, he appointed a sanitarista and PMDB counterpart, Dr. Darilo Tavares, as SES secretary. Tavares had also occupied that position during the 1970s when the Montes Claros program arose. In 1983, Tavares took an initial step toward health-sector municipalization in Belo Horizonte by supporting the creation of the city's municipal health secretariat (SMS) as its own stand-alone entity.[3] And following Neves's eventual appointment of his fellow *pemedebista* (PMDB member) Rui Lage as Belo Horizonte's mayor, Lage appointed Borges as the first SMS director in 1984. In Borges's own description, Lage offered initial support for the sanitarista agenda of decentralizing the health sector: "In no moment did he question the fact that we were discussing a new model or fail to approve resources that so that this model could be put into motion; on the contrary, he gave substantial support for this" (J. M. Borges, interview, 2010).

Thus, with sanitaristas controlling both the SES and SMS in 1984, the two agencies signed one of Brazil's first Integrated Health Actions (AIS) contracts with the Ministry of Health (MS). Pushed through on the national level by the sanitarista planning director Eleutério Rodriguez Neto, the AIS was the quintessential pre-SUS reform program for the health sector nationwide. The AIS had a somewhat more blunted immediate effect on service provision in Belo Horizonte than it had in other cities, such as São Paulo, with more capable municipal public health states at the time (Falleti 2010b). Due to deficits in its administrative capacity, the city's fledgling SMS struggled to transform already sparse new revenue streams created by the AIS into large increases in service delivery (J. M. Borges, interview, 2010). Nevertheless, health-sector municipalization got off to an early start in Belo Horizonte because two sanitaristas—Borges and Saraiva—came to hold both of the most powerful offices atop the subnational public health state in Belo Horizonte.

These cooperative ties laid the groundwork for the unfolding of more fundamental municipalization processes later in 1991. That year, after Hélio Garcia won his first election as Minas Gerais's governor, he appointed Saraiva as SES director. Saraiva quickly began a campaign to municipalize the health sector across the state. These efforts gained traction in Belo Horizonte in large part because Borges again occupied the post of SMS secretary in 1989, having been appointed by the PSDB mayor Pimenta da Veiga. Da Veiga had won the 1988 election in a second turn by a thin margin of only 28,000 votes in a município of over two million residents (TSE, 2016) and faced the prospect of governing with a city council whose seat shares were nearly deadlocked between the PSDB and PT, with the PT holding a narrow advantage. This, combined with the fact that polling found health to be the top social concern of horizontinos, gave Da Veiga strong incentives to expand primary-care provision, a project for which Borges, his eventual appointee as SMS director, had been previously lobbying him to take up (J. M. Borges, interview, 2010). With Borges and Saraiva united in their primary goal of fostering localized control of the health sector, the stage was set in Belo Horizonte for one of the country's earliest health-sector municipalizations.

In 1991, Belo Horizonte's SMS assumed a large number of basic health units from federal agencies and the SES of Minas Gerais. The vast majority—112 of 123—of these SMS facilities were rudimentary primary health clinics.[4] In contrast to some other major capitals, Belo Horizonte managed only one hospital during this period. In part, this was because the state of Minas Gerais had already spun off many of its hospitals within the município's territory to a state-owned company (*autarquia*) called FHEMIG. Thus, Belo Horizonte's município was not immediately burdened with managing an expensive and complex network of hospitals. This allowed office-holding sanitaristas such as Borges and, later, Tonón to focus more squarely on expanding access to basic services as well as to prenatal and neonatal programs (L. Tonón, interview, 2010). Yet most of these inherited facilities were poorly staffed and in an ill state of repair. These facilities included both hospitals and urgent-care units (PAMs) previously managed by the federal INAMPS as well as more primitive health units (US) previously managed by the federal health ministry. Borges described them this way:

> In truth, the PAMS were in a very precarious condition and had tiny staffs of office managers and assistants, and doctors and their assistants with little available time. There were doctors who were contracted for four hours a day but in practice only delivered appointments for two . . . and the great majority delivered services only to formal sector workers. The USs . . . were even more precarious than the hospital network, were terribly equipped and had poorly-trained staff and basically focused their attention on disease control (J. M. Borges, interview, 2010).

Clear problems arose from this almost-immediate inheritance of physical infrastructure not being accompanied by adequate increases in new resources for hiring health professionals to adequately equip and staff them. Although Belo Horizonte later become one of the few capitals in the country to nearly comply with Constitutional Amendment 29 of 2000, which required municipalities and states to spend 25% of their budgets on health, this proportion was closer to 7% in the early 1990s (L. Tonón, interview, 2010). Further, many of the health workers who populated these hospitals and clinics remained employees of the state or federal government agencies that previously managed the facilities. In part, this was due to reticence on the part of some health-worker unions, particularly the powerful Belo Horizonte Doctors' Union, to negotiate contracts with a new employer, the SMS, that they feared would offer lower salaries and worse benefits. As Borges said, "We had internal difficulties with our own group of health workers, with the unions, including the Regional Doctors' Council, which was very reactionary" (J. M. Borges, interview, 2010). Amid these disputes, "many of the health posts remained empty" (P. C. Perreira, interview, 2010) during the early 1990s, something that Borges's administration aimed to ameliorate through the opening of public concursos but struggled to accomplish immediately.

But despite the precarious state of the physical infrastructure it inherited and such major staffing shortages, Borges's SMS implanted a nascent primary-care model that was then ahead of its time for urban Brazil. Among its most important features were the creation of health regions within the city and more systematic efforts to gauge epidemiological risks along with the existing capacities on hand in each region to address them. Given the state of the facilities and staffing of the clinic network and of its administrative headquarters in downtown Belo Horizonte, this project had necessarily humble origins. The SMS that Borges took over was, in his words, "small and chaotic . . . the SMS at first referred to whatever religious institution was hosting a clinic (*corão*) inside of it as a health center . . . there just were no administrative jurisdictions, no regionalization, no sense of the distribution of services being provided" (J. M. Borges, interview, 2010). To address this state of affairs, Borges convened a team of sanitaristas, most of whom hailed from outside of the SMS, including Saraiva, Machado, and Eugenio Vilaça, a Brazilian consultant from the Pan-American Health Organization (OPAS).

The team's approach to creating a new primary attention model combined a technocratic approach to gathering epidemiological information with more democratic methods of integrating the expressed preferences, critiques, and demands of the communities in the regions surveyed. The group first divided the city spatially into regions "so that we could get to know in greater detail the circumstances that were aggravating health in each microspace and change the type of attention offered in each. This allowed us to create maps of the risks in each of Belo Horizonte's regions so that we could have inductively derived information about the specificities of each area, the distribution of certain disease and extreme poverty, and in that moment, we were especially preoccupied with premature births" (J. M. Borges, interview, 2010). The SMS also began taking inventories of its clinics and their equipment in a more systematic matter that echoes the approach of Fortaleza's SMS director, Dr. Anamaria Cavalcante e Silva, at about the same time. With a better sense of such needs throughout the city's health facilities, Borges's team "divided the município of Belo Horizonte into administrative regions, and into each local administration we looked to channel the budget more strategically. This way, we were able to develop a more purposeful budget that allowed us to begin renovating the health units to create minimally functional conditions in each of the regions" (J. M. Borges, interview, 2010).

Yet compared to other capitals like Curitiba and Fortaleza, Belo Horizonte's group more systematically established democratic procedures for gathering inputs into the SMS's risk mapping, assessment, and inventory work. "We created a Municipal Health Council (CMS) before the advent of such councils [as bodies required to exist by the federal Organic Health Laws of 1990] so that we would be able to incorporate the thinking and the complaints, especially the critiques and needs brought by their own population that had a certain leadership in the community. . . . From the standpoint of citizenship, it was an important moment because the council began to grow, express itself politically, channel its anxieties, and began to be heard in a democratic fashion" (J. M. Borges, interview, 2010). Such protodemocratic moments of participatory governance foreshadowed the relatively early legal creation of Belo Horizonte's CMS in 1991 via Law 5,903.[5] And these initial efforts paved the way for the later establishment of subsidiary health councils of residents, patients, and caregivers within each clinic that remained in sustained dialogue with the city's CMS.

This approach of Borges to combining democratic and technocratic elements in the early establishment of Belo Horizonte's primary-care model helps explain the city's early progress in expanding health care delivery. Most tangibly, the agency's interventions paved the way for an immediate and substantial broadening of primary-care delivery. Borges's SMS used the data from its inventory to undertake modest renovations to the city-wide network primary-care clinics and to give small salary increases that supported longer shifts for the doctors and other health professionals working in those clinics. By the early 1990s, the SMS had also instituted a training program for community health employees that worked in the decentralized network of primary-care clinics throughout the city. And by 1992, the SMS had created a new Municipal Health Fund that did not immediately operate as intended but nonetheless received federal transfers for the express financing of the health sector, theoretically untouchable by mayors for any other purposes (L. Tonón, interview, 2010). Perhaps most importantly, Borges's team had "sought to implement a model of attention in which a network of health clinics were organized into regionalized administrations that could repeatedly receive that citizen who lived in the area and, in some form, monitor their lives and the development of their needs in the area of health and—for people who fell ill—to be able to treat them and refer them to other facilities. . . . I think this was an important moment in Belo Horizonte" (J. M. Borges, interview, 2010). As these transformations began opening new access points to the local public health state, they likely contributed to the impressive reductions in IMR witnessed during Borges's tenure. Compared to its IMR of 57.57 five years earlier in 1988, Belo Horizonte's infant death rate in 1993 had fallen about 28% to 41.32.[6]

The interventions of Borges also offer instructive lessons for theories of the state-society dynamics and state-building processes that can foster inclusive social development transformations. Scholars of coproduction and the twentieth-first-century developmental state such as Peter Evans have argued that "to create effective state-society linkages, the state must facilitate the organization of counterparts in 'civil society'" and that channeling the civil societies with often "conflicting particular interests" into participatory democracy can be one effective way of doing so (Evans 2010, 49). But the account that Borges offered for having instituted new participatory venues to democratically engage neighborhood-based civil societies highlights a distinct driver of such coproduction: his own lineage as an activist from a social movement with an already cohesive ideology of health equity and universalism that nevertheless resonated with a wide variety of other civil-society actors. Most obviously, Borges sought to implant a new primary-care model that he and his activist collaborators believed would foster Sanitarist Movement ideologies of universal and equal access to basic forms of primary health care. Nevertheless, he credits former interactions with erstwhile Trotskyites in the Mineiro Sanitarista Party (PMS) with having inspired the desire to do so in a democratic fashion by creating a health council (J. M. Borges, interview, 2010).

In this sense, the episode suggests that, even when acting in formal capacities as state officers, the activist profiles of individuals such as Borges dramatically altered the tenor and content of their interventions in ways that, as scholars like Wolford and French (2016) highlight, complicate simplistic notions of the Brazilian state. The early interventions by Borges are especially instructive because of his expressed sense that occupying the office of SMS director entailed democratic responsibilities that had not yet even been codified in Brazil's 1988 Constitution. Even before the formal establishment of the democratic office of SUS manager, the civil-society lineages of officers such as Borges inspired a sense of public responsibility for engaging local communities in an accountable manner. This demonstrates how communicative institutions of civil society like Belo Horizonte's PMS propagated such responsibilities in ways that prefigured their more formal codification into the civil-society regulative institutions of office, as was the case with the subsequent creation in 1990 of the SUS manager's office on a nationwide basis. It also suggests that such normative obligations can contribute to the tangible, material success of such interventions by civil-society actors, who leverage state positions to advance universalizing ideologies like the universal and equal right to health.

In terms of the material effects of such dynamics, Borges's nine intermittent years as SMS director (1984–1992) launched a process of slow but pathbreaking institutional change within Belo Horizonte's SMS. The process had delayed effects on mortality reduction that were perhaps more impressive than its immediate ones. IMR reduction was considerable during his actual tenure, but Borges was even more influential for having instituted a primary-care model that would have long-lasting significance locally and nationally. Dr. Helvécio Miranda Magalhães Jr., Belo Horizonte's future SMS secretary and president of the National Council of Municipal Health Secretaries (CONASEMS), emphasized the period's longer-term effect of implanting a primary-care model based on sanitary reform ideologies of universality and equity for the first time. As he put it, "Belo Horizonte has a strong tradition of primary care that began in the 1980s and preceded the SUS by many years and instituted local, professionalized management districts earlier than anywhere else in Brazil except São Paulo" (H. M. Magalhães, interview, 2010). In this sense, Borges introduced institutional changes that had relatively small immediate effects but prefigured the future of Belo Horizonte's public health sector in fundamental ways.

3.2. CONSISTENT SANITARISTA OFFICE HOLDING, STATE-BUILDING, AND ROBUST IMR DECLINE, 1993–1996

The four years from the beginning of 1993 to the end of 1996 featured a continuous episode of sanitarista office holding that helped dramatically lower IMR during that time from 41.32 to just under 30. These impressive reductions owed much to an elaborate phase of sanitarista-driven state-building that initially sought to establish basic administrative capacities of the SMS, then still a fledgling agency. Initial efforts in this regard focused on redistributing existing municipal health workers into city regions in which residents faced the gravest epidemiological risks of premature mortality. In these efforts, sanitarista directors of the SMS such as Dr. Cézar Campos (1993–1996) drew on the regionalized structure of health-management districts and relatively primitive inventories that Borges had previously developed to begin this process. A major result in terms of municipal capacity was a gradual but palpable redistribution of existing health workers to city regions characterized by disproportionately high risks of infant mortality.

There can be little doubt that in addition to sanitarista office holding, other dimensions of Belo Horizonte's participatory-programmatic mode of health democratization contributed to the city's impressive IMR reductions during this time. For one, a newly competitive electoral environment called greater attention of political elites to the fact that horizontinos during the early and mid-1990s named health as their single top public concern (Folha de São Paulo 1995). Although urban violence was then the social ill for which Brazil was perhaps best known internationally, public opinion regarding the primacy of health in Belo Horizonte mirrored that in other major capitals such as Rio de Janeiro and São Paulo. But the response of elected political leaders in Belo Horizonte differed dramatically, particularly when compared with the response of leaders in Rio de Janeiro. On the level of policy discourse, all three mayors of Belo Horizonte between 1993 and 2008 declared at various points that public-health-care provision was a top political priority of their administrations (Folha de São Paulo 1997; Estado de Minas 2000a).

On the level of policy action, too, political leadership clearly mattered. Although less explicitly focused on the primary public health sector per se, Belo Horizonte's PT mayor from 1993 to 1996, Patrus Ananias, pursued a Brazil-wide strategy of the party to "invert priorities" of government toward the party's base in mobilized civil society—lower and working classes. Existing scholarship emphasizes how Mayor Ananias introduced Participatory Budgeting and established new arenas for the city's participatory publics to engage the state in rule-bound, institutionalized forms of demand making.[7] Additionally, Patrus's administration also expanded food security programs in schools and favelas along with the creation of a public policy management council for the food security sector roughly similar to that of the SMS (Machado, Meniucci, and de Souza 2009). To be sure, the public health sector benefited from these efforts to invert priorities through participatory institutions. As in Porto Alegre, the OP began channeling municipal funding from the capital construction budget into renovating existing health centers and breaking ground on new ones. Further, the CMS assumed its formal authorities to develop and approve new health-policy programs, although it typically lacked the power to play these roles in practice.[8]

Yet both of these participatory institutions lacked the necessary influence to address one of the most vexing problems then facing the city's public health sector: shortages and misallocation of trained primary public-health-care providers. As in other major capitals, a center-periphery pattern of spatial inequality left Belo Horizonte with a relative dearth of health clinics and health professionals in the peripheral regions of the city where health risks were highest but with a relative plethora of both in central regions with generally lower health risks. While Belo Horizonte's OP was a pathbreaking institution that meaningfully contributed to authoring the city's capital construction budget, it mirrored counterparts across urban Brazil in its lack of tangible ability to reduce such inequality through the hiring and management of public employees. And given the fact that the SMS director doubled as the CMS's de facto president, the council during this period and thereafter struggled to exert its comanagement authorities, particularly as they pertained to questions about human resources. Indeed, the SMS director and de facto president of the CMS during the Patrus administration was Dr. Cézar Campos, a PMS veteran with stronger ties to the PT's new unionist current than to the Trotskyite current of participatory publics that occupied the CMS and the city's OP process (L. Tonón and P. C. Perreira, interviews, 2010). In this regard, the CMS itself was (by default) led by a sanitarista, whose most muscular state-building powers emanated from his position as SMS director, not from his role as CMS president.

This, too, suggests that a more consequential factor in Belo Horizonte's early state-building for primary health was continuity in sanitarista office holding atop its SMS. Campos, the first SMS director of the Patrus administration, was a respected psychologist, who had been more strongly connected during the 1980s to PC do B currents than to PT ones. Campos was offered the position partly on the strength of his wide appeal as a consensus candidate primarily interested in health reform with few discernable ties to any one tendency within the PT (L. Tonón and P. C. Perreira, interviews, 2010). Indeed, Campos's appointment owed much to his movement lineage outside of the PT as well as to his prior experience working alongside Saraiva, Machado, Borges, and other sanitarista veterans of the PMS inside Minas Gerais's SES during the 1980s (J. M. Borges, interview, 2010). Patrus also appointed Dr. Lídia Tonón, the onetime PMS organizer, petista, and former colleague of Campos's, as second in command of the SMS. Tonón assumed the day-to-day work of transforming the SMS into a bureaucratic agency capable of expanding the inherited primary-care model given a resource-constrained environment in which the country's hyperinflation crisis "seriously limited what we could with our already limited capacities. When I started in 1993, we had four 386 computers and that was it" (L. Tonón, interview, 2010).

Occupying the two most powerful offices at the nonbureaucratic top of Belo Horizonte's public health state, Tonón and Campos assembled a team that in 1993 began improvising a pathbreaking series of prenatal and neonatal programs. The team did so by launching the BH Vida project in 1994, and the related Intake project (*Acolhimento*) the following year (Campos et al. 1998; Junqueira et al. 2002; Malta et al. 2000). Far from constituting the mere adoption of federal programs hypothesized by diffusion theorists of Brazilian health care reform (Weyland 2009; Borges Sugiyama 2012), the programs constituted Belo Horizonte's tailored reactions to the shifting nationwide landscape of the SUS. In 1994, the city officially became one of only twenty-four municipalities nationwide to assume the partial (*semi-plena*) management mode specified by SUS Basic Operating Norm of 1993 (NOB-93), which then represented the most advanced level of municipal responsibility vis-à-vis the federal health ministry (Heimann et al. 1998). In addition to the 121 clinics it was already managing, Belo Horizonte observed the relatively limited, preordained requirements of assuming partial status when it took control of fifty-eight hospitals with nearly eight thousand beds, three emergency rooms, and a panoply of other facilities of varying levels of sophistication (Junqueira et al. 2002).

Belo Horizonte's SMS took the step (then optional in the eyes of the federal MS) of assuming these new responsibilities at an early moment in 1994 mostly because of pressures that Tonón and Campos applied on federal health ministry and municipal officials from inside their offices atop the SMS (L. Tonón and P. C. Perreira, interviews, 2010). Also, the SMS sought to manage the new and more sophisticated network of facilities it assumed in a way that would foster the team's overarching goal of reducing infant mortality. In particular, the BH Vida and Uptake projects installed a more systematic approach to channeling SUS users into the municipal health system in a manner that improved early identification of patients, particularly pregnant women, facing urgent health risks. Furthermore, there is little evidence that the team's formulation of this priority emerged from downwardly disseminated federal perquisites or from elected politicians such as Mayor Patrus, who had generally prioritized the expansion of participatory governance during this early moment. Rather, the focus emerged from an alchemy of improvisational problem solving and normative convictions on the part of office-holding sanitaristas who controlled the SMS. Tonón put it this way:

> We functioned in a totally informal manner. We invented jobs among us that didn't exist. Somebody would say, "Oh, I think we should create an epidemiological unit." And then we would get to work on it, but the computer or the phone wouldn't work. . . . But we had nothing in the way of the most important services, including a neonatal program. And so we started to address the question of uptake and evened out the distribution of our personnel and clientele. We made up a prenatal and neonatal program because it was possible and because it had to be done" (L. Tonón, interview, 2010).

On the one hand, the sanitaristas in charge of the SMS improvised their approach to assuming a large network of more sophisticated medical facilities and staff in a largely unscripted and surprisingly unguided manner reminiscent of Deweyan pragmatism. On the other hand, however, their problem-solving orientation toward doing so was hardly reducible to a technocratic exercise devoid of guiding normative principles. Indeed, overtones of sanitary reform ideology inflected the response with its central-most purpose of universalizing and equalizing access to a notion of health with meanings that they conceptualized in terms of infant survival, speaking once again to the importance of these actors' lineages as movement activists.

The resulting interventions sought to reallocate the SMS's human and infrastructural resources toward city regions with residents facing the most severe risks of premature death. During this episode, the SMS continued municipalizing health care professionals, who previously worked in federal- and state-run hospitals located in the city's center. As it did so, Campos and Tonón reallocated them away from hospitals and clinics located in wealthier central regions of the city with relatively low health risks and toward clinics located in generally poorer outlying regions with much higher risks of infant mortality. The SMS particularly sought to increase staffing for a new neonatal monitoring program that flagged and offered additional doctor visits to illiterate mothers, adolescent mothers, and mothers whose newborns weighed under 2,500 grams (about 5.5 pounds). By 1996, the SMS had also created an obstetrics center that increased the total number of hospital beds available for newborns and mothers in the capital to 117, compared to 70 in 1994 (Junqueira et al. 2002). Ultimately, such measures helped increase the proportion of live births occurring in hospitals (L. Tonón, interview, 2010) as well as the proportion of mothers giving birth after seven or more prenatal visits, which would grow to nearly 70% by 2004 (World Bank 2006, 39). These efforts helped considerably reduce IMR more than 27% in only four years, from 41.32 in 1993 to 29.85 by 1997.

3.3. A SANITARISTA MAYOR, EXTENSIVE STATE-BUILDING, AND ROBUST IMR DECLINE, 1997–2002

The Sanitarist Movement achieved an impressive victory when Dr. Célio de Castro (PSB) won two consecutive mayoral elections that saw him occupy the city's highest elected office for nearly five uninterrupted years between 1997 and November of 2001. As a cofounder of the Mineiro Sanitarista Party (PMS), Castro was a local standard-bearer for Sanitarist Movement ideologies, and his tenure amounted to the longest and most sustained episode of sanitarista office holding in the mayorship ever recorded in a major capital of Brazil to that point. Castro didn't merely ride the momentum of prior mayors' state-building efforts in the public health sector; he eclipsed them by dramatically increasing health spending to nearly 18% of all municipal expenditures and rolling out new primary health programs with unprecedented reach. Ultimately, the human consequences of Castro's office-holding tenure in the mayorship were considerable. IMR during Castro's less than five years as mayor fell at nearly twice the rate (60%), from 29.85 in 1997 to just 12.17 in 2002, that it had fallen during the four years of Patrus's mayorship (27%, from 41.32 in 1993 to 29.85 in 1997). In office only a few months longer than Patrus, Castro's record of social development was especially impressive since IMR reductions at lower levels are generally more difficult to achieve than at higher levels.

Castro's electoral victories and his corresponding record of expanding Belo Horizonte's public health state clearly reflect the context of the coalitional party politics in which he captured the mayor's office. The vice mayor during Patrus's administration, Castro won a plurality of votes against his PT and PSDB rivals in the first turn of the 1996 election before defeating his PSDB rival with 76.6% of votes in a second turn (TSE 2016). The victory was all the more impressive because although Patrus was unable to run for reelection that year due to constitutionally mandated term limits, Castro still had to defeat a PT candidate. Although the PT and PSB had previously formed a coalition that yielded the successful 1992 ticket of Patrus and Castro, the PT abandoned a 1992 commitment to support Castro's 1996 mayoral campaign (Wampler 2015, 87).[9] Thus, Castro ultimately overcame the daunting challenge of having to defeat both a PT and PSDB candidate, all amid the disintegration of an electoral coalition that would have otherwise greatly improved his prospects of victory.

In this regard, it was hardly incidental that Castro's victories emerged amid cohesive sanitarista efforts to establish electoral campaigns, elections, democratic offices, and other regulative institutions of civil society as outposts within the state for its ideology of health universalism and equity. During the dictatorship, Castro had been a militant in the same current of Belo Horizonte's PC do B that produced other office-holding sanitaristas such as Borges. In fact, the capital's Mineiro Sanitarista Party (PMS) "was led by Célio de Castro, who had a more radical insertion in politics" than other members like Machado, Saraiva, and Campos (J. M. Borges, interview, 2010). Beyond just his professional medical background, Castro's impressive mayoral victories owed much to the fact of this activist pedigree in such Sanitarist Movement associations. Although Castro had long espoused commitments to the Sanitarist Movement ideologies of universal and equal access to health, the mobilization of public opinion and the framing of his electoral campaigns around such issues brought an even sharper focus on health than that of his predecessors in the mayor's office.

Castro's campaigns mobilized public opinion by offering a candidate biography as well as a topical public discourse that directly addressed the central concern with health that Belo Horizonte's voters consistently expressed. In both 1992 and 1996, polling suggested that the electorate viewed health as the principle challenge facing the capital, outpacing even concerns with crime (Estado de Minas 2000a). In part by using a campaign jingle that touted him as "Doctor BH," Castro's campaigns carefully accentuated his background as a medical doctor. But such publicity also counterbalanced that professional background with his demonstrated record as an activist, union leader, and sanitarista committed to improving public health services by redeeming the SUS's promises of universal and equal access. Furthermore, he carried this discourse far beyond the campaign trail and into his swearing-in to the office of mayor. Following his first oath of office, Castro extolled the importance of localized efforts to "offer concrete alternatives to the neoliberal project underway [in Brasília]," proclaiming that "health will be Priority #1 of my new administration" (Folha de São Paulo 1997).

In material dimensions, Castro's administrations matched such ideologically infused proclamations by appreciably expanding, not just maintaining, the continuity of prior commitments put in place by his PT predecessor. Indeed, Castro's administrations increased the proportion of all municipal expenditures dedicated to the health sector by greater degrees than Patrus's administration did. During the early 1990s, this proportion hovered around 7% (L. Tonón, interview, 2010), had modestly increased to no higher than 12% by the end of the Patrus administration, and most likely hovered around only 10%.[10] By the time Castro left office in 2001, however, Belo Horizonte was dedicating 17.57% of all municipal spending on the health sector (SIOPS 2017). Equally striking is the fact that the SMS had gone from possessing four 386 computers and hardly any employees in

1993 to having a comparatively sophisticated bureaucracy and 14,145 employees by 2003 (SMS-BH 2008, 38).

To be sure, the two mayors operated in different contexts vis-à-vis pressures and incentives for spending imposed by federal laws and agencies. Yet Castro's expansions were all the more impressive given that his administration faced arguably more severe federally imposed spending constraints during the lion's share of his administration. In particular, the passage of the federal Kandir Laws of 1996 severely limited the ability of municipalities to hire public employees. Nevertheless, Castro's administration found ways to move ahead, opening public concursos to hire health professionals and sizably expanding both the sheer magnitude of the health budget and the proportion of all municipal spending that it represented. Despite challenging nationwide circumstances, the single largest proportional increase in Belo Horizonte's expanding financial commitment to health occurred with a sanitarista in the city's mayorship.

Among other destinations, Castro's administration funneled these resources into the hiring of approximately 1,500 municipal health workers associated with a new primary-care program called BH-Health (*BH-Saúde*). The program was a localized adaptation of the nationwide PSF model, and its overriding purpose was to deepen the clinic-based primary-care model by expanding entry points into the SUS through a larger and still more decentralized network of facilities and health professionals in outlying regions of the city. One dimension of this plan involved simply expanding delivery of preventative care in extant primary-care facilities through the already existing federal platform, the Community Health Agents Program, that was pioneered in Fortaleza and then advocated nationwide by the federal MS. But a subtler dimension of it involved localized modifications to accommodate the demands of organized labor and more explicitly reduce premature mortality. One major difference between BH-Health and the more general PSF model was that Belo Horizonte's version prioritized stronger labor contracts for health workers. In this regard, the city differed considerably from Porto Alegre, where PT mayors not steeped in the norms and traditions of the Sanitarist Movement initially adopted the PSF by hiring its workers to emergency contracts with little job security and none of the benefits of municipal workers. By contrast, Belo Horizonte's SMS explicitly developed agreements in this regard with increasingly powerful health-worker unions such as SIND-SAÚDE and SINDIBEL. In particular, the SMS agreed to hire workers for the program through public concursos in which successful candidates became public employees of the municipality (P. C. Perreira, interview, 2010). Not surprisingly, however, the negotiations over the terms of these agreements proved to be time-consuming, helping explain why it was not until 2002 that the SMS fully expanded the program.

Thus, BH-Health began in 1998 as a pilot project in only 22 of Belo Horizonte's 130 health clinics. The SMS also focused on more extensive training of workers in these twenty-two clinics. In 2000, Castro himself gained federal support to expand the project from José Serra (PSDB), who, as the federal health minister, was then zealously pursuing PSF expansion. Castro said, "I went to Brasília and showed [the pilot program] to José Serra and he was enthusiastic, so we signed an agreement to expand it with 6.6 million reais" (Estado de Minas 2000b). Thus, far from simply becoming a pass-through for federal or state financing, BH-Health was tailored by Castro as a larger framework in which to apply multiple sources of local and federal funding on terms agreed on by organized health workers, SMS planners, and the mayor himself. Although BH-Health was just a modest pilot project, it would prove to be precedent setting in laying an institutional foundation for expanding this tailored version of the PSF on an unsurpassed scale in urban Brazil.

Although in 2001 Castro restructured the city's bureaucracy in ways that likely weakened the SMS directorship,[11] this mattered relatively little immediately since the mayor himself had already begun facilitating efforts to build the SMS's capacities for expanding BH-Health. During Castro's first term, he tasked the SMS director, Dr. Marílio Malagutti, and the agency's Division of Planning and Development (GPLD) with developing more sophisticated technical competencies for targeting BH-Health teams to city regions facing the most severe health risks. The GPLD was then led by Paulo Cesar Perreira, a former PC do B activist who had organized in clandestine dictatorship-era unionization campaigns alongside Castro and Dr. Evilázio Tuebner, Castro's appointee as SMS director (2001–2002). Perreira oversaw the development of more sophisticated technical and spatial tools for assessing health risks in different city regions. These assessments were then used to create a Health Vulnerability Index (IVS) for assigning teams to city regions and microregions served by particular clinics.

In 2001, when the GPLD rolled out 382 PSF teams, it employed the IVS to make these allocative decisions. The IVS also became a central tool for deciding the service and infrastructure rollout strategies outlined in the Municipal Health Plan for 2001 to 2004 and for 2005 to 2008. Under the directorship of Perreira, the GPLD also began authoring annual budgetary reports for the upcoming year, spending summaries for the preceding year, and four-year strategic plans for all of the secretariat's new infrastructure construction and service-provision plans. Although the GPLD routinely presented these documents to the city's health council for deliberation and approval, the main decisions they described were ultimately ones proposed by teams of sanitaristas within the SMS and approved by the SMS director and Castro himself. And by 2001, SMS-BH had evolved the technical tools within the GPLD to allocate to health clinics and professionals within city tracts according to the most serious health risks of infant mortality. The GPLD liaised with an epidemiological unit within the SMS that tracked vital statistics, and infant mortality prevention became an overriding priority in these allocative decisions (P. C. Perreira and E. Tuebner, interview, 2010). Although Belo Horizonte's massive expansion of the program did not occur until 2002, such major planning decisions about its rollout had been made while Castro was still in office.

Due to his own failing health, however, Castro stepped away from the mayorship in November 2001. Fernando Pimentel, his PT vice mayor and director of the city's powerful planning agency, then assumed the office of mayor. And while this change eventually induced personnel shifts atop the SMS in early 2003, it had relatively little immediate bearing on the underlying processes of state-building for primary health care expansion that Castro had already set in motion. On a larger cross-sector level, by 2001 Castro had already increased the health budget to the biggest single destination for municipal spending of any policy sector, at 17.57% (SIOPS 2017). And in narrower terms of the BH-Health expansion that Castro had already negotiated with the federal health ministry, little of relevance changed.

In particular, Tuebner remained in the SMS directorship for a year and a half thereafter and oversaw the preplanned deployment of 382 teams, who reached over 1.3 million residents, or about 58.3% of the population, by the end of 2002. Unlike in other major Brazilian capitals, the city's already established network of basic health units (UBS) hosted these teams, in part because their locations more seamlessly matched Castro's and Tuebner's earlier prioritization of city regions facing the highest risks of premature mortality. Interestingly, this goal conflicted somewhat with a goal that was of arguably greater interest to the health ministry, which promoted municipal adoption of the PSF at the time to maximize the proportion of the population covered by the program (even if doing so meant dedicating fewer resources to high-risk areas). It is a testament to the enduring influence of Castro's localized adaptation of the model that the SMS continued prioritizing IMR reduction when it maintained the severity of health risk as its primary criterion for allocating teams to regions. It is additionally notable that the SMS initially maintained its commitment to hiring all PSF workers as municipal employees. Although it reflected persistent difficulties in hiring doctors and pediatricians, this decision also contributed to having adequate capacity to staff only 382 of the 504 teams that the MS had authorized the SMS to implant (P. C. Perreira and E. Tuebner, interviews, 2010). When Tuebner left its directorship in March of 2003, the SMS had hired additional staff for another 48 teams, raising the total to 430, and had begun opening concursos that would populate another 43 teams by December, raising the total to 473.

It is difficult to overstate the human consequences of institutional changes in the municipal public health sector overseen by office-holding sanitaristas in Belo Horizonte, especially Castro himself. Despite beginning the episode in 1997 as a middling performer at best, Belo Horizonte had, by 2002, reduced its IMR by 60% (to 12.17), effectively tying Curitiba (11.62) for the lowest level in urban Brazil. This achievement was especially impressive given the intense demands for health services emerging from citizens well beyond Belo Horizonte's municipal borders in the nearly three dozen other municípios that constitute its encompassing metropolitan area. Thus, Belo Horizonte achieved most of its reductions in IMR by 2002 (in 2015, for example, Belo Horizonte's IMR of 10.34 had changed relatively little). It is especially notable that this accomplishment predated the beginning of Brazil's PT presidencies, the post-2003 incarnation of Bolsa Família, and a PT mayorship that lasted longer than four years. And while local participatory politics contributed important oversights of the city's health sector, the more thoroughgoing processes of state-building that drove IMR reduction during this episode emanated from office-holding sanitaristas atop the public health state and in the highest democratic office in the capital, the mayorship itself.

3.4. CONTINUED SANITARISTA OFFICE HOLDING AND LOW IMR, 2003–2016

Although Belo Horizonte's public health state continued expanding after 2003, these changes had far less effect on IMR reduction than those of the antecedent episode, for several reasons. One was that the reach of primary health care had already been extended so broadly that additional expansions began to reach the point of diminishing marginal returns, placing a new focus on public access to more sophisticated types of health care. And in this regard, office-holding sanitaristas such as Tuebner became victims of their own success in ways that underscore how health democratization was predicated on an expansion in accountability of officeholders to citizens. Most basically, the relative success of office-holding sanitaristas in universalizing and equalizing access to the most basic forms of care had generated new demands for other, more sophisticated health services. Expansion of the reach of primary-care entry points into the city's SUS had begun generating demand overload on the city's larger network of public health facilities. Indeed, high-profile failures of the system and associated public complaints played no small role in the resignation of Tuebner in March 2003 (Giovanella et al. 2008, 100; E. Tuebner, interview, 2010). Although Mayor Pimentel quickly replaced him with a sanitarista SMS director, Dr. Helvécio Miranda Magalhães Jr., the earlier successes of his predecessors had expanded democratic claims-making such that another SUS principle, integrality of care, came to assume a growing importance.

Part of a younger generation of sanitaristas more attuned to shifting citizen demands for higher-quality care, Magalhães was broadly respected as a petista as well as a sanitarista, and he soon also became president of the nationwide CONASEMS at a moment in which the PT held Brazil's presidency for the first time. Magalhães's circulation in nationwide networks of other officeholders atop the public health state instilled in him the importance of creating new and more vertically integrated systems of care delivery that could meet the various needs of a generally healthier population (H. M. Magalhães, interview, 2010). Yet his focus turned to expanding the wider variety of secondary and tertiary services required to complement primary health in delivering more integral forms of care. In advancing this loftier and more expensive goal, the proportion of all municipal spending dedicated to health expanded significantly under Magalhães, from 19.3% in 2003 to 22.89% by 2008, a level rarely witnessed in urban Brazil. During his last year as director, the SMS spent over 1.18 billion reais, had 16,908 employees, and hired thousands of other contracted workers (SMS-BH 2008).

None of this, however, prevented Magalhães from executing the Castro-era plan to expand the PSF or from later expanding its coverage even further. By 2008, Belo Horizonte had a much better-equipped network of nearly 145 municipally run health clinics that delivered over four million primary-care appointments (SMS-BH 2008). Additionally, he reorganized the program to focus on hiring and training health professionals more specifically attuned to roles in service provision through a PSF-specific work process (Magalhães 2010; Pereira Lopes and Gesteira e Matos 2010). Initially, this involved providing financial incentives for the SMS's existing primary-care workers to convert their assignments into new positions with job descriptions that listed responsibilities particular to the PSF work process. Throughout this process, Magalhães remained committed to Castro's practice of hiring workers for the program as municipal employees. Between 2003 and 2008 alone, however, Magalhães succeeded in opening five concursos, which helped increase the number of municipal health professionals from 14,145 employees in 2002 to a total of approximately 16,908 in 2008 (H. M. Magalhães, interview, 2010; SMS-BH 2009). By the end of his directorship in 2008, these concursos had helped expand the PSF to 497 teams that reached over 1.7 million residents, or about 71.5% of the population, by far the highest rate of any major Brazilian capital and nearly double that of the second-place city. In 2009, the year after Magalhães's directorship ended, the city's IMR—already at the low level of 12.17 in 2002 before he took office—had fallen modestly to 10.84.

In 2008, the PT agreed to support a successful telecommunications executive as the PSB's mayoral candidate, and Marcio Lacerda won the first of two elections that saw him occupy the mayorship for eight consecutive years. Winning both the 2008 and 2012 elections representing the increasingly centrist PSB, Lacerda became known for his technocratic, performance-based approach to improving the quality of public-service delivery. But after appointing Marcelo Gouvêa Teixeira, a PSDB member and business administration expert as SMS director, Lacerda's first term saw a near flatlining in the PSF's coverage rate, which hovered around 502 teams by the end of 2012. After Gouvêa left the position during the first year of Lacerda's second term, however, Lacerda appointed his second in command, Fabiano Geraldo Pimenta Jr., as his replacement. A public health expert with a research and professional background in epidemiology and infectious disease prevention, Pimenta and his SMS expanded the PSF by additional 72 teams, bringing the city's total by the end of 2014 to 574 teams covering nearly 1.98 million residents, or 82.66% of the population, at which this level remained well into 2016. By 2015, however, the city's IMR of 10.34 had remained effectively unchanged from its 2009 level. Indeed, while these historically low levels persisted in Belo Horizonte, the city's most consequential strides in reducing premature death had been achieved nearly a decade and a half earlier.

4. Conclusion

Even as Brazil returned to formal democracy, few could have predicted that a city like Belo Horizonte, with IMRs resembling those in northeastern cities such as Recife and Salvador, would become one of urban Brazil's top performers in this regard less than fifteen years later. In the more than three decades after the restoration of local democratic elections in Brazil, Belo Horizonte witnessed nothing short of a historic transformation in the capacities of its municipal state to prevent premature death, and locally rooted sanitaristas were at the heart of this shift. This chapter has argued that, alongside other conditions, a central cause of this outcome was a participatory-programmatic trajectory of health democratization in which ideologically motivated sanitaristas helped establish and then capture new democratic offices atop the municipal state. In turn, municipal state capacities expanded to more broadly deliver basic forms of health care.

Although it is thus difficult to explain the city's monumental IMR reductions without reference to the local civil-society agents that propelled these shifts, this chapter pointed to a distinct type of civil society—pragmatist publics—as the prime animator of this overall dynamic. Epitomized by the city's sanitaristas, pragmatist publics differ considerably from the city's participatory publics, who focused more centrally on making the OP and CMS into citizen-driven monitors of the local public health sector. To be sure, sanitaristas often worked alongside these other civil-society actors and left-leaning PT mayors to establish a Participatory Budgeting (OP) process and its CMS at notably early moments in the early 1990s. Such processes clearly deepened health democratization in Belo Horizonte by institutionalizing transparent, rule-bound, and citizen-driven modes of monitoring the public health sector that eclipsed what participatory publics were able to establish in otherwise similar cities such as Curitiba and Fortaleza. But, although the achievements of these other civil societies should not be minimized, this chapter emphasized important limitations of their practical effects on the state-building processes that are most essential for maximizing IMR reduction. Although Belo Horizonte's well-organized participatory publics built the capacities of the city's participatory-democratic institutions for engaging political elites in health-policy debates, its CMS has generally lacked sufficient power to fully exert its formal authority as a cogovernor with the SMS of the public health sector. This is a generally accepted fact among councillors themselves (Ferreira, personal communication, 2010; Wampler 2015), but such stark realities nevertheless have important implications for how and what kinds of civil societies can maximize democracy's effect on social development outcomes, a topic to which I return in the book's conclusion. The chapter's within-case analysis suggested that these more deeply democratic processes in Belo Horizonte have been less relevant than other factors have been in propelling the discreet state-building processes that are most consequential for improving delivery of primary health care and thus reducing infant mortality.

By contrast, more cohesive groups of office-holding sanitaristas in the SMS directorship and at the city's nonbureaucratic top sought (with much success) to leave their imprint on service-delivery arms of the municipal public health state by aggressively seizing control over state-building in a remarkably early and sustained manner. In particular, this pragmatist public exercised substantial control over the city's multiple impressive hiring waves of primary health care professionals. One of the most important dimensions of capacity-building for IMR reduction, meritocratic hiring of primary health care providers came to be overwhelmingly directed by sanitarista officeholders atop Belo Horizonte's SMS and in the mayor's office itself. It is also an especially telling indicator of these actors' state-building influence that sanitarista office holding in the SMS directorship stretched across the administrations of mayors from three distinct political parties (PSDB, PT, PSB). As in other capitals such as Fortaleza, these parties included the PSDB organization of Pimenta da Veiga (1989–1990) and Eduardo Azeredo (1990–1992), which remained open to and enacted the modest state-building proposals of office-holding sanitaristas despite being a generally less progressive party than the PT or PSB. Perhaps more importantly, Belo Horizonte's most important expansion of the state capacity to deliver morality-reducing health care occurred during a moment in which a party alliance between the PT and PSB had effectively disintegrated and a sanitarista occupied the mayor's office. In short, the infusion of sanitary reform ideology into this notably wide variety of political parties and democratic offices—not just the mere fact of political rule by such parties per se or the separate contributions of participatory publics—better accounts for Belo Horizonte's impressive state-building record in the public health sector as well as for its robust development outcomes.

FIVE

Porto Alegre

I was a militant, a PT founder and militant, but I had a
double-militancy. . . . I had a militancy in public health, as
well as militancy in unions and parties.

—*Dr. Lucio Barcelos, sanitarista director of Porto Alegre's SMS*
(1998–2000)

Porto Alegre, the capital of Brazil's southernmost state of Rio Grande do
Sul, is the country's tenth-largest município, with a population of nearly
1.5 million residing in the geographic core of the country's fifth-largest metropolitan area. As with the capitals of the states of Minas Gerais and São
Paulo, Porto Alegre is one of Brazil's historic power centers in national politics, having produced arguably the country's single most influential poli-
tician of the twentieth century, Getúlio Vargas. For students of contemporary politics, the city is best known as the birthplace of Brazil's now famous
and oft-emulated Participatory Budgeting (OP) process. But even before
Porto Alegre witnessed the rise of such pathbreaking institutional experiments or the advent of the health-democratization period, it had already
become urban Brazil's top performer in minimizing premature death. In
1988, the city's IMR of 30.06 was by far the lowest of any major Brazilian
capital, outpacing even other high-performing, southern-region neighbors
such as Curitiba. Furthermore, Porto Alegre largely maintained this status
well into the 2010s, after tying Curitiba as Brazil's first capital city to record
an IMR below 10 (9.95) in 2006.

The chapter traces Porto Alegre's record of robust social development to
both a relatively privileged starting point and a participatory-programmatic
trajectory of health democratization. The city's history of less-damaging colonial legacies and greater independence from national power structures
differed from all other Brazilian capitals in ways that fostered stronger ini-

tial conditions. Yet initial conditions alone cannot account for additional progress achieved in mortality reduction after Brazil's return to democracy. Indeed, Porto Alegre's continued improvement owed much to a participatory-programmatic trajectory of health democratization that transformed the subnational capacity to broadly deliver primary public health care. Two dimensions of this trajectory particularly stand out. First, Porto Alegre's participatory publics established and transformed the city's Municipal Health Council (CMS) and its Participatory Budgeting (OP) process into civic arenas in which citizen-participants routinely monitored the public health sector and influenced certain state-building processes, especially the construction of physical infrastructure such as health clinics. Additionally, the city's office-holding sanitaristas helped expand the city's ranks of public health professionals in ways that mattered especially for broadened access to primary care and, ultimately, for robust development.

Thus, the chapter argues that a key mechanism by which the participatory-programmatic democratization of health yielded robust development involved sanitarista officeholders building new local state capacities to deliver mortality-reducing primary health care. As in other cases of robust development, the capital witnessed several episodes of office holding in its SMS directorship by sanitaristas such as Maria Luiza Jaeger (1989–1992), Dr. Henrique Fontana (1997), Dr. Lucio Barcelos (1998–2000), and Dr. Sandra Fagundes (2003–2004). Jaeger also held the office of SES director (1999–2002) of Rio Grande do Sul state during an especially consequential moment of state-building for health in Porto Alegre. And although all these sanitarista office-holding episodes occurred under PT mayors, not all PT mayors appointed sanitaristas to the SMS directorship. This is particularly notable, because when they didn't—as was the case both from 1993 to 1997 and from 2001 to 2002—such state-building largely stalled, suggesting more than just a spurious relationship. This complements the chapter's within-case analysis in suggesting that a subset of civil-society actors (that is, office-holding sanitaristas), not political-society actors like PT mayors, most animated state-building for public health in Porto Alegre. Indeed, such episodes suggest that the PT was hardly immune from insulating itself from sanitarista-driven reformist influences.

Within-case analysis reveals that office-holding sanitaristas particularly leveraged the SMS directorship to expand the city's ranks of municipally employed health professionals in the primary-care sector. Although Porto

Alegre's SMS eventually embraced the PSF model, the office-holding sanitaristas at its helm also preserved a parallel, homegrown model of primary-care delivery that most resembles that of Curitiba. In this sense, Porto Alegre's stronger starting point—particularly an especially large network of formerly federally and state-run hospitals and clinics—meant diminished urgency for more fully adopting the PSF model, helping explain why robust development coincided with low PSF coverage rates. Nevertheless, the primary source of efforts to expand mortality-reducing primary care through Porto Alegre's bifurcated primary-care model—namely, office-holding sanitaristas atop the SMS directorship—was essentially the same as in all other positive cases of robust development. None of this nullifies how Porto Alegre's participatory publics accumulated considerable power to monitor the health sector through a continual presence within the CMS and OP. But the inability of the CMS to independently exert its formal authority to cogovern the sector was a recurring theme throughout the period. In this respect, another dimension of participatory-programmatic health democratization—namely, considerable expansion of the municipal public health state's service-delivery arms by office-holding sanitaristas—constituted a more central driver of the state-building processes by which Porto Alegre became one of urban Brazil's most robust developers by the early 2000s.

1. Pre-SUS-Era Civil and Political Society in Porto Alegre

True to the global reputation it would later earn as a hotbed of radical social movements and host of the World Social Forum, Porto Alegre entered the health-democratization period with some of Brazil's most highly organized and militant civil societies. During the military dictatorship, the city's health movement was especially connected to the city's famously radical neighborhood associations. As early as 1978, activists in the neighborhood movement created decentralized committees focused on improving access to health and sanitation infrastructure, citing poor access to both services as a central cause of the poor public health conditions of the city's population. When such activists in the Grande Cruzeiro region discovered a stockpile of sewer pipes sitting idle in the city's sewage department late in that year, they seized and installed them within the neighborhood, launching a popular health movement that eventually helped found the city's CMS in 1992 (Avritzer 2009, 127; Réos 2003). These early experiences in Porto Alegre played no small role in rallying the city's health activists around more radically decentralized models for comanaging the public health sector, including deep extensions of the CMS into a dense network of community-based health clinics (P. G. B. Carvalho, J. Pillar, and H. Scorza, interviews, 2010). In contrast to Belo Horizonte, then, early movements for public health more clearly resembled those observable in other major capitals such as São Paulo, where the more broad-based Popular Movement for Access to Health (MOPS) exerted greater influence earlier on in the municipal politics of health.

As was the case with the city's participatory publics and civil society more generally, Porto Alegre's early sanitarista associations were unevenly distributed across the city, maintaining stronger presences in certain neighborhoods than in others. In part, this reflected how a few state-run public health clinics clustered in some city regions became especially important organizing spaces for the city's sanitaristas. The early importance of such clinics to the rise of sanitarista activism in Porto Alegre mirrored similar dynamics in Belo Horizonte. In Porto Alegre, sanitarista organizing also began at a notably early moment at the beginning of the 1970s within clinics operating on a precocious, territorially oriented primary-care model that loosely resembled the Cuban model of the time. Created by early, epidemiologically trained leaders of Rio Grande do Sul's health secretariat such as Dr. Clovis Heitor Fernandes Tigre, Dr. Airton Fischmann, and others, clinics in Porto Alegre's Partenón and Santa Cecília neighborhoods constituted two such hubs of sanitarista organizing. Santa Cecília's Murialdo Health Clinic became an important nexus that influential *gaúcho* (residents of Rio Grande do Sul) sanitaristas often credit as the birthplace of their militancy during the dictatorship (L. Barcelos, M. L. Jaeger, and H. Scorza, interviews, 2010).

Equally important in the early rise of the movement in Porto Alegre was the dual militancy of many sanitaristas as student and union activists. Here, while the early establishment of clinics such as Murialdo played many important roles in the local rise of the movement, the fact that its workers were state employees (L. Barcelos, interview, 2010) proved especially salient because of the political opportunities this created for proto-union organizing. At the time, however, Brazil's military dictatorship also posed severe threats of violence, undermining any simplistic explanation of sanitarista organizing merely as the product of such political opportunities. The activist lineage of Dr. Lucio Barcelos, a venerable gaúcho sanitarista who would later serve as Porto Alegre's SMS secretary and the state's health council's president, offers an instructive example of this. Even amid an environment in which threats seemed to outweigh opportunities, the considerable individual commitments and persistence of activists such as Barcelos were of paramount importance.

For instance, while Barcelos was still earning a medical degree from Porto Alegre's Federal University of Rio Grande do Sul (UFRGS), the dictatorship jailed him for one month in 1970 along with other political prisoners on Gunpower Island, outside of the city. In 1976, after he had begun work as a public servant organizing within clandestine proto-unions and federations in the state health secretariat's (SES) Murialdo clinic, the military again captured and imprisoned Barcelos for a year. Facing the likely threat of such repression during the most violent period of Brazil's dictatorship did little to dissuade Barcelos from continuing to organize health workers in such proto-unions. These efforts included his presidency of a state health workers' association known as the Center for Civil Servants of the State Health Secretariat as well as of the Federation of State Civil Servant Associations (FASPES), which linked health workers with other public servants of the state bureaucracy. Also a cofounder of the PT in Porto Alegre, which he would later leave over dissatisfactions with the party's weak commitment to public health financing,[1] Barcelos described his activist lineage as "a double-militancy . . . I had a militancy in public health as well as militancy in unions and parties" (L. Barcelos, interview, 2010).

The biographies of other venerable sanitaristas such as Maria Luiza Jaeger also show how the convergence of proto-union, political party, and public health militancy emerged within state-run universities as well as the state health secretariat's clinics and headquarters. After graduating with a social science degree from UFRGS, where she began her militancy in public health and proto-union struggles, Jaeger began working for the SES in 1973. As a public servant of state government, she not only helped implement dimensions of the AIS and SUDS programs that focused on infant mortality reduction but also helped found an SES chapter of the Central Única dos Trabalhadores (CUT), Brazil's most important confederation of worker unions. Although she returned to work in Rio Grande do Sul's SES before being able to complete her thesis at the University of São Paulo's (USP) prestigious public health school in 1975, Jaeger became increasingly connected to nationwide sanitarista organizations such as CEBES and ABRASCO during this time (M. L. Jaeger, interview, 2010). In 1986, her stature as a public health activist grew to a new level upon being named to the National Health Commission (CNS), which, under the leadership of Dr. Sergio Arouca, would eventually draft passages in Article 196 of the Brazilian Constitution of 1988, codifying a universal citizenship right to health.

The pre-SUS-era landscape of political society in Porto Alegre was notable for the strong ties of dominant parties to unions and neighborhood associations. The Democratic Labor Party (PDT), initially known as the Brazilian Labor Party (PTB), was one of the first and most enduring parties to have cultivated such ties in the city (Baiocchi 2005, 13). Establishing connections to urban social movements well before the 1964 military seizure of power, the PTD was a populist party with a strong discourse of citizen empowerment that nevertheless governed in a traditional, patronage-fueled mold typical of Brazilian politics at the time (Conniff 1981; Cortés 1974). After a name change that echoed the rising salience of democratic ideals throughout Brazil, the PDT continued to be an influential actor within the city's powerful Neighborhood Association Movement (UAMPA) and the Municipal Employees Union. It continued, however, to gravitate around a few charismatic leaders, such as the party's founder, Lionel Brizola, and, later, Alceu Collares (Goldfrank 2011). The PDT was still a major force in local politics as the health-democratization period arose, although the nascent PT soon supplanted it as the dominant party in electoral politics.

Although the rise of the PT during the 1980s transformed Brazilian party politics in well-documented ways (Abers 2000; Avritzer 2009; Baiocchi 2003; Keck 1992), its coalescence in Rio Grande do Sul did not always foster enactment of nationwide sanitarista agendas within Porto Alegre itself. This was particularly the case for the sanitary reform project of strengthening municipal control of the health sector within the capital. The reasons for this are many and complex. One is that the agenda that sanitarista cofounders of the PT aimed to infuse into the party's local organization prioritized health-sector municipalization in rural municípios across Rio Grande do Sul more so than in Porto Alegre itself (M. L. Jaeger, interview, 2010). Additionally, many politically active sanitaristas had begun and continued their professional careers as public health workers not within Porto Alegre's municipal health department (SMS) but within a state-level health secretariat (SES) that had proven early on to be reasonably effective at delivering primary health services within certain city neighborhoods. Indeed, these sanitaristas helped design that state-operated model, which used an early precursor of the territorially based clinic approach to health care that would later become the dominant mode of service delivery under the federal PSF. Further, although prominent local sanitaristas such as Jaeger and Barcelos had helped cofound the PT locally, their militancy had been more vigorously focused on labor union organizing than on reforming the municipal public health state per se, contributing to a relegation of such sanitarista agendas beneath other PT priorities like instituting OP (L. Barcelos, M. L. Jaeger, and J. Kliemann, interviews, 2010).

Thus, the generally low priority that sanitarista agendas assumed within the Rio Grande do Sul's PT cannot be attributed to the absence of a local sanitarista network, which was so dense and connected to political society that its members helped cofound the PT in the city. But with no analog of Belo Horizonte's cohesive Mineiro Sanitarista Party (PMS), Porto Alegre's sanitaristas lent their support to separate proposals of popular health activists and participatory publics for OP and neighborhood-based control of health care provision. And because the city's sanitaristas were professionally rooted with the state-level SES that managed such facilities, their advocacy for municipalization in the primary health sector was not as early or as strong as that of the sanitaristas in Belo Horizonte. One result was that health-sector municipalization within the capital itself never became a similarly high priority (L. Barcelos, M. L. Jaeger, and J. Kliemann, interviews, 2010). And during the 1980s and 1990s, "health policy, in general, was never taken on or understood by the party, as such," as Dr. Joaquim Kliemann, a PT cofounder and future SMS secretary, put it (Kliemann, interview, 2010).

The PT did, however, maintain the strongest connections of any other locally influential party to municipal health workers' unions, such as the FASPES, as well as to municipal employees' unions and the CUT more generally. But in part due to its close ties with the popular health movement and participatory publics that integrated into the socialist democratic current of the party more deeply than into a new unionist current, the Sanitarist Movement permeated the former faction of the PT far more completely than it did the latter (L. Barcelos, M. L. Jaeger, J. Kliemann, and H. Scorza, interviews, 2010). The implications of the pattern for health democratization would reverberate throughout the subnational state-society politics of public health in the capital for decades to come.

2. *Participatory-Programmatic Democratization of Health in Porto Alegre*

Porto Alegre's participatory-programmatic trajectory of health democratization shared three baseline qualities with all other cities in this study. First, although reformist political parties would not immediately capture either Porto Alegre's mayorship or Rio Grande do Sul's governorship, the restoration of direct local elections for both offices was especially consequential because it ended an unsurpassed period of dominance by the military-endorsed ARENA party. While the ARENA party held the mayor's office for nearly twenty uninterrupted years between 1964 and 1983, it also dominated the mayorship during the eighteen years between 1966 and 1983 (TSE 2016). As was the case throughout urban Brazil, the end of the military's control of subnational governance through the ARENA party had far-reaching implications for democratizing the health sector. Not the least of these was how the newly competitive playing field in the mayoral (1985) and gubernatorial (1982) races permitted parties such as the PT to contest these increasingly influential offices.

Second, when Porto Alegre formally assumed constitutional and legal responsibilities for enacting the right to health after 1990, the presence of local sanitarista networks in the capital lent this nationwide victory a special local resonance. Although enshrinement of a right to health was not a factor that meaningfully differed across any of the major capitals examined in this study, it was a clear normative and political victory for locally organized sanitarista networks in Porto Alegre. This symbolic relevance created meaningful political opportunities for sanitaristas activists, who came to enjoy wider recognition among progressive party elites as a result. In particular, locally active sanitaristas enjoyed normative recognition within center and especially left parties such as the PT as influential defenders of a then-new right to health. They also garnered heightened political attention as promising candidates for occupying the new democratic offices of the SUS that assumed responsibility for enacting the right to health (M. L. Jaeger, interview, 2010).

Third, as in the rest of urban Brazil, Porto Alegre witnessed far-reaching political, fiscal, and administrative decentralization processes after 1982 that left state and municipal government with new responsibilities (and eventually more resources) for managing the public health sector. Although the state-level government of Rio Grande do Sul was an early mover in assuming responsibility for administering former federal health facilities, it tended to focus its efforts on decentralizing funding and responsibilities to municípios in rural parts of the state more than on the município of Porto Alegre itself. With this considerable rural focus of the state health department (SES) continuing well into the mid-1990s, it was especially salient that Porto Alegre's municipal government eventually assumed greater responsibility for administrating public health services within the capital's boundaries. Thus, while municipalization of the primary health sector occurred later in Porto Alegre than in other capitals such as Belo Horizonte and even Fortaleza, its eventual occurrence shifted the nexus of public responsibility for health to municipal officeholders in ways that consequentially deepened lines of democratic accountability for administering the sector to local citizens.

Nevertheless, Porto Alegre's participatory-programmatic trajectory of health democratization differed in other respects from the minimalist variant observable in Rio de Janeiro and Salvador. After 1988, Porto Alegre's state-society politics shifted away from a tutelage regime that had suppressed civil-society inputs into public decision making by selectively incorporating certain groups according to their political allegiances to a few party elites (Baiocchi 2005). Although the city's encompassing state of Rio Grande do Sul experienced no such similarly entrenched or extreme pattern of coronelismo as that witnessed in Bahia, Ceará, or Minas Gerais (Cortés 1974; Hagopian 2007), the implications of the shift were stark, even if increased electoral competition did not immediately spell the end of rule by populist politicians such as Alceu Collares of the PDT. To win the 1985 election for Porto Alegre's first directly elected mayor since 1964, Collares had to defeat opponents from four parties, including the PT (TSE 2016), bringing demands for more institutionalized modes of civil society–state intermediation to the fore. Thus, even if the new reality of electoral competition did not immediately stop Collares's mayoral administration (1986–1988) from generally continuing a pattern of tutelage that was heavier on populist rhetoric than on genuine political opportunities for civil society to influence local governance (Baiocchi 2005, 31–33), it did contribute to a playing field in which candidates ignored such demands at their own peril. And such increasing civil-society demands played no small part in the subsequent election of the city's first PT mayor, Olívio Dutra (1988–1992), on a platform centrally focused on such demands.

Existing research persuasively shows how the PT mayorships of Dutra, Tarso Genro (1993–1996, 2001–2002), Raul Pont (1997–2000), and João Verle (2002–2004) helped replace Porto Alegre's prior tutelage mode of governance with a participatory-democratic mode that created new state-society spaces in which participatory publics influenced the city's budget for physical infrastructure (Baiocchi 2005). But while political society in Porto Alegre (and Belo Horizonte) particularly sought to include diverse participatory publics in local governance through institutions like the OP (Avritzer 2009; Goldfrank 2011) and the CMS (Wampler 2015), the more general feature of openness to civil society in governance was a quality that both cities shared with the contrastingly nonparticipatory variants of programmatic health democratization witnessed in Curitiba and Fortaleza. As will become clearer later, specific reforms pursued in the primary public health sector depended to a considerable extent on these distinct ways that political societies in different cities sought to include civil society. In Porto Alegre, political-society elites routinely included participatory publics through the OP and CMS but were somewhat less open to including pragmatist publics such as office-holding sanitaristas through new democratic offices like the SUS directorship. Porto Alegre's institutional experiments with OP and the CMS clearly show how its political elites opened the state-society interface of public health politics to an especially broad extent by integrating civil-society actors into authorship of the city's physical infrastructure budget and monitoring of the public health sector through the CMS. But in the more general respect of opening governance processes to civil society, Porto Alegre's political-society elites shared such basic receptivity with all other cities in this study except for Salvador and Rio de Janeiro. And while this reflected how Porto Alegre's PT managed to disrupt the prior monopoly on local political power held by conservative elites from right-leaning parties, that achievement owed much both to the party's strong connections to a broad range of civil-society actors and the considerable organization of the city's participatory publics and its pragmatist publics.

After 2003, Porto Alegre's participatory-programmatic trajectory also reflected an unsurpassed penetration of Bolsa Família (BF) within the city. Generally thought to emanate from national-level actors, the city's broad implementation of BF nevertheless suggests that local conditions may well have made a difference in expanding the reach of such programmatic social-policy reforms, even one that is ostensibly federally run and supposedly less reliant on effective local governments. Compared to all other cities in this study, Porto Alegre achieved the highest proportion of eligible families who actually received transfers through the program (its targeting rate) in 2016. Cumulatively speaking, it recorded an average targeting rate of 96.78% between 2004 and 2016, which was the highest in all of urban Brazil. Furthermore, despite constituting one of the most economically developed capitals in Brazil's southern or southeastern regions—a factor that necessarily limits the reach attainable by a means-tested program such as BF—Porto Alegre recorded the highest coverage rate of any major capital in either region. Capturing the 2004–2016 average proportion of families enrolled in BF to total families in the city, Porto Alegre's coverage rate of 61.6% reemphasizes how programmatic interventions such as BF had a particularly broad reach in the city that outpaced what even Curitiba (47.75%), Rio de Janeiro (48.32%), Belo Horizonte (49.43%), and São Paulo (40.86%) witnessed. Although analysis of Porto Alegre's high coverage and targeting rates is largely beyond the scope of this study, these rates show that far-reaching programmatic interventions in social-policy sectors were not confined to the health sector but also included Brazil's premier antipoverty program.

An especially decisive quality that Porto Alegre shared with Curitiba, Fortaleza, Recife, and Belo Horizonte (but not with Salvador or Rio de Janeiro) was how it precociously and consistently expanded the subnational public health state's service-delivery arms. Although Porto Alegre's infrastructure for delivering primary public health care through the PSF was never as sophisticated as Belo Horizonte's, its SMS accumulated considerable service-provision capacity outside the PSF platform. Porto Alegre was most like Curitiba in this regard, with health facilities originally run by the SES of Rio Grande do Sul within Porto Alegre's borders that employed a similar territorially based and team-based platform for delivering primary care that proved to be quite sticky, even after the SES transferred these facilities to the município in 1996 (M. L. Jaeger and O. Paniz, interview, 2010; H. Alencar [president of CMS's Technical Commission,

SETEC], personal communication). All things considered, Porto Alegre accumulated impressive combined state capacities to deliver primary care through this homegrown model as well as through the PSF. Yet the unexplored question of which social actors drove such fundamental changes remains an important topic that the chapter addresses later. The foundation of this impressive capacity was an especially extensive network of health facilities and primary-care workers that initially clustered in the city's geographic core but slowly expanded outward into peripheral city regions as the period progressed. In per capita terms, the city featured one of urban Brazil's most prolific networks of public health facilities at nearly all times between the early 1990s and 2016. In 2016, its SMS delivered primary-care services in 141 health facilities. The PSF platform delivered primary care in 112 of these clinics, leaving 29 units that delivered such services according to Porto Alegre's non-PSF model of attention (SMS-PA 2016, 111, 477). Also in 2016, the SMS employed 208 PSF teams that achieved over 50% populational coverage, or about 717,600 residents, with each PSF team serving an average of about 8,200 exclusive SUS users. Porto Alegre's slow uptake of the program reflected one of the lowest average coverage rates for the 2005 to 2012 period at only 21%. But when considering its combined delivery of all primary services to exclusive SUS users through both PSF and non-PSF platforms, the city ranked well above the median for large Brazilian capitals.

Finally, and as intimated above, it is impossible to speak of Porto Alegre's health-democratization period without reference to its sophisticated participatory institutions in the public health sector and beyond. As in Belo Horizonte, civil-society actors who were connected to but distinct from Porto Alegre's sanitaristas established an elaborate set of participatory-democratic institutions for monitoring the local public health sector. In particular, Porto Alegre is home to an especially well-organized Municipal Health Council (CMS) and the oft-noted OP process that its first PT mayor, Olívio Dutra, introduced in 1989. Existing work establishes how both institutions have created spaces quite apart from the city's sanitaristas for participatory publics to monitor operations of the municipal public health state (Avritzer 2009; Baiocchi 2005; Heidrich 2002). Such institutionalized experiences of participatory governance have undeniably deepened the democratization of health in Porto Alegre, perhaps more so than anywhere else in urban Brazil. In sharp contrast to Rio de Janeiro, Salvador, Curitiba, and Fortaleza until much more recently, there can be little dispute that Porto Alegre's CMS and OP created rule-bound, institutionalized spaces in which citizens and neighborhood-based collectives can make demands on local government for public-service expansions, including in the primary health sector.

Nevertheless, there are limits to what participatory publics and citizens in participatory governance institutions can achieve with respect to statebuilding for primary-care delivery and mortality reduction, even in Porto Alegre. On the most basic level, even the formal authorities of CMS councillors and OP participants to direct municipal state-building in the public health sector are simply more limited than the more concentrated authorities at the disposal of SMS directors. Porto Alegre's CMS mirrors others across urban Brazil in that Brazil's Organic Health Laws (Federal Republic of Brazil 1990a, 1990b) formally assign it authority to cogovern the public health sector alongside the SMS. While this authority could in theory certainly extend to major state-building actions such as the hiring and firing of municipal public health workers, actual practice has been a different story. Despite their considerable organizational and technical competencies to exercise such rule, CMS councillors have generally lacked the power required to exert such authorities alongside mayors and SMS officials in anything like an equal fashion. Such power deficits were particularly conspicuous between 2005 and 2016, when the city's mayors hailed from more conservative political parties with little connection to the participatory publics that traditionally animate the council. For example, despite possessing the authority to veto proposed budgets of the SMS, meeting minutes and resolutions passed by the CMS between 1992 and 2012 offer no evidence that its councillors ever exercised this veto in ways that suspended federal transfers for the sector. In part, this reflects how councillors often perceive such vetoes and the suspensions of funding they can theoretically trigger to undermine the public interests of health system users (P. G. B. Carvalho, O. Paniz, and H. Scorza, interviews, 2010).

Perhaps more importantly, state-building proposals in the primary health sector have typically emerged from office-holding sanitaristas atop the city's SMS rather than from participatory publics within the CMS, whose main role in this regard has often been relegated to (at best) approval of such proposals rather than sustained or genuinely equal coauthorship of them. This was especially the case before Porto Alegre's council began selecting its own coordinator during the mid-1990s. Before this, the SMS director filled the position in a de facto manner. Such lack of coauthorship is particularly conspicuous in matters of hiring public-health-service workers, although it extends to other forms of state-building, such as proposals to build new health clinics or renovate existing ones. Although plans that emerge from Porto Alegre's SMS (for example, prospective four-year Municipal Health Plans) often reflect inputs of the CMS, SMS directors and their staff typically author their content, whereas a technical commission of CMS (SETEC) reviews the plans (L. Barcelos, J. Kliemann, and O. Paniz, interviews, 2010). Further, because Porto Alegre's most significant reductions in childhood mortality had already been achieved by the mid-1990s, it is difficult to argue that deepening institutionalization of the CMS thereafter had a sizable influence on mortality reduction per se. In sum, although such participatory institutions clearly deepened the quality of health democratization and established rule-bound ways for civil society to monitor the public health sector in Porto Alegre, the causal importance for the social development outcomes examined in this is far from obvious.

3. Sanitarista Office Holding and Expansion of Porto Alegre's Public Health State

Although Porto Alegre witnessed a period of participatory-programmatic health democratization that was roughly similar to that of Belo Horizonte, its far lower initial level of premature mortality fundamentally differed from the level seen in Belo Horizonte. Indeed, Porto Alegre's IMR of 30.06 in 1988 was by far the lowest of any major capital city in Brazil. On the one hand, this makes it difficult to argue that the city's subsequent trajectory had as profound an impact on its robust development outcomes as in otherwise similar cases. Indeed, a principal question surrounds why and how Porto Alegre began the period with such low levels of premature death at all, a topic addressed later. On the other hand, within-case analysis of Porto Alegre's trajectory thereafter still provides theoretically rich insights into the dimensions of participatory-programmatic democratization of health that mattered most for mortality reduction. As in all other cases of robust development, sanitaristas held key offices atop the SMS with remarkable consistency from 1989 to 2004. Indeed, the analysis that follows traces nearly all consequential moments of health-related state-building throughout the period to the political influence of sanitarista SMS directors. Porto Alegre also experienced two contrasting episodes in which even PT mayorships yielded tepid state-building of this kind, in part because the city's SMS lacked office-holding sanitaristas at its helm.

Expansion of the subnational public health state in Porto Alegre during the 1980s initially reflected sanitarista-driven changes to federal- and state-level health institutions more than to municipal ones. Entering the health-democratization period, Porto Alegre hosted one of urban Brazil's most sophisticated networks of public health facilities. Yet much of it was initially managed not by Rio Grande do Sul's state-level SES or by Porto Alegre's SMS but by a federal autarchy created by the military dictatorship in 1977, the National Institute for Medical Assistance in Social Security (INAMPS). This state of affairs began changing to dramatic effect in the capital after a series of national-level reforms started eroding the control of INAMPS over this network (Falleti 2010a). Porto Alegre's SMS absorbed none of this physical infrastructure initially (M. L. Jaeger, interview, 2010). Founded in 1963 as a joint Municipal Health and Social Service Secretariat (SMSSS) project, the SMS would not even become a stand-alone entity dedicated solely to the health sector until 1994. In the absence of such organizational capacity on the level of municipal government, Rio Grande do Sul's SES formally inherited most of the capital's INAMPS-era hospitals and clinics in 1987.

While the initial subnational absorption of the federal INAMPS network in Porto Alegre was partly the result of sanitarista interventions on the national level that have been documented elsewhere (Falleti 2010a, 2010b; McGuire 2010), local politics also played a role. The most important federal reform to begin decentralizing control during the episode was the 1984 Integrated Health Actions (AIS) program, for which sanitaristas had been the prime advocate on the national level. In Porto Alegre, however, the AIS quickly induced greater cooperation between the rapidly eroding INAMPS and both subnational health agencies in the capital. In August of that year, the state and município jointly created the Inter-Institutional Municipal Health Commission of Porto Alegre (CIMS-Porto Alegre). In 1985, the CIMS signed an agreement known as a *Convênio AIS* to begin jointly coordinating delivery of basic and emergency health services with the INAMPS and other bodies (CMS-PA 2017). Although systematic data are not available for this episode, gaúcha sanitaristas inside the SES such as Maria Luiza Jaeger helped along Porto Alegre's AIS reforms in ways that almost certainly expanded primary public-service provision within the capital (M. L. Jaeger, interview, 2010).

Institutionally, the general effect of Porto Alegre's CIMS was to decenter decision-making power away from INAMPS bureaucrats so that public access to basic public health services within the city began expanding. Not all major capitals formed as robust a CIMS or adhered as fully to the AIS prescriptions as Porto Alegre did. And observers generally agree that cities that formed a CIMS and adopted the AIS during this episode began shifting the kinds of health services delivered from those that were complex and privately consumed to those that were less complex and publicly consumed (M. Coelho 2006; Escorel 2008). A central mechanism of this effect was disruption of control by INAMPS bureaucrats, who were widely recognized as having thrived on lucrative patronage ties to private sector hospitals and insurers that could be billed for expensive, high-complexity services with little public oversight (Hochman 1998). In September 1985, a technical committee of Porto Alegre's CIMS began weekly meetings to collectively strategize ways of improving the quality of health-service provision in the capital (SMS-PA 2016). The AIS reforms more fully involved the inputs of both sanitaristas and popular-health-movement activists in the commission's decisions and actions. Although the additional funding for primary service provision that it made available was limited, AIS adherence explicitly tasked the CIMS with making public hospitals and especially clinics more publicly accountable to users within the município (Cortes 2002; Escorel 2008, 422). State-driven implementation of the AIS most likely contributed to Porto Alegre's considerable reduction of infant mortality from 39.27 in 1984, the first year of AIS, to 30.06 by 1988, the year after the project decentralized its first set of health care institutions to Rio Grande do Sul's SES.

Thus, national- and state-level activism by sanitaristas within the SES was initially more consequential for mortality reduction in Porto Alegre than were actions of municipal politicians or civil-society actors seeking to mold its health-sector interventions. Indeed, although Alceu Collares of the PDT (1986–1988), the city's first directly elected mayor since 1964, maintained ties to neighborhood associations and participation activists, he was better known for his populist rhetoric and governance than for any programmatic interventions to improve public health conditions in the city (P. G. B. Carvalho and M. L. Jaeger, interviews, 2010). Unlike PT mayors who followed him, Collares exhibited little discernible commitment as mayor to enacting the proposals of civil society to institute participatory governance measures that would devolve actual budgetary control to citizens (Baiocchi 2005, 31). Public health politics hewed to a similar discourse-heavy line, with the administration drafting a preliminary Municipal Health Plan (M. L. Jaeger, interview, 2010) that precipitated few noticeable improvements in municipal state capacity for service delivery. By the end of Collares's term, the city's popular-health movement and sanitaristas alike had lost whatever initial belief they may have previously had in his administration's ability to improve public health conditions in the city.

Activism by those in similar popular-health movements played an important role as well. In late 1988, discontent with municipal health governance boiled over into the familiar, disruptive pattern of militancy commonly pursued by popular-health-movement activists in the Vila Cruzeiro region (P. Ribeiro, interview, 2010). A major flashpoint in this mobilization was the popular-health movement's reaction to the closure of the pediatric emergency wing of the city's largest emergency room, the INAMPS-run "PAM-3" facility in the Vila Cruzeiro neighborhood. Health activists organized an occupation of the facility on September 14, 1988, that continued to have symbolic resonance for Porto Alegre's health councillors nearly a quarter century later (CMS-PA 2012, 9–17). The president of the state's doctors' union (Dr. Flávio Mouro Agosto) and the *petista* (member of the PT) president of the state assembly's health commission (Selvino Heck) joined the occupation, which was coorganized by Heriberto Back, the president of Porto Alegre's neighborhood association union. Back called the occupation an attempt to "call the attention of authorities to problems of health and the generally precarious situation of this health post, which is among the best in Porto Alegre" (Jornal Brasil 1988). It is notable that among the group's demands was greater local control of the facility, a theme that would characterize much of Porto Alegre's state-society politics for the next decade. The protestors specifically demanded the municipalization of the pediatric emergency room by the SMSSS and acceleration of the transfer of local control to the SES of the rest of the PAM-3 facility (CMS-PA

2012, 15). Yet their occupation precipitated only a reaffirmation by the federal representative of Porto Alegre's CIMS to continue an already ongoing devolution of control of the facility to the SES. Demands for greater municipal control of the PAM-3, the protestors were told, had become a matter for Porto Alegre's SMSSS to negotiate with the Rio Grande do Sul SES. Nevertheless, the ongoing discontent among such health-focused popular movements and participatory publics as well as sanitaristas would soon count on new democratic institutions of the SUS to contribute their inputs into health-policy-making.

3.2. SANITARISTA-DRIVEN STATE-BUILDING
AND ROBUST IMR DECLINE, 1988–1993

After codification of a constitutional right to health and the election of Porto Alegre's first PT mayor, a consistent episode of municipal-level sanitarista office holding from 1989 to 1993 helped reduce IMR during this period by a third, from 30.06 to 20.03. Although a central mechanism of this reduction was sanitarista-propelled state-building, the full array of advocates and adversaries of such state-building differed somewhat from those in otherwise similar cities such as Belo Horizonte. Although Olívio Dutra's mayoral victory precipitated the appointment of the venerable sanitarista Maria Luiza Jaeger as Porto Alegre's SMSSS secretary, her proposals to municipalize actual primary health facilities and hospitals met with stiff resistance from the federal health ministry and the successive PMDB and PDT governors of Rio Grande do Sul. Nevertheless, Jaeger still managed to improve service-delivery capacities through modest renovations to the SMSSS's small network of facilities, the deployment of a new territorialized model of health-service provision within eleven health-management districts, and increased CIMS-organized cooperation between SMSSS and SES health workers within each district (M. L. Jaeger, interview, 2010; SMS-PA 2016).

That such state-building and related mortality reductions occurred at all was impressive given that sanitaristas and petistas in Porto Alegre's SMSSS could not count on the sanitarista control of the state-level SES that had facilitated health-sector municipalization in Belo Horizonte. Upon gaining control of the municipal SMSSS, Jaeger had to contend with PMDB and PDT governors, who insulated the nonbureaucratic top of the SES from control by sanitaristas and other civil-society actors pursuing municipalization. Among its other effects, this yielded comparatively weaker commitments to immediate health-sector municipalization than arose in Belo Horizonte. Indeed, by the time Jaeger's efforts to municipalize the health sector began gathering momentum in 1991, the PDT's Collares had won the state's governorship. And given his rivalry with Dutra, who had defeated Collares's PDT counterpart in the 1988 mayoral race, the public health sector became something of a political football in which Collares's administration consistently rejected Jaeger's and Dutra's municipalization requests (M. L. Jaeger, interview, 2010).

Jaeger's appointment as SMSSS director paradoxically confirms how *sanitarista* ideologies and political projects for reforming the public health sectors were generally low priorities for Porto Alegre's PT, starting with its early days in power (L. Barcelos, M. L. Jaeger, and J. Kliemann, interviews, 2010). By Jaeger's own account, Dutra's appointment of her to the office reflected their long-standing relationship and background in union militancy as much as it did her local and national reputation as a *sanitarista* who had sat on the 1986 National Sanitary Reform Commission and was helping design the institutional architecture of the SUS. She put it this way:

> So Olívio is the mayor, and Tarso Genro is named his vice mayor. Creating the government was entirely a process of negotiation between various tendencies of the PT. The name that they first arrived upon was [Dr. Rogério] Amoretti, who ran the GHC and was a person connected to Tarso. There was a meeting of the directorate in which Olívio presented Amoretti's name, and Amoretti went home to celebrate his having become secretary. Only the meeting continues, and people who came more from the health and union movements proposed my name. Olívio ended up accepting it because he had known me since the days of the union movement . . . when I was president of the sociologists' union and he was president of the Bank Employees' Union. So we had known each other for a long while through the PT, the CUT, etcetera (M. L. Jaeger, interview, 2010).

Thus, although Jaeger came to control the SMSSS, this appeared not to emanate from any similarly purposeful or unanimous conviction among political-society elites of the importance of instituting sanitary reform, as was evident in the early appointments of *sanitarista* SMS directors in Belo Horizonte and Fortaleza. Rather, personal ties forged in union and labor struggles are what sealed Jaeger's appointment.

In this context, it is less surprising how the small network of SMSSS fa-

cilities that Jaeger came to oversee grew relatively little during her directorship. She said, "The secretariat we assumed was a miniscule thing that included only one emergency room hospital, twelve or thirteen clinics [health
units, US], and the emergency room of the PAM-3 hospital in Cruzeiro"
(M. L. Jaeger, interview, 2010). Taken together, these facilities absorbed
about 90% of the SMSSS's budget at the time (Leite 2010, 124), leaving little financing for major expansions or renovations of the network. Effectively blocked from annexing state facilities and hamstrung without major
budgetary increases to hire new municipal health workers, Jaeger instead
aimed to reorganize the SMSSS's existing clinics to better address patient
needs with a new system of local councils. To do so, she tasked Soraya Cortes, her close confidant and planning coordinator within the SMSSS, with
most operational aspects of this work during 1989 and 1990 (M. L. Jaeger,
interview, 2010; S. Cortes, personal communication, 2009).

Jaeger and Cortes introduced a new, territorialized system of health-
management districts to organize patient uptake into the city's health facilities. This system effectively built on the Santa Cecilia neighborhood's
long-standing model of territorialized primary-care provision in the Murialdo clinic. Yet it dramatically expanded the model to encompass the entire município and added new institutional mechanisms for expanding
local participation in the management of each region's health facilities. Reflecting Cortes's sociological training and background in the local PT's socialist democratic current, these institutions included strong participatory
governance components that were designed to dovetail with the city's then
emergent Participatory Budget process (J. Pillar, interview, 2010; S. Cortes,
personal communication). Deepening the preexisting CIMS framework
to the regional level, the CIMS formed local health commissions (CLIS)
within each of the eleven new districts in 1989 (SMS-PA 2016). Consisting of service providers, health workers, SMSSS and SES representatives,
and neighborhood association leaders, each CLIS was tasked with identifying service-provision gaps in their jurisdictions and seeking ways to improve the quality of health-service delivery on that smaller scale (M. L. Jaeger, interview, 2010). Among its other institutional legacies, the CIMS and
its subsidiary network of CLISs became a strong institutional forerunner of
the city's Municipal Health Council, founded officially through Municipal
Law 277 in 1992 (CMS-PA 2017).

Beyond these administrative reforms, Jaeger paved the way for future municipalization of the public health sector and fended off proposals to privatize public facilities. Under her direction, the SMSSS also tasked its employees with shadowing and beginning to work alongside their SES counterparts in clinics and hospitals that her management team anticipated would eventually be decentralized to the município. To begin planning for this inevitable shift, SMSSS managers also started coordinating with former INAMPS bureaucrats whom the SES had absorbed as state employees (Leite 2010, 124). Thus, even amid the hostility of state-level political elites to municipalization, the SMSSS still accumulated modest capacities to broaden delivery of primary care through the new regionalized model of service delivery, even if the SES continued to deliver most of those services within that model. Jaeger also fought and won key defensive struggles such as helping defeat a proposal to privatize the largest network of public hospitals in the city, the Conceição Hospital Group (GHC). Specifically, she contended with this privatization attempt by securing Dutra's support for a counterproposal to the federal health ministry that would have resulted in the SMSSS assuming control of the GHC instead. Jaeger commented on the process:

> Olívio didn't have this preoccupation about finances, so much so that he agreed to propose municipalizing GHC, which would have been absolute madness for us. When I went to him with this proposal, I thought, *There is no way he will accept this.* He accepted it. . . . Our [first] proposal for municipalization was to get everything, hospitals included. It was very much like, "Let's go; let's do this." And the secretariat that would have been left to do everything was a tiny thing. But the idea was, "Let's do this now and see how it turns out later" (M. L. Jaeger, interview, 2010).

Although rejected by the health ministry, Jaeger's proposal helped induce Rio Grande do Sul's SES to eventually take control of the GHC, effectively blocking the privatization proposal.

Among its other insights, the episode demonstrates how sanitarista office holding atop the SMSSS dovetailed with certain aspects of the participatory governance model then being pursued throughout the city through institution such as the CIMS, its subsidiary CLISs, and eventually the CMS. Interestingly, however, office-holding sanitaristas were key actors in establishing these participatory governance institutions in the health sector. And although broadly sympathetic to the stronger ideological convictions of the city's participatory publics that authority for managing the health sector should be decentralized on its own democratizing merits, these institutions' practical benefits for improving actual service-delivery and social development outcomes were a major inducement for activists like Jaeger to pursue the office in the first place. Indeed, Sanitarist Movement ideologies of universalizing and equalizing access to health services were central motivations for these officials' support of a participatory-democratic model that deepened cooperation between public-health-care providers, citizen users of the SUS, and managers of the city's health care bureaucracy. Interviews with public health managers and officeholders suggest that such coordination likely increased subnational delivery of mortality-reducing primary health care and improved its targeting to neighborhoods, such as Vila Cruzeiro, that faced disproportionately high risks of premature death. Systematic statistical data on service provision are not available to complement this theory, however. At a minimum, adoption of Porto Alegre's regionalized model of public-health-service delivery reflected a deepening of public accountability among both municipal-level and even state-level health agencies like the SES that still delivered most primary health services within the capital. Such shifts continued to echo in subsequent efforts to municipalize the health sector.

3.3. SIDELINED SANITARISTAS, LIMITED STATE-BUILDING FOR PRIMARY CARE, AND IMR DECLINE, 1993–1996

Despite continued PT mayoral rule between 1993 and 1996, sanitaristas lost control of the SMS directorship during this episode, undermining the creation of new municipal state capacities needed for further expansion of mortality-reducing primary care within the capital. After the PT won its second mayoral election, Mayor Tarso Genro began his term (1993–1996) by appointing Dr. Luiz Henrique de Almeida Mota, a nonsanitarista expert in hospital management, to direct the SMSSS. The exit of Collares from Rio Grande do Sul's governorship after 1994 had helpfully removed a major veto point, permitting Mota greater leeway for municipalizing public health facilities and workers from the state of Rio Grande do Sul during 1994 and 1996. But despite the on-paper increases this generated in capacity for health-service delivery, expansions of Porto Alegre's network paradoxically yielded few increases in usable capacity for IMR reduction. Indeed, municipalization imposed growing pains that temporarily undermined existing capacities for primary-care delivery through the previous regionalized model that the state's SES had operated in the capital. Amid such short-term constraints, IMR actually increased from under twenty during the last year of Jaeger's directorship in 1992 to about twenty-two by the end of Mota's directorship in 1996.

Porto Alegre's SMS during this episode faced a difficult environment in which to further reduce infant mortality. Most obviously, IMR had already reached the lowest level of any major capital in urban Brazil during 1993, leaving somewhat less room for improvement than was the case in previous episodes or in other large capitals at the time. After all, the SES had already developed, with reasonable effectiveness, formidable capacities for delivering primary public health care in the capital through a regionalized model that already targeted service delivery to areas of greatest epidemiological risk. Further, national-level changes such at the Kandir Law of 1996 imposed greater constraints on the abilities of municipal governments to hire state employees during the last year of Mota's directorship, when hiring needs were especially acute. And it was not until 1999 that Porto Alegre would experience a pattern of simultaneous gubernatorial and mayoral control by sanitarista-influenced political elites that was similar to what Belo Horizonte had enjoyed continuously since the mid-1980s. Nevertheless, certain elements of Porto Alegre's stalled record of state-building and IMR reduction during this episode are at least partially traceable to state-society dynamics.

For one, the public health sector continued to be a relatively low political priority for a PT mayoral administration that insulated itself from sanitarista demands in a manner not unlike that witnessed in negative cases of minimalist health democratization. With Dutra unable to run for reelection due to term limits, the 1992 mayoral victory by Genro (Dutra's former vice mayor) began solidifying what would eventually become a sixteen-year period of electoral hegemony in the city. But it also brought important changes to the nonbureaucratic top of the municipal public health state. In appointing Mota, a doctor who had previously worked in hospital management under Jaeger's SMSSS, Genro elevated a doctor better known for his ties to Genro's new unionist current of the PT than for any demonstrable commitment to sanitary reform ideology that was similar to his predecessor. Mota also lacked strong roots in the socialist democracy tendency that had influenced Jaeger and Cortes, and his administration somewhat predictably proved generally less concerned with primary-care expansion or with devolving significant or autonomous cogoverning power to the CMS (L. Barcelos and M. L. Jaeger, interviews, 2010). After 1990, when the Organic Health Laws mandated the creation of a CMS in every município, Porto Alegre's committee benefited greatly from absorbing the already existing organizational infrastructure of the CIMS and its subsidiary CLIS. With CMS members pressing for further reaching reforms, Mota's SMS revisited and revised previous proposals to municipalize the state-run network of hospitals and clinics in the capital.

In 1994, however, Mota took the much more modest initial step of declaring only an "incipient" (rather than a partial or full) management status within the SUS (Leite 2010; O. Paniz, interview, 2010). The process of becoming an incipient manager meant slower-moving change, and initially this generated little in the way of new dedicated financing for the primary health sector. Somewhat surprisingly—or unsurprisingly for scholars like Hunter (2010) who have highlighted an unwillingness among many PT executives to assume the major financial burdens associated with further-reaching reforms of the public health and education sectors—cost concerns among the state's PT leaders impeded the SMS from adopting a more committed, "partial" (*semiplena*) management status within the SUS that could have freed up additional funding. In particular, Mota's administration found itself hamstrung by concerns among the PT's Genro-affiliated directors of the treasury and of finance that assuming deeper service-provision responsibilities would require hiring new municipally employed health workers, which would correspondingly impose untenable long-term financial commitments on the city (L. Barcelos, interview, 2010; Leite 2010, 128). Although not unfounded, such concerns belie the image of a PT that was willing to spend liberally on social policy, instead foreshadowing the financial conservativism detectable within its coming presidencies of Brazil (Hunter 2010).

Thus, when prompted by the federal health ministry's promulgation of SUS Basic Operating Norm of 1993 (NOB-93) to assume a deeper level of responsibility for the health sector, Mota's SMS opted in 1994 for an incipient status within the SUS that considerably limited such new commitments. The biggest institutional change that this ushered in was the 1994 creation of a Municipal Health Fund (FMS) that was in theory solely dedicated to public health and unusable for purposes other than those approved by the SMS director and the city's CMS (Carvalho de Noronha, Dias de

Lima, and Vieira Machado 2008). Yet in something of a catch-22, the unwillingness of PT authorities to approve the hiring of health-service professionals as municipal employees led to federal contributions to the FMS remaining unusable, a phenomenon that became a persistent pattern in years to come. A central reason for this was that PT elites in charge of municipal finance and the treasury remained uncertain about whether federal sources of funding placed into the FMS would be sufficiently large, consistent, and dependable enough to be counted on in defraying the costs of salaries for municipal health workers in perpetuity (L. Barcelos and O. Paniz, interviews, 2010; Leite 2010, 129–30). During the final year of Mota's directorship, the SMS adopted the somewhat more committed partial management status that placed fuller responsibility on the city to begin delivering primary care itself, further ratcheting up pressures on Mota and city managers to institute a staffing plan of some kind.

In lieu of any proactive agreements about how to staff the primary health sector, a haphazard initial implementation of the federal PSF in the capital precipitated the SMS's first improvised foray into hiring municipal health workers. Upon implanting the program in 1996, Mota's SMS first placed neighborhood association presidents—not trained public health bureaucrats or SMS officeholders—in charge of hiring and managing PSF teams. Thus, instead of the SMS directly overseeing PSF implementation, as was standard practice in Belo Horizonte and more common throughout much of urban Brazil, Porto Alegre's neighborhood association presidents became de facto managers of PSF's teams of health care professionals. This unorthodox arrangement worked as follows:

> So the neighborhood association there in Lomba do Pinheiro [a neighborhood in southeastern Porto Alegre] employed the PSF teams that worked in Lomba do Pinheiro. And the município had a contract with the association. It passed funds to the association, and the association hired the teams. So the president of the association was the employer of the PSF team. This was a crazy arrangement! For better or worse, the guy who was president of the association—he thought he was the owner of all the equipment, but not everyone, not every community leader, had a good head for this work. These guys thought they were the boss and that they could fire workers and order the teams around. So this created a tense situation (L. Barcelos, interview, 2010).

This unconventional surrendering of state responsibilities for the program to neighborhood leaders quickly became controversial in the sanitarista cir-

cles that had not been fully integrated into the SMS under Mota's administration. As codified in the Organic Health Laws and SUS Basic Operating
Norms (NOBs), the primary health sector constituted a major programmatic responsibility of municipal government and particularly of the SMS.
Among its other consequences, the way that Mota's SMS devolved those
public responsibilities to neighborhood association presidents led to an in-
auspicious and seemingly ineffective beginning for the PSF. It also offers
insights into the social actors, particularly neighborhood associations and
their presidents, that influenced Porto Alegre's public health politics when
office-holding sanitaristas held less sway atop the SMS.

Indeed, how the city's primary health sector came to be governed in
such a manner speaks to an odd conglomeration of structural and other
factors that converged in a particular moment in the city's state-society politics of health. For one, these factors reflect how the luster of the PT's initial participatory governance innovations had begun wearing off for some
popular-health-movement activists and participatory publics. Dr. Humberto Scorza—a longtime petista, a progressive Catholic priest, a sanitarista, and the first non–SMS director to become coordinator of Porto
Alegre's CMS—described this moment as one in which the initial buzz
and novelty of Participatory Budgeting was beginning to wear off. As he
put it, "When people started to participate, the novelty of OP was that they
felt, to a certain point, validated in their efforts. With the passage of time
and with all that kept disturbing the process—people started to encoun-
ter delayed projects, projects that never actually arrived, you know—people
started to, in quotes, I won't say tire, but to not participate as effectively"
(H. Scorza, interview, 2010). For some, a palpable sense had emerged that
participatory policy-making control through the OP was not always as effective for influencing the health sector as it was for influencing other sectors in which physical infrastructure was a more central concern than in
the service-dependent health sector.

For example, Heverson da Cunha, a longtime popular-movement and
health activist who sat on the city's CMS in 2010, pointed out that OP offers participants no control over a fundamental organizational problem of
effective health-service delivery: the ability to hire new health professionals
to work in clinics. He said, "Whenever citizens begin to make more fundamental critiques of the government's provision of, say, primary health
services in health posts, the reply is always the same: go to Participatory

Budgeting to make your claim. But in Participatory Budgeting, you can advocate for a health post to be built where you live, but it doesn't work for solving more complex problems like opening concursos for the doctors and nurses who work in the health post—you know, making sure there are actual professionals working in clinics" (H. da Cunha, personal communication, 2010). Activists like da Cunha acted on such sentiments by gravitating to less broadly inclusive (than OP) but more empowered participatory institutions such as the city's CMS, although the CMS similarly struggled to practically influence human resource dimensions of state-building. Even popular health activists such as da Cunha who became councillors expressed growing frustrations with the inability of the CMS to exercise its comanagement authorities in moments of greatest tension with the SMS. Such frustrations reached more acute levels after the end of PT electoral control in 2005. More immediately, the CMS still struggled to carry out its comanagement functions independently of the SMS, whose director still served as de facto head of the CMS throughout most of Mota's tenure (P. G. B. Carvalho and O. Paniz, interviews, 2010).

From the standpoint of many sanitaristas, such limitations in the power of Porto Alegre's otherwise robust participatory institutions contributed to a weaker-than-hoped-for beginning of the PSF in Porto Alegre. Serving as de facto president of the CMS, Mota secured the council's approval on September 21, 1995, for an SMS plan to establish twenty-nine PSFs in neighborhoods that it had determined to be most in need of access to primary care based on infant mortality and epidemiological data (Gue Martini 2000, 73). Yet the SMS did not hire these health professionals as municipal employees with regular contracts and benefits. Rather, in relinquishing oversight of the PSF to neighborhood association presidents, the SMS laid the groundwork for hiring these workers on precarious six-month emergency contracts. This led to neighborhood association leaders—important actors within the PT's electoral coalition—assuming considerable powers to effectively govern the primary health sector as the managers of these workers. Systematic data on service provision are not available for this period, but SMS officeholders and CMS councillors converged in the view that these dynamics considerably undermined the actual delivery of primary care through the PSF well into the 2000s (L. Barcelos, M. L. Jaeger, and H. Scorza, interviews, 2010).

Among other insights, this episode demonstrates how even an otherwise progressive party such as Porto Alegre's PT may well have inadvertently undermined primary health care delivery and mortality reduction by shielding sanitaristas from control of key offices atop the SMS. To be sure, structural constraints also played a role, including the 1996 Kandir Law and jurisdictional confusions about financing in the early moments of health-sector decentralization. Yet amid the PT's conservatism about hiring municipal employees, insulation of sanitaristas from control of the SMS yielded a decidedly nonprogrammatic implementation of the country's first major primary public-health-care program. More specifically, when sanitaristas were relegated to the sidelines of the SMS, a different configuration of actors filled the gaps they left, and not always in ways that produced programmatic change in the health sector. This was particularly true of neighborhood association presidents with no health-management experience and of participatory institutions such as the CMS that played monitoring roles but lacked sufficient power to cogovern the sector. One intermediate outcome was persistent deficits in service-provision capacity, especially inadequate staffing of the PSF and of primary care more generally, that lingered into subsequent SMS administrations.

3.4. SANITARISTA OFFICE HOLDING, MAXIMAL STATE-BUILDING,
AND ROBUST IMR DECLINE, 1997–2001

Following the 1996 mayoral victory of Raul Pont (1997–2000), sanitaristas reclaimed control of the SMS directorship during four brief but consequential years in which they helped to reduce IMR by nearly 40%, from 22.06 in 1996 to 13.9 in 2001. Unlike in the previous Genro administration that had excluded sanitaristas from the SMS directorship, office-holding sanitaristas such as Dr. Henrique Fontana and Dr. Lucio Barcelos occupied and leveraged the office to make considerable strides in permanently staffing the PSF. Additionally, Barcelos negotiated multiple arrangements with the federal health ministry that both increased Porto Alegre's municipally employed health workers and municipalized the largest infant and children's hospital in the capital. Thus, a main mechanism through which sanitarista office holding helped reduce IMR during this episode was the mobilization of political elites' support for new hiring waves that significantly expanded the SMS's ranks of primary-care workers.

The control that Fontana and Barcelos exerted atop the SMS between 1997 and 2000 in part reflected how sanitaristas had more fully penetrated Pont's socialist democratic current of Porto Alegre's PT compared to the faction from which Genro hailed (L. Barcelos, M. L. Jaeger, and J. Kliemann, interviews, 2010). Although it would clearly be an exaggeration to suggest that the PT operated as two parties, well-documented factionalization within the party (Avritzer 2009) created palpable organizational hurdles for sanitaristas trying to mobilize party support for their proposals to hire large numbers of public health workers. Despite few strong objections within the party to amorphous sanitary reform principles of universal and equal access to health, Porto Alegre's sanitaristas struggled to secure active support from both PT factions for their political program to advance those principles by expanding the municipal public health state. Here, Genro's wing particularly subsumed sanitarista preferences for hiring large numbers of municipal health workers beneath separate concerns with cost minimization, as Mota's tenure demonstrated. But especially in 1999, when Pont was already mayor, the PT's Olívio Dutra began a concurrent governorship (1999–2002) by appointing Jaeger as director of Rio Grande do Sul's SES. With a governor and mayor from the same party faction that sanitaristas had more fully rallied around this political project for advancing sanitary reform, the stage was set for major programmatic changes to the health sector in the capital.

Yet even if the stage was set as such, actual state-building required office-holding sanitaristas in the SMS to successfully mobilize governing elites in the PT to enact such proposals, an endeavor in which success was never guaranteed. Here, the office of SUS manager proved a helpful tool for sanitarista efforts to do so, in part because of the access it provided to executives and the key state-building levers they wielded. Particularly instructive in this regard was Barcelos's three years as SMS director (1998–2000), which precipitated the single largest three-year period of expansion of tenured municipal health workers seen in the city to that point. At the beginning of 1999, the SMS employed a total of only 4,119 workers, only 1,995 of whom were health professionals working in the decentralized network of primary-care clinics scattered across city districts (CMS-PA 1999).[2] By the end of 1999, after Barcelos's interventions, around 2,795 municipal employees worked in the regionally decentralized primary-care network of facilities. Comparing this increase to such levels in 2010, when the SMS employed only 5,250 total workers, suggests that in the eleven years following Barcelos's 1999 interventions, the number of SMS employees had expanded by only 27% (1,131 employees). By contrast, Barcelos's tenure produced a one-year increase that amounted to over 70% of all new hires made in the next eleven years. In short, his tenure was the single most prolific SMS directorship in the city's history to that point.

These increases resulted from two discreet mobilizations by Barcelos during his SMS directorship. Both were likely consequential for Porto Alegre's impressive IMR reductions during the 1997 to 2000 episode. The underlying constraints that both interventions had to confront was enduring reticence among PT elites to assume the considerable costs of hiring health workers as municipal employees. Barcelos said, "There was always a strong tendency to not want to open public concursos. This was true of Tarso before and after my administration, and true of João Verle's [PT] administration" (L. Barcelos, interview, 2010). Untying this Gordian knot required a pragmatic approach to inventing new forms of state capacity for delivering basic health services in a more programmatic fashion than had been the case when Mota's administration first introduced the PSF to Porto Alegre. A first mobilization occurred in 1998, when Barcelos began his tenure as SMS director. Upon entering the office, one of his first priorities was to convert all PSF workers, then under the control of neighborhood associations and precariously employed with temporary six-month contracts, into municipal employees. Barcelos made the following comment about the process:

> When I entered, there was this widespread commotion and an ongoing battle between [the PSF] teams and the neighborhood associations. Some had a good relationship, but most were in serious disarray. So what did I do? There was a political discussion. I tried to negotiate with the treasury secretary for us to employ all the PSF team workers. But despite also being from the PT, that guy only thought about money. So he arrived at the following conclusion: "Listen, we can't hire everyone, since this will create a very large expense for the município when these people retire as municipal employees and the município will have to continue paying them a full salary. So, no, we can't hire them" (L. Barcelos, interview, 2010).

With his proposal initially rejected, Barcelos went back to the drawing board with little guidance about how to solve the problem of hiring the PSF workers to stable contracts. Some months later, Barcelos improvised a solution for permanently employing the PSF workers through a foundation associated with an actual state institution and his alma mater, UFRGS.

He explained that "the alternative I found was to remove these workers from their linkages to the neighborhood associations and to negotiate with FAURGS [the University Foundation of the State of Rio Grande do Sul] to become their employer. So instead of remaining with that scattered arrangement of having these ten teams here contracted by the [neighborhood] association, we negotiated and made a contract with FAURGS, passed them the resources, and they started to employ everyone according to CLT requirements" (L. Barcelos, interview, 2010).[3] Thus, solving the problem of how to hire PSF workers into permanent positions ultimately required an end around the PT-run municipal government entirely and Barcelos's proactive enlistment of other state institutions more willing to accept the burdens of managing new workers.

In 1999, during a second successful mobilization, Barcelos secured the support of PT elites to hire about eight hundred municipal health care workers through another improvised arrangement. A prime motivation for Barcelos was to again replace the precarious "emergency" contracts on which the Mota administration had hired the workers with permanent ones that he believed would contribute to more consistent and broader service provision (among other benefits). This time, Barcelos negotiated an impressive agreement with the federal health ministry (MS) according to which the MS agreed to pay all the retirement expenses for these eight hundred new municipal employees in perpetuity, most of whom were due sizable pensions as former MS and SES employees. Although this impressive deal, the only one he knew of nationwide, freed the SMS of major cost burdens, getting approval for it still required a major political effort to gain support of reluctant PT elites. Here, Barcelos secured PT support for the deal only by raising the contracts as a potential electoral liability in the 1998 election for state governor, which the party (successfully) aimed to capture for the first time ever in the state. Barcelos put it this way:

> In truth, during my administration, we were able to [hire the 800 workers as permanent employees] because of a political interference that occurred—not naturally or due to conviction alone but because when I was [SMS] secretary there was an election for state governor and the PT's candidate was Olívio Dutra. So I negotiated with the treasury secretary, another cabinet-level position which was also ours [held by the PT], and said, "Look, my friend, let's do the following: let's nominate these 700, 800 precariously employed guys. Let's open concursos and nominate them, because we can use this as a cam-

paign tool, right, you know, saying we are going to hire doctors, nurses, psychologists, audiologists, blah, blah, blah." So, because of this specific situation, which involved a state election in which we could use it as a campaign tool, we nominated and wiped the slate clean of the emergency contracts in the health sector during that period (L. Barcelos, interview, 2010).

In short, Barcelos successfully reframed a sanitarista-inspired hiring project then being pursued by the movement's activists across urban Brazil as a political tool for advancing the PT's electoral strategy at the time.

Among their other insights, such episodes show how pragmatist publics such as Porto Alegre's sanitaristas can skillfully occupy and wield democratic offices like the SUS manager's office to pursue universalistic social movement ideologies through decidedly pragmatic means. Barcelos's unconventional scheme to hire the PSF workers as FAURGS employees particularly echoes the Deweyan notion of evolutionary learning that scholars such as Christopher Ansell have highlighted as a defining feature of "pragmatist democracy" (2011). Yet far less has been said regarding the types of civil-society actors that might cultivate pragmatist democracy. Barcelos's approach in both episodes demonstrates how pragmatist publics uncommonly combine critiques of existing power structures with microlevel efforts to leverage democratic offices to devise and advance discreet solutions for ameliorating the policy blind spots of ruling parties with whom they align. On one hand, Barcelos vigorously criticized the first Genro mayorship and Mota's SMS directorship for having persistently used the emergency contracts at all, which he understood to be both ideologically vacuous and practically ineffective for broadening access to basic public health services. Barcelos said, "When I entered the secretariat, there were practically eight hundred workers, who had been contracted to work on an emergency basis [through a six-month contract] four years ago. . . . So where's the emergency? This was the policy, a policy that should never have been made by the PT, no, but it was the policy that the central administration of the state-level PT applied in that era" (L. Barcelos, interview, 2010).

On the other hand, if Barcelos intervened in a way that presented a solution with pragmatic appeal to party elites then contesting the state's highest democratic office, his main motivation for doing so was the solution's fit with the core sanitarista ideology of enacting a universal and equal right to health. Here, the democratic office of SUS manager became an essential tool for improvising such solutions to pressing public problems like how to absorb the high costs of adequately staffing public health facilities. For one, the fact that Barcelos held the office at all owed much both to his reputation as a knowledgeable and medically trained problem solver with intimate knowledge of the SUS and his movement lineage as a veteran of sanitarista struggles to establish and enact a constitutional right to health, a rare combination for any activist at the state-society interface. And although PT administrations such as Pont's exhibited an openness to campaigns by sanitaristas to occupy the office and then leverage it for their modest state-building campaigns, this was hardly a unique quality of the party. Rather, it was a generic, not especially proactive feature that the PT shared with many left, center-left, center, and, occasionally, center-right parties across urban Brazil at the time. Given such underlying openness, however, Barcelos's ability to capture the office and then wield it to secure support for the hiring plan cannot be separated from his activist lineage. As an activist who had sacrificed much to codify the right to health and establish the SUS and its high-level democratic offices in the first place, Barcelos personified the very normative responsibilities enshrined in the SUS manager's office. To be sure, Barcelos applied his more generic skills as a savvy negotiator to emphasize the political dividends of his state-building stratagems when pitching them to executives primarily concerned with their electoral prospects. But his activist lineage was a central reason he was in the office to begin with.

Such mobilizations by office-holding sanitaristas in the SMS directorship yielded tangible, material results for Porto Alegre's municipal health state and its ability to further reduce premature mortality by expanding primary public-health-care delivery. By 1999, the SMS managed ninety hospitals and clinics that employed nearly three thousand health workers. The presence of the PSF within these facilities, however, remained quite limited. In part, the program's small footprint reflected ongoing resistance among many of these workers and their unions to converting to the PSF work regime and accepting the possibility of being subjected to the looser standards for contracting then allowed by the federal MS. Through the arrangement that Barcelos brokered with FAURGS, only twenty-nine PSF teams worked in the capital, reaching just over 120,000 residents, or 8.79% of the city's population, by the end of 2000. Indeed, a more important platform for the SMS's delivery of primary care remained a modified version of the regionally decentralized model instituted in the Murialdo clinic nearly two decades earlier (H. Alencar and C. Freitas, personal communication,

2010). Key to maintaining this model, however, had been Barcelos's successful interventions to convert the network's public health workers into municipal employees. Ultimately, these interventions contributed to one of the single largest five-year reductions of IMR in Porto Alegre's history.

3.5. INFREQUENT SANITARISTA OFFICE HOLDING
AND PRESERVATION OF LOW IMR, 2002–2016

For purposes of demonstrating the effects of health democratization on robust development outcomes, considerably less remains to be shown about Porto Alegre's outcomes after 2002, when IMR declined only modestly but the city remained highly ranked vis-à-vis other capitals. By 2002, Porto Alegre's IMR of 12.17 left the city effectively tied with Curitiba and Belo Horizonte as urban Brazil's nationwide leaders in minimizing premature death, a ranking it would maintain over the next fourteen years. By 2015, Porto Alegre's IMR of 9.87 remained one of the lowest in urban Brazil, despite only two years of sanitarista-led SMS directorships after 2001. This suggests that, although consistent pragmatist public office holding was necessary for maximizing IMR reduction, it was perhaps less important for maintaining already low levels of premature death. Still, the episode reconfirms the central finding of the case throughout the period: that pragmatist public office holding continued to be a core mechanism of health-related state-building and that even Porto Alegre's PT mayors did not propel robust infant mortality declines without sanitarista office holding.

In 2001, upon beginning the PT's third consecutive term in the office, Mayor Tarso Genro appointed Dr. Joaquim Kliemann to an SMS directorship that he would hold only until 2003. Although Kliemann was a former director of the PAM-3 emergency room, he mirrored Genro's 1993 appointee to the office (Mota) in his lack of involvement with Sanitarist Movement political struggles. Kliemann brought significant experience working within the SMS, however, having served in two subcabinet-level SMS offices during the directorships of Jaeger, Mota, Fontana, and Barcelos. Indeed, Kliemann had been appointed to two ephemeral "substitute" terms as SMS director following the departures of Fontana and Barcelos from the office. But like Mota, Kliemann came to the position largely because of his close personal friendship with Genro and because he lacked strong ties to either of the most dominant factions within the party (J. Kliemann, interview, 2010). Ultimately, this reflected in a directorship in which Kliemann struggled to channel significant new resources into the primary health sector. There were reasons for this beyond just Kliemann's lack of a Sanitarist Movement lineage. Operationally, Porto Alegre's SMS mirrored Belo Horizonte's in that it had become increasingly focused on advancing sanitary reform principles in the SUS other than just universality and equality, especially the principle of integrality in care provision. This translated into greater emphasis on increasing coordination between primary and more sophisticated forms of health-service delivery, which contributed to increasing the city's share in 2002 of all spending on the health sector above the 20% level for the first time. Kliemann's directorship also suffered from a major circumstantial setback, with federal election rules requiring Genro to resign as mayor in mid-2002 to (unsuccessfully) run for governor that year.

Yet the powerlessness that Kliemann suffered as SMS director was not unrelated to his lack of a sanitarista lineage. Because Kliemann was a personal appointment of Genro with none of the various factional allies within the party that sanitaristas such as Jaeger and Barcelos had cultivated through their militant histories, Kliemann's efficacy declined markedly after Genro's departure from the mayor's office to run for governor. Here, it benefited Kliemann little that he had maintained internal harmony within the SMS between his highest-subcabinet-level appointees, who prioritized hospital management, and lower-level sanitarista-filled offices responsible for primary care. He said, "In debates about the search for more resources for the sector, I always hit a brick wall because I was seen as Tarso's personal appointment. Coming from no real internal current of the party meant that I had little support or assistance, and that hindered our agenda a lot" (J. Kliemann, interview, 2010). The episode reiterates how Genro's faction of the PT, whose impermeability to sanitarista infiltration diverged sharply from the more open non-PT administration of Castro (PSB) in Belo Horizonte, exacerbated other circumstances to effectively stall state-building in the primary-care sector. As Kliemann exited the office in 2003, the SMS indirectly employed only sixty-three teams that reached about 15.71% of residents, or 217,350 of them. Not surprisingly, IMR reductions from 2001 (13.9) to 2003 (11.8) were similarly modest.

Indeed, the post-2003 period was one in which IMR plateaued for the next fourteen years, despite the advent of Bolsa Família, national PT rule in the presidency, and the persistence of Porto Alegre's CMS and its world-famous OP. This was also a period of almost no sanitarista office holding in the SMS, with the exception of Dr. Sandra Fagundes, a sanitarista who replaced Kliemann as SMS director from late 2003 to 2004. Indeed, it was

Fagundes's SMS who worked alongside FAURGS to open the largest public concurso in the primary-care sector of the next decade, leading to a total of over eighty PSF teams that achieved populational coverage of over 20% by 2005, a level beyond which the program would expand little until 2013. But in terms of Porto Alegre's more general trajectory of health democratization, considerable atrophy set in after 2005. Upon winning the mayorship, the city's new PMDB mayor (José Fogaça) appointed an SMS director, Eliseu Santos, with little detectable concern for either the CMS's cogovernance authorities or sanitarista state-building agendas. These limitations became especially conspicuous when, for the first time in its history, the CMS had to contend with unsympathetic non-PT mayors and SMS directors with little prior connection to either popular-health or sanitarista circles. Correspondingly, deep frustrations also arose for activists in these spaces (O. Paniz, J. Pillar, H. Scorza, and H. da Cunha, interviews, 2010). In 2010, Maria Letícia de Oliveira Garcia, the elected CMS coordinator, successfully worked with the state public prosecutor's office (Minsterio Público-RS) to solicit a denunciation of the SMS by the National Accounts Tribunal of Rio Grande do Sul (TCU-RS) for failing to fully present the council with sufficiently detailed financial accounting of its 2007 and 2008 spending. Until 2010, the city witnessed nearly systematic exclusion of sanitaristas from high-level office atop the SMS and a generalized pattern of insulating both sanitaristas and participatory publics from governing the health sector. After actually increasing by the end of that episode, IMR had recovered to its 2006 level of 9.95 by 2015 (9.87). But with no overall improvements in ten years, the period of health democratization in the city reached a near standstill.

4. Conclusion

Although it began from a much more favorable starting point than other capitals with similar trajectories, such as Belo Horizonte, Porto Alegre witnessed a major transformation in the subnational public health state's capacity to reduce premature mortality after the mid-1980s. On the most general level, an overarching cause of robust development in the capital was its participatory-programmatic trajectory of health democratization. Although relatively favorable initial conditions of political, social, and economic development worked alongside the city's famous participatory institutions and PT mayors in fostering these changes, the chapter's within-case analysis of this trajectory pointed to a distinct, deeper-seeded feature of this path that propelled Porto Alegre's social development strides. Specifically, office-holding sanitaristas atop the city's SMS played a decisive but often overlooked role by equipping service-delivery arms of the subnational public health state with considerable new capacities to tangibly enact the universal right to the most basic forms of health care in a programmatic, rights-based fashion.

Somewhat less important for Porto Alegre's robust development outcome but nevertheless notable for how they helped broaden the state-society interface of local health politics were the popular-health activists and participatory publics who coconstituted Porto Alegre's path of health democratization alongside pragmatist publics. Especially when compared to cities such as Rio de Janeiro, Salvador, and even Curitiba and Fortaleza, all in which CMS councillors found their monitoring overtures stonewalled, obstructed, or otherwise circumvented even more consistently, Porto Alegre's trajectory represented perhaps a deeper expression of health democratization than almost anywhere else in urban Brazil. This is all the more apparent when we also consider the influence of OP participants in directing considerable portions of public spending toward physical infrastructure for the health sector (Marquetti, Ariano de Campos, and Pires 2008). Nevertheless, from the narrower standpoint of what explains the city's impressively robust IMR reductions, office-holding sanitaristas played at least as crucial a role. Indeed, the chapter traced nearly all major expansions in state capacity to deliver IMR-reducing primary care in Porto Alegre to the state-building interventions of office-holding sanitaristas, who sought to build new municipal capacities for operating the sector in a programmatic manner. Whereas participatory publics in Porto Alegre's CMS vigorously and consistently monitored SMS interventions in the health sector after the mid-1990s, they lacked sufficient power to comanage the public health sector, especially when the hiring of actual health care providers was involved. Further, the chapter's findings also complicate efforts to trace such improvements solely to the initiative of ruling left parties such as the PT, which expressed little appetite for such state-building when not otherwise pressed by office-holding sanitaristas like Jaeger, Fontana, and, especially, Barcelos. Such dynamics call attention to the possibility, explored next in the critical cases of Curitiba and Fortaleza, that democratic office holding by pragmatist publics such as Brazil's sanitaristas could propel such state-building, even when such alternative factors were contrastingly absent.

SIX

Curitiba

> Your mission [as an SUS director] is a sacred one. . . . You
> cannot just do what you want, but what the law requires, and
> this imposes obligations that must be met. . . . You must do
> your duty. . . . Health is a public good. . . . You must always
> observe this public mission of serving society!
>
> —*Dr. Armando Raggio, sanitarista director of Curitiba's SMS*
> *(1989–1992) and Paraná's SES (2001–2006; my translation)*

Although other Brazilian capitals built stronger reputations for their ruling left parties and participatory governance institutions, none achieved a lower IMR or wider access to primary health care by the end of the health-democratization period than Curitiba. The capital of Paraná state and nucleus of Brazil's eighth-largest metropolitan region, Curitiba is perhaps best known in national and global policy-making circles for its state-directed forays into the public transportation and environment sectors (Adler 2016). Academic observers and civil-society actors alike have highlighted the urban planning processes that Jaime Lerner, arguably the city's most influential political-society elite during the health-democratization period, introduced and sustained over nearly five decades.[1] Less emphasized, however, has been the fact that the city also achieved urban Brazil's strongest social development record by the end of the period. More specifically, despite recording an IMR that ranked outside the highest-performing third of major Brazilian capitals in 1988 (39.96), Curitiba had by 2003 become urban Brazil's top performer in this regard, and it maintained that status well into the mid-2010s.

The chapter traces these impressive strides to a pattern of programmatic health democratization through which sanitaristas consistently occupied and leveraged subnational offices atop the public health state to build new capacities for reducing IMR. Curitiba witnessed a particularly sustained period of office holding in its SMS directorship with sanitaristas such as Dr. Armando Raggio (1989–1992), Dr. Luciano Ducci (1999–2000, 2006–2007, 2009–2010), and Michele Caputo Neto (2001–2005) all holding the post for considerable durations. Raggio (2001–2006) and Caputo Neto (2011–2012, 2017–) also occupied Paraná's SES directorship for sustained periods. Thus, even though PT-affiliated politicians have never won Curitiba's mayorship, sanitaristas held the office of SMS director during two-thirds of the twenty-four years between 1988 and 2012. Indeed, Ducci become such a widely recognized protagonist of public health reform and programmatic policy reform that he also went on to hold Curitiba's offices of vice mayor (2004–2008) and mayor (2011–2012). This pattern of consistent office holding reflected sanitarista success in institutionalizing core principles of sanitary reform, especially universal and equal access to basic health services, as a dominant set of guidelines for enacting health-sector reform among a variety of powerful subnational political elites from multiple parties.

A defining feature of Curitiba's programmatic trajectory of health democratization was the outsized and enduring role of these actors in leveraging such offices to expand the city's network of primary service clinics, build its ranks of meritocratically recruited municipal health professionals, and institute effective models for delivering mortality-reducing variants of health care. While office-holding sanitaristas sizably expanded the PSF's reach and that of a parallel, homegrown model of primary-care delivery, they also pioneered more unique programs, such as the Curitiban Mother Program (*Programa Mãe Curitibana*, PMC), that later became the template for Brazil's nationwide *Rede Cegonha* (Stork Network) program. Compared to other capitals, like Salvador, that witnessed only minimalist trajectories of health democratization and nonrobust development outcomes, Curitiba had sanitaristas that propelled the city's programmatic trajectory by more consistently occupying subnational democratic offices of the SUS and similar protodemocratic offices that predate the SUS.

Thus, this chapter argues that it was neither participatory-democratic institutions nor ruling left-party mayors nor the mere local presence of a sanitarista network that most fostered programmatic health democratization and robust social development in Curitiba. Indeed, Curitiba never established Brazil's most iconic participatory institution, Participatory Budgeting (OP). Further, its Municipal Health Council (CMS) exhibited persistent deficits of institutionalization that relegated it to predominantly consultative rather than more empowered roles when it came to matters of constructing new state capacities for primary public-health-care delivery. Additionally, policy diffusion accounts struggle to explain robust development in Curitiba because their core theorized driver—the mere local presence of a *sanitarista* network—hardly guaranteed that these actors gained access to actual control of the state-building levers that mattered most for IMR reduction. It is also not possible to attribute Curitiba's impressive social development outcomes to subnational rule by the PT, which never captured the city's mayorship or Paraná's governorship during the period examined. National-level PT rule also cannot be credited with Curitiba's improvements, since most of the city's progress in reducing IMR occurred before the party took power in 2003. To instead examine how *sanitarista* office holding better explains Curitiba's trajectory and outcomes, it is first necessary to assess the initial conditions in which their interventions arose.

1. Initial Conditions of Civil and Political Society in Curitiba

Unlike roughly similar cases such as Fortaleza, institutional change in Curitiba's public health sector responded to the fact that its dictatorship-era political leaders prioritized systematic approaches to urban planning from an early moment, especially in the realms of public transportation, environment, and public space. The small number of elites who controlled Curitiba's mayorship and Paraná's governorship during the period aimed to make their public planning efforts compatible with the dictatorship's state-directed efforts to foster economic growth and cultivate new industries. Curitiba's mayors and governors correspondingly sought to foster governmental efficiency and public planning strategies, especially those for advancing the business interests of entrepreneurs in the real estate, construction, mass-transit, and industrial sectors. In the notably early year of 1965, the municipality opened a public competition for a city master plan (*plano diretor*) that eventually highlighted economic growth, industry promotion, and improvement of environmental quality as key objectives to be achieved through major urban design and infrastructure projects.

One of the plan's key legacies was that the 1966 creation of its chief implementing agency, The Institute for Urban Research and Planning of Curitiba (IPPUC), catapulted its first president, Jaime Lerner, into an enormously influential, five-decade political career that spanned three mayoral and two gubernatorial terms. As an urban planner and architect whom the dictatorship helped install as Curitiba's mayor in 1971, Lerner personified the IPPUC's marriage of political power to technocratic planning as well as its bypassing of both city bureaucracies and the larger citizenry to accomplish planning objectives when necessary (Irazabal 2009, 213–14). Although commonly criticized for this cohesive approach to formulating and executing planning goals, Lerner and his contemporaries' aggressive pursuit of this urban planning agenda unfolded over multiple decades, spanning the divide between Brazil's era of military dictatorship and its redemocratization. And despite its considerable deficits in establishing more democratic processes for guiding planning processes, the Curitiban political elite epitomized by Lerner evolved a reputation for a planning ethos and panoply of state-driven transformations in policy sectors of greatest interest to them. Although the public health sector was not initially among these sectors, the emergence of Curitiba's sanitaristas amid dictatorship-era struggles for democracy gradually changed this top-down approach to public planning by infusing it with sanitarista-supplied ideological notions of a democratic right to health. Especially after the creation of the SUS, state health agencies that were established during this previous era, including the precursor of Curitiba's SMS, became subject to regulative institutions of civil society such as laws and democratic offices. Indeed, the Organic Health Laws of 1990 eventually assigned the public officials who oversaw these agencies with responsibilities of the SUS manager for enacting principles of universality and equity in access to health.

At first, however, the capital's status as a major urban hub of Paraná served to reinforce the ingrained, top-down planning ethos of multiple city governments. Key to this ethos was the fact that Curitiba hosted large and important public and private universities that produced many of the relatively well-educated *técnicos* (technocrats) who helped operate the IPPUC-headed public planning apparatus of Lerner and his colleagues. These included the Federal University of Paraná (UFPR), the State University of Paraná (UESPAR), and the Catholic Pontificate University of Paraná (PUC-PR). But the city's institutions of higher education did more than simply produce técnicos. They also produced university and postgraduate students, who built local organizations and framed demands for improved access to health as a democratic right of all Brazilian citizens. As in the rest of urban Brazil, the city's sanitaristas were important student activists in the capital throughout the dictatorship. Especially after the 1964 seizure of power by Brazil's military dictatorship, the city's sanitaristas mirrored the nationwide movement in gradually adopting a more clearly prodemocratic frame for their health-focused demands during the 1970s. Amid the dictatorship's waning repression of progressive social movements, Curitiba's sanitaristas increasingly voiced more politically charged demands for health reform. Among the city's sanitarista activists were medical students and residents, who had been forced underground because of their affiliations with the banned National Student Union (UNE).

The efforts took on a more consolidated and organized character when networks of sanitaristas began founding localized communicative institutions of the Sanitarist Movement in the capital. At first, these were loosely connected to Rio de Janeiro's Brazilian Center for Health Studies (CEBES), which began organizing meetings called Community Health Studies Weeks (SESACs) in the medical schools of major universities and university hospitals throughout urban Brazil. In 1976, Curitiba became one of the first meeting sites for SESACs within the Federal University of Paraná (UFPR), which also drew participants from medical students and residents in the Catholic Pontificate University of Paraná (PUC-PR; Escorel 2008). As in much of urban Brazil, Curitiba's SESAC largely evaded repression due to its decentralized character and corresponding lack of an easily detectable connection to the UNE, the military's main target for undermining student organizing. Additionally, sanitarista organizers skillfully concealed the antidictatorship tenor of SESAC discussions within official agendas that specified more benign issues of parochial interest to medical professionals (L. Tonón, interview, 2010). Under this cover, core ideological principles of sanitary reform emerged from the SESAC, including demands for a thoroughgoing democratization of the country's polity and the public health sector as well as resistance to any role for capitalist interests in the health sector.

Although initially militants in the international and Brazilian student, communist, socialist, and prodemocracy movements of the era, prominent Curitiban sanitaristas soon became primary public-health-care providers as well as activists for a right to health. To be sure, the involvement of individual sanitaristas in the Brazilian student movement served as a springboard into political activism for venerable Curitiban sanitaristas such as Dr. Luciano Ducci, Dr. Armando Raggio, and Michele Caputo Neto. For instance, Ducci—later an SMS director, vice mayor, and, eventually, mayor of Curitiba—initially organized within Freedom and Struggle (*Liberdade e Luta*, LIBELU), a group within Brazil's student movement that was connected to Socialist International and embraced Trotskyite ideologies. By the 1980s, however, Ducci was mobilizing within nationwide sanitarista struggles to democratize and municipalize the public health sector in Curitiba while also working as a pediatrician in the Cajuru neighborhood's municipally run Trindade public health clinic (Ducci 2017). Dr. Armando Raggio—a Curitiban sanitarista who eventually went on to become one of the city's longest-running SMS directors—had by 1978 become the city's representative to the *Saúde em Debate* journal of the CEBES, the movement's main mouthpiece. Yet Curitiba was not alone among major capitals in its dense network of politically active sanitaristas, who were then mobilizing for universal rights to health and a state responsibility for ensuring such a right through civil-society communicative institutions of dictatorship-era Brazil. As such, these networks alone cannot adequately account for the city's exceptionally early, sustained, and robust expansion of the municipal public health state.

Rather, what set Curitiba's sanitaristas apart from their peers in other major capitals such as Salvador and Rio de Janeiro was their early and sustained success in founding and wielding regulative institutions of the movement—including protodemocratic and democratic offices like the municipal office of SUS manager—atop the subnational public health state. For instance, after working as a doctor in several of Curitiba's first municipal public health clinics, Raggio became Curitiba's SMS director in the late 1980s and, in this capacity, served as president of yet another regulative institution of the movement, the National Council of Municipal Health Secretaries (CONASEMS). Particularly in the years immediately following the 1990 founding of CONASEMS and its legal recognition in Law 8,080 of 1990 as an organization with legitimate authority for enacting the SUS, the body's presidency became one of the movement's most influential offices for strengthening municipalities' efforts to implement the new right to health. Beyond serving as director of Curitiba's SMS (2001–2005) and Paraná's SES (2011–2012), Caputo Neto and other activists like him also occupied leadership roles within the state-level counterpart of CONASEMS, the National

Council of State Health Secretaries (CONASS). Thus, following their earlier, more radical activism, Curitiba's sanitaristas often wore several hats as primary public health providers, organizers in seminal communicative institutions of the Sanitarist Movement, and prime agents within regulative institutions that increasingly sought to orchestrate local state interventions for enacting the universal, equal right to health. These efforts would prove to be of far-reaching consequence in molding the city's distinctively programmatic path of health democratization, which I turn to next.

2. Curitiba's Trajectory of Programmatic Health Democratization

Curitiba's impressive strides in IMR reduction and primary public-health-care expansion emerged from a programmatic trajectory of health democratization characterized by multiple qualities. This path included generic, nationwide qualities such as the restoration of free and fair local elections of mayors and governors through universal suffrage, the ratification of constitutional responsibility for establishing a universal and equal citizenship right to health, and decentralization of political, administrative, and fiscal management of the health sector. Following agreements made in its first Municipal Health Conference in 1991, Curitiba further decentralized the health sector by creating health-management districts in which clinics assumed new roles as primary health care providers for specified jurisdictions (Ducci et al. 2001).

Yet additional qualities of Curitiba's path were specific to programmatic health democratization and thus differ from the minimalist variant observable in Rio de Janeiro and Salvador. For one, Curitiba's electoral politics featured a relative dearth of monopolistic local political rule by patronage-oriented, regional hegemons initially installed into subnational power during the dictatorship.[2] On one hand, Brazil's dictatorship helped initiate the political career of Jaime Lerner, arguably the single most influential subnational executive in the state's contemporary history. Officially part of the military-backed ARENA political party for his first two mayoral terms (1971–1974, 1979–1983), Lerner subsequently won three direct elections, including one for Curitiba's mayorship (1989–1992) and two for Paraná's governorship (1995–1998, 1999–2002). On the other hand, Lerner faced more concerted competition from political adversaries in such elections, including from Roberto Requião de Mello, who in 1986 defeated him in Curitiba's first directly elected mayor's race of the postdictatorship era (TSE 2016). More importantly, however, Curitiba's subnational executives generally exhibited less extreme records of patronage than did the coronels who dominated the mayorship and governorship in Fortaleza, Belo Horizonte, and Salvador. Even though mayors Rafael Greca and Cassio Taniguchi, Lerner's one-time colleagues in the PDT and later the PFL, combined with Lerner to hold the mayorship for fifteen consecutive years from 1989 to 2004, Curitiba experienced nothing like the patronage-fueled raid on public-service sectors that characterized cities such as Salvador under ACM's political machine. Rather, a collection of subnational executives in multiple political parties remained at least somewhat open to pragmatist publics with proposals for solving trenchant public problems like endemic childhood mortality. These parties included the PDT (and later the PFL) of Jaime Lerner, Rafael Greca, and Cassio Taniguchi as well as the PMDB of Àlvaro Dias and Roberto Requião de Mello and the PSDB of Beto Richa.

Curitiba's programmatic trajectory also maximized the reach of nationwide, pro-poor social programs like Bolsa Família (BF) after 2003. In general, the program has contributed to nationwide improvements in health outcomes such as IMR both by providing direct cash transfers to participants and by mandating receipt of regular medical care as a condition for receiving them (Rasella et al. 2013). Yet Curitiba exemplifies how local capacities of the democratic state also matter for maximizing these programmatic qualities. The federal social development ministry (MDS) administers the program in a nationally standardized manner by drawing on multiple data sources to determine eligible beneficiaries and by stipulating and monitoring conditions with which participants must comply to gain access. Those are but a few of its key roles. Nevertheless, it is likely that qualification of candidates for receipt of benefits can improve when municipal administrations are more capable. For instance, Borges Sugiyama argues that municipal state authorities constitute the entry point for the program insofar as they interact with applicants and enter families' information into a nationwide registry (2016, 1194). In broader respects, too, the ability of participants to meet conditions required to access transfers—particularly the requirements that parents demonstrate regular attendance of their children in school and at medical checkups—depends on subnational governments that can deliver such public services, with health service constituting a particularly likely bottleneck. And across the major capitals examined in this study, the ratio of families enrolled in the program to those who are eligible for it varied considerably. Using an additive index that sums this "targeting" rate with a "coverage rate," capturing the proportion of enrolled families to total families, Curitiba was surpassed only by Recife in its 2004 to 2012 average for BF coverage (103.1) across major capitals. Given that other bottlenecks in program administration can emerge from uneven local capacity of the municipal offices that update the program registry, Curitiba's considerable, well-known competencies in planning and bureaucratic effectiveness have likely helped improve BF delivery.

Another decisive quality of Curitiba's programmatic trajectory was early and sustained expansion of the subnational public health state's service-delivery arms. By 2014, the city had seen impressive expansions of municipal capacity to deliver primary health services. During the 2005 to 2012 period, each PSF team served fewer than 5,900 exclusive SUS users, a record that was eclipsed only by Belo Horizonte's ratio of 2,513. And by 2014, Curitiba's SMS had assembled 236 PSF teams that achieved over 45% populational coverage, an impressive achievement given that the city operated the PSF model alongside a homegrown model for providing additional primary health services not reflected in these numbers. In per capita terms, the city featured one of urban Brazil's most prolific networks of public health facilities, with 109 health units (US) principally oriented around primary-care delivery. Although Curitiba's SMS operated all of these clinics itself, it organized service provision in only 66 of them according to the work regime associated with the federal health ministry's Family Health Program (PSF). Thus, given that PSF-organized units accounted for only 60% of the city's overall primary-care clinics, it is notable that the city's ratio of approximately 3,229 exclusive SUS users (726,016) per PSF team (236) was the second-lowest in urban Brazil by 2014. The remaining 41 clinics instead followed a homegrown platform developed by sanitaristas and other public health professionals working inside Curitiba's Municipal Health Department (SMS; SMS-Curitiba 2016). In this sense, Curitiba diverged from most other major capitals (except Porto Alegre) that organized primary-care delivery solely according to the PSF model. As a result, its modest 2014 rate of populational coverage through the PSF (44.04%) considerably underestimates the actual reach of primary public-health-care delivery in the municipality, necessitating other measures for a more accurate estimate. Assessing the combined output of primary health services in both the PSF and non-PSF clinics shows that Curitiba outpaced all other major capitals in Brazil by 2014.[3]

Finally, in contrast to these far-reaching transformations of the subnational public health state's service-delivery arms, Curitiba's participatory-democratic spaces for citizen monitoring of those arms played at-best peripheral roles in such state-building throughout the period. By 2017, Curitiba had never instituted any kind of Participatory Budgeting (OP) process, unlike other major capitals such as Porto Alegre, Belo Horizonte, and Recife that instead witnessed participatory-programmatic trajectories of health democratization. Such a lacuna is particularly nontrivial given that OP participants nationwide have often emphasized the primary public health sector.[4] The absence of OP in part reflects how civil-society advocates for the process have generally relied more exclusively on left parties with stronger commitments to participatory democracy than on the generally more center and sometimes center-right parties that have controlled Curitiba's mayor's office. The tendency for otherwise well-organized participatory publics to depend on local rule by one party (the PT) that has never held mayoral or gubernatorial power in Curitiba or Paraná has likely undermined the emergence of an OP process, drawing a sharp contrast to how pragmatist publics have injected their core ideologies and projects into a wider array of parties.

Also indicative of the generally weaker state-building processes that characterized Curitiba's participatory-democratic institutions for overseeing the health sector were early and significant challenges to the autonomy of its Municipal Health Council (CMS), the body with the greatest formal authority in this regard. In 1991, Curitiba complied with the nationwide requirement to establish a CMS as mandated by federal legal specifications of the Constitution. Nevertheless, the municipal executive has repeatedly undermined fundamental qualities of the CMS specified in Law 8,142, including the requirement that SUS users compose at least 50% of its seats, the requirement that council members autonomously nominate and choose the organizations that comprise the 25% of seats reserved for civil society, and the ability of civil society and users to contest the presidency of the council (Albertini 2002, 2, 83–84). Indeed, community, neighborhood, and union activists in Curitiba were more active in fostering popular mobilization in defense of the right to health. In 1991, such groups joined state and municipal health councillors to form the Popular Health Forum (FOPS), a more deeply democratic precursor of Curitiba's SMS that aimed to influence the city's public health politics through more disruptive interventions.

Thus, it is difficult to defensibly argue that Curitiba's CMS was as influential or effective at monitoring and informing state-building in the primary public health sector as was the CMS in either Porto Alegre or Belo Horizonte. But this clearly did not result from any absence of participatory publics or total lack of influence on their part. Rather, mobilizations of the FOPS and other manifestations of the city's popular health movement clearly indicate the presence of a participatory public that consistently attempted to influence the city's health sector, occasionally with success. For instance, FOPS members within Curitiba's CMS even managed to defeat particularly extreme proposals to privatize health-service provision advocated in 1998 by nonsanitarista directors of the city SMS such as Dr. João Carlos Gonçalves Baracho. By holding a series of council-wide votes in 1998, FOPS councillors on the CMS halted a proposal to institute a version of private-sector Health Organizations (OSs) for contracting out health care provision in the city (Albertini 2002, 84). Yet Curitiba's participatory publics wielded precious little influence in more proactively building capacities of the municipal public health state's service-delivery arms, particularly when compared to how the city's sanitaristas wielded the office of SMS director to open concursos for hiring municipal health care professionals. Indeed, participatory publics often struggled to act independently of SMS directors, as in 1998 when Curitiba's CMS rubber-stamped a proposal from SMS leaders to introduce an otherwise unpopular incentive program for primary health workers (World Bank 2006, 41). But even though Curitiba's programmatic trajectory of health democratization featured fewer institutionalized mechanisms of influence for participatory publics, the city witnessed impressive primary health-sector state-building and IMR reductions anyway. Next, I turn to the more central drivers of these shifts.

3. Sanitarista Office Holding and State-Building in Curitiba's Primary Public Health Sector

Well before the Sanitarist Movement's iconic national victories of 1988, its activists were expanding Curitiba's public health state in subtle but important ways that began lending their reformist visions for the sector a privileged place among the plans of subnational political elites. Although Curitiba eventually gained less international acclaim than other positive cases of robust development such as Fortaleza, its trajectory of subnational state-building for public health was as precocious and sustained as any other major Brazilian capital during the period. As in all other positive cases of robust development examined in this study, the main agents of such reforms during these earlier moments in Curitiba were sanitarista occupants of various subnational positions atop the public health state. Indeed, it is striking that nearly all of the most sweeping and consequential state-building interventions in Curitiba's primary health sector are traceable to the office-holding interventions of just three sanitaristas: Dr. Armando Raggio, Dr. Luciano Ducci, and Michele Caputo Neto.

3.1. SANITARISTA-LED STATE-BUILDING FOR PRIMARY HEALTH CARE REDUCES IMR, 1979–1988

A defining feature of Curitiba's programmatic trajectory of health democratization was a pattern of state capacity-building that consistently expanded the size and sophistication of the municipal public health sector earlier and more significantly than in otherwise similar cases of robust development, such as Fortaleza. Indeed, the very municipal public health institutions that underwent significant expansion after 1986 were themselves products of earlier sanitarista interventions to establish humble new primary health programs that embraced principles of universal and equal access to such services. These efforts had significant institutional precursors in the 1964 creation of Curitiba's Department of Education, Recreation, and Health (DEROS), which opened the city's first municipally run health clinic in the Cajuru neighborhood the following year (SMS-Curitiba 2016). Even more important was a later set of municipal state agencies that Curitiban sanitaristas such as Dr. Armando Raggio helped Jaime Lerner to establish beginning in the late 1970s. Up until this point, the renowned Curitiban planning model epitomized by the *plano diretor* had been dutifully pursued and implemented in urban policy making for over a decade by mayors such as Lerner himself (1971–1975) and his successor, Saul Raiz (1975–1979). Yet before the interventions of sanitaristas, public health had occupied a far less important place within these public planning efforts.

During the late 1970s, Curitiban sanitaristas such as Raggio began changing this state of affairs in subtle but consequential ways. In addition to simultaneously establishing a local presence of key communicative institutions of the movement such as CEBES, Raggio also helped found pivotal institutions of the municipal state for public health promotion. Prime among them was the municipal forebear of Curitiba's municipal health secretariat (SMS), the Department of Social Development (DDS), which Lerner founded in 1979 during his second appointed term as mayor. Intended to pursue social policies targeting low-income residents, the DDS had three divisions: a Community Development Directorate that coordinated the work of urban service centers such as childcare facilities, a Social Promotion Directorate that served residents of favelas and other communities with irregular housing in the city's geographic periphery, and a Health Directorate (DS) that delivered basic medical and dental services (SMS-Curitiba 2016; Ribeiro 2009, 113). Serving as both the DS's director and a key CEBES representative for Paraná, Raggio encountered a golden opportunity in 1979 to mold the DS in the image of sanitary reform principles.

After being appointed as the DS's director by Luiz Carlos Zanoni, the head of the DDS, Raggio seized this opportunity by recruiting a brain trust of local sanitaristas and public health experts, who crafted a proposal for founding the DS around a primary health care model (Curitiba, Prefeitura Municipal 1979; Ribeiro 2009, 113–16). Included in the group he recruited was Paulo Gustavo de Barros Carvalho, a doctor, erstwhile Popular Action (AP) member, and fellow student movement activist at UFPR, who had previously been jailed by the military regime for his involvement with the then clandestine Communist Party of Brazil (PC do B). Members of the group were also embedded in international public health circles that were then advocating for aggressive pursuit of various primary-care models globally. As with the nascent sanitary reform ideology then crystallizing at the core of the movement more generally, this local proposal for crystallizing Curitiba's early public health model drew heavily on the propitiously timed and influential set of ideas and proposals emerging from the 1979 Alma-Ata Declaration on Primary Health Care. In addition to the inputs of sanitaristas in other major Brazilian cities like Campinas that were then also developing municipal primary health systems, Alma-Ata principles such as universal access to health featured prominently in the group's proposal for founding Curitiba's Health Directorate. It also emphasized municipal investment to establish a network of primary-care facilities in poor geographic peripheries of the city populated by groups long excluded from access to health services (M. L. Jaeger, interview, 2010; Ribeiro 2009).

Crucially then, it was Raggio's group that shaped the mission of the first public health agency to be created within the formidable architecture of municipal planning institutions overseen by Lerner and IPPUC.

It was thus crucial that the new decentralized, primary-care-based model dovetailed with the logic of strategic planning and of the actual state planning agencies that Lerner established from an early moment as the dominant force in public policy making within Curitiba (Raggio and Giacomini 1996). In this regard, Raggio's interventions added modest new capacities to the municipal public health state that nevertheless had longer-lasting relevance because they created momentum and state-society spaces in which sanitaristas continued to pursue state-building. Indeed, the most important consequence of Raggio's role in helping found the DS was not the relatively meager local capacities for primary health care delivery it generated, per se. By 1982, the DS had opened just six health clinics with very limited capacities.[5] Doubling as community centers, these clinics provided only a modest suite of preventative services and laboratory exams and distributed vaccines and medications provided by the state-level Secretariat of Health and Well-Being for Paraná (SESB-PA).

Rather, the larger importance of the intervention was that it harnessed a decentralized, primary-care-oriented project for public-health-sector reform to the considerable political will of Lerner and the all-powerful public-planning apparatus. Thus, small and seemingly unimportant expansions that Raggio undertook during these early moments shaped the city's future public health system in ways that were greater than the modest size or relatively limited immediate importance of the expansions themselves. Prime among these interventions was his introduction of a team-based model of public-service provision first adopted in Curitiba's Cajuru health clinic and later in the São Pedro, Santa Amélia, and Santo Inácio clinics (SMS-Curitiba 2016). Based on a clinical model, doctors joined nurses, dentists, sanitary engineers, and community health workers in addressing some of the diverse factors—including high disease burdens and scant access to functional sewage and sanitation systems—that influenced the health of residents (Ribeiro 2009, 104). These teams prioritized contact with infants, children, pregnant women, and new mothers, and they focused on vaccination and prevention of diseases such as tuberculosis and Hansen's disease among adults. Raggio's team also established general guidelines for these clinics that included coverage expansion, holistic medicine, community participation, hierarchical organization of attention levels, and the democratization of medical attention, all subtle rejections of the exclusive curative model centered in state and federal health facilities of the era (Curitiba, Prefeitura Municipal 1979; Ducci et al. 2001). Further, when Curitiba channeled federal resources associated with the AIS program into the addition of fourteen health centers and three dental clinics in 1985, it did so in conjunction with competitive public concursos that hired the new workers for these clinics as public employees (SMS-Curitiba 2016). In this respect, Curitiba's early institutionalization of a primary health model also foreshadowed the community-based, territorially focused, and team-oriented approach to fostering health that the ACS and PSF models operationalized on a nationwide basis nearly fifteen years later.

Additional office-holding episodes by Raggio in the SMS directorship during 1986 and 1989 precipitated the decade's two largest single expansions of Curitiba's primary-care network. During Raggio's directorship in 1986, Curitiba expanded its network to forty-two primary health clinics and twenty dental clinics that began operating according to a territorialization strategy by which clinics focused service provision on residents within their catchment area. By 1989, the network had further climbed to fifty-three primary clinics and thirty-four dental clinics (Ribeiro 2009, 123). Among the mechanisms of the earlier expansions was the signing of agreements through the federal, nationwide AIS program that facilitated federal transfers to the município for building new clinics, renovating existing ones, and improving their capacities for laboratory testing and distribution of basic medications. Furthermore, between 1983 and 1987, Raggio also directed the Caetano Munhoz da Rocha Foundation (FCMR), with which Paraná's SES had partnered to advance the training of health professionals working in such clinics. Thus, Raggio's continued interventions throughout the 1980s further entrenched the primary-care model for the public health sector that he had previously made legible to Curitiba's political elite by integrating into the city's larger network of urban planning institutions (Ribeiro 2009, 123).

To be sure, other, more generic factors within Curitiba's ongoing democratization process conditioned the success of Raggio's interventions during this phase. In particular, Municipal Law 6,817 of 1986 created greater autonomy for municipal state-building for public health by effectively transforming the DS into its own stand-alone agency—the municipal health secretariat (SMS) of Curitiba that endures today. Most prominently, it was no accident that these interventions gained considerable strength during the first democratically elected mayorship in Curitiba since the military's

1964 seizure of power. Indeed, Requião de Mello's 1985 mayoral victory benefited from his embrace of the newly democratic context of party competition, which rewarded successful articulation of platforms that addressed
ubiquitous voter demands for social service expansion, including in the
health sector (Ribeiro 2009, 123). Yet there are limits to the argument that
such expansions are solely traceable to the return of democratic electoral
politics. Although both of Curitiba's PMDB mayors of the 1980s—Maurí-
cio Fruet (1983–1986) and Roberto Requião de Mello (1986–1988)—increasingly challenged the *plano diretor* on grounds that it excluded public inputs
into planning,[6] they also generally preserved the powerful and technically
driven planning institutions that the plan precipitated. Ultimately, however, this helped preserve the nontrivial place of the decentralized primary-
care model of public health that Raggio and other sanitaristas had carved
out within Curitiba's infamously top-down urban planning institutions.

One intermediate result of these early developments was that Curitiba
entered the heyday of the health-democratization period with a considerable head start on its IMR vis-à-vis other major capitals. Indeed, in 1988
only Porto Alegre recorded a lower IMR (30.06) than Curitiba's 39.96. Further, this low level reflected a substantial 44% reduction during the decade
from a level of 53.23 in 1980. Some of the main reasons for Curitiba's relatively strong performance for urban Brazil were straightforward. For one,
the city began the period with a larger (in per capita terms) network of
primary health clinics than that of nearly any other major capital. These
clinics were relatively well targeted to city regions with residents facing especially high risk of premature death due to poverty and otherwise poor
access to basic public services. Additionally, Curitiban sanitaristas such as
Raggio had instituted training programs for primary health care providers that attuned health professionals working in these clinics to the challenges of serving residents in neighborhoods facing this disproportionately
high risk. Thus, in many crucial dimensions of state-building that would
continue to matter greatly for IMR reduction in coming decades, office-
holding sanitaristas had initiated a subtle process of change in Curitiba's
public health sector at a notably early moment. This local process had already begun institutionalizing core tenets of sanitary reform such as universality and equity in access to health nearly fifteen years before their crystallization into the nationwide SUS.

3.2. STATE-BUILDING LED BY SANITARISTA OFFICEHOLDERS
FURTHER REDUCES IMR, 1989–1993

If earlier sanitarista-driven state-building established the localized primary-care model that propelled Curitiba's precocious IMR reductions, subsequent refinement, expansion, and deepening of that model further reduced mortality over the next five years. Indeed, Curitiba had reduced IMR an additional 37%, to 25.32, by 1993, in part by considerably expanding the territorially oriented primary-care model that Raggio had previously implanted in select regions (SMS-Curitiba 2016). These improvements undoubtedly benefited from nationwide dynamics such as the restoration of formal democracy, codification of a right to health, and creation of the SUS, all of which heightened local accountability of elected leaders to citizens seeking access to health services. Yet it is notable that Curitiba made considerable strides in establishing a primary health network of facilities and workers before other such factors took practical effect. In this sense, the SMS's municipalization of the primary public health sector was an already ongoing process that gained additional momentum through the signing of formal agreements with the federal MS and Paraná's SES in 1992.

By then a recognized public health authority among Curitiba's political elites, Raggio was the prime agent of this process as SMS director from 1989 to 1993 under Lerner, the city's newly elected mayor. Raggio again moved quickly to enhance municipal capacities to expand primary-care delivery over the short term and to deepen the primary-care model by setting in motion institutionalization processes that continually evolved for decades thereafter. Raggio's shorter-term expansions included ten additional health centers and fourteen dental clinics, raising Curitiba's total to fifty-three and thirty-four, respectively, by the end of his first year in office (SMS-Curitiba 2016). By 1993, Raggio had expanded this network to eighty-five clinics. All told, his interventions during only four years as SMS director accounted for a doubling of Curitiba's already considerable network of primary-care facilities. He accomplished this sizable expansion through both old and new tactics made possible by the creation of the new SUS. Raggio in 1992 again municipalized existing clinics previously under the control of the state and federal governments. This time, he did so by signing official agreements with both specifying the município's control over primary-care and public health operations within the capital's borders more generally. But in 1991, he also capitalized on the changing nationwide landscape of SUS institutions to attract new federal funding for such expansions. For instance, Raggio signed a Pro-Health (*Pro-Saúde*) agreement with the federal MS that provided access to federal block grants for expanding, renovating, and building new health clinics, including the city's first twenty-four-hour emergency health clinic. Thus, in large part due to Raggio's initiative, Curitiba had begun securing federal resources to support its primary-care model well before the federal MS's issuance of various SUS Basic Operating Norms (NOBs) created an official process for doing so (Carvalho de Noronha, Dias de Lima, and Vieira Machado 2008, 459).

Although they bore less immediate fruits, Raggio formed partnerships with international organizations such as the Pan-American Health Organization (OPAS) to train the health professionals of clinics like the Pompéia Health Center in the care-provision and human resource management challenges introduced by the newer and more clearly defined territorialized model (Albertini 2002, 41–42). Among the most important longer-term projects was an effort to more explicitly focus on reducing child and maternal mortality in the capital. For instance, Raggio immediately created a Municipal Committee on Maternal Mortality, whose purpose was to analyze causes of maternal mortality in the capital and devise prevention measures to be implemented by the SMS (Albertini 2002, 43). The SMS also began publishing an epidemiological bulletin of the new SMS that brought renewed attention to the ways in which the capital's primary-care model could be modified to better address premature mortality (Pedotti and Moysés 2000). Such interventions created a foundation on which the city's pathbreaking PMC would later be built.

Subsequent efforts to infuse the SMS directorship with new SUS manager responsibilities for universalizing access to health clearly benefited from Raggio's previous successes in instituting primary health programs of the Health Directorate (DS). Early programs of the DS set a precedent for expanding primary health care delivery through the deployment of medical teams working on a family health model in high-risk city regions. It helped that the neighborhood-based clinical model of care already implanted by Raggio and other Curitiban sanitaristas enjoyed considerable and early support from actors in a variety of communicative institutions, including civil-society associations linked to the Sanitarist Movement (Ribeiro 2009). Among these groups were neighborhood associations in peripheral regions such as Cajuru and Vila São Pedro, in which territorially based forerunners of the PSF's community health model had been implemented years before the SUS's codification of such responsibilities or the arrival of the PSF on the national scene. Even when voicing demands for renovations to community health centers in such neighborhoods, such groups rarely contested the clinic-based primary-care model itself.[7] Other communicative institutions such as Curitiba's biennial Municipal Health Conference played a role as well. The first edition of the conference in 1991 convened approximately six hundred delegates to guide Curitiba's municipalization process and lay groundwork that established still other regulative institutions such as the city's Municipal Health Council (CMS; SMS-Curitiba 2016; Ribeiro 2009). Yet the presence of such communicative institutions of the Sanitarist Movement ideologies was hardly unique to Curitiba. Rather, what separated the capital from others that struggled to enact sanitarista state-building proposals articulated by communicative institutions of the movement such as CEBES was their establishment and occupation of regulative institutions like the SUS manager's office and its precursors. In particular, Curitiban sanitaristas such as Raggio ultimately wielded the SUS manager's office to construct material state capacities for enacting the ideological principles of universality, equity, and community vigilance articulated by such communicative institutions.

The primary-care-oriented model for universalizing and equalizing access to health that Raggio instituted had longer-lasting effects. This model had three main qualities that were meant to orient care provision in the city's primary health clinics: "districtization," the creation of neighborhood-based "sanitary authorities," and the refinement of a family-health model. Raggio first divided the city into seven health districts that would each be monitored by an appointed manager, and then he instituted a "health vigilance" system within each whereby appointed sanitary authorities at each clinic assumed responsibility for monitoring service provision therein. Adapting a more refined version of the community-and family-based model of primary-care provision he had installed earlier in the Cajuru clinic, Raggio first implanted the new model in the Pompéia Health Center on the city's poorer south side. Whereas the Cajuru clinic had been founded on the loose principle that local professionals, residents, and patients would jointly manage its operations through joint consultation, the new health vigilance system outlined for the Pompéia clinic prescribed more clearly delineated local responsibilities of sanitary authorities, who were intended to be neighborhood residents drawn from civil society (Raggio and Giacomini 1996). In this respect, the primary attention model implemented in the Pompéia clinic anticipated SUS Basic Operating Norm of 1993 (NOB-93), which specified the pursuit of such "sanitary and epidemiological vigilance" by local communities as a requirement for receiving federal funding (see Paim 2008, 559–60). Serving as a prototype that facilitated Curitiba's later embrace of the PSF, Pompéia's service-delivery model featured a team of pediatric, gynecological, dental, and general-practice doctors along with nurses and nurses' assistants. Other clinics such as the São José clinic in Curitiba's western region quickly followed by adopting the model in 1993 (SMS-Curitiba 2016; Ducci et al. 2001). Studies of São José have found that, in addition to improving prenatal care, child nutrition, and the frequency of infant examinations between 1993 and 1998, the clinic generally reduced IMR, in part due to its integration with an adjoining nursery that, through its milk and meals programs, diminished the number of underweight and under-height children (Sant'Ana, Rosser, and Talbot 2002). This revised model of care provision became an essential feature, if not the dominant feature, of the city's public health system in later years. Additionally, Curitiba's model of primary-care provision both foreshadowed and prepared the SMS's clinics to adopt the PSF model that the federal MS began encouraging on a nationwide basis only three years later (Pedotti and Moysés 2000; Raggio 1992).

At first glance, such material expansions in Curitiba's primary-care network might appear to be the result of factors other than the agency of office-holding sanitaristas. Some might argue, for example, that Curitiba's seminal moments of state-building for primary-care expansion were nearly automatic by-products of the movement's codification of a right to health. But the movement's victory in codifying its core principles of universal and equal access to health into laws and the Constitution did not automatically guarantee their local enactment. To be sure, Curitiba's expanding primary-care network during this phase clearly benefited from the establishment of key movement-regulative institutions on the national level and even the deepening of its communicative institutions in Curitiba. In particular, the network drew on the movement's central-most regulative institutions on the national level, particularly the SUS as the master institution for enacting the new right to health. Even further, creation of the SUS deepened the prestige of sanitarista SMS directors such as Raggio by codifying laws with underlying normative principles—especially the sanitary reform tenet of universal and equal access to health—for which sanitaristas were staunch, publicly recognized advocates. Still, actual enactment required subnational agents to build state machinery for implementing the right to health, and sanitaristas such as Raggio achieved the greatest success in this regard through office holding itself. While such office-holding forays benefited from these actors' reputations and histories as framers of the right to health, they are not solely reducible to them. Rather, they emerged from sanitaristas' strategic, purposeful, and sustained occupations of those local offices.

Others might argue that such enactment was the result of bureaucratic entrepreneurship by individual *técnicos* acting in narrowly technocratic capacities or even the product of such individuals simply belonging to particular social or policy networks. Still other accounts would suggest that the origins of such reforms were in political parties rather than in civil-society actors and institutions. In general, however, such accounts discount how the power of office-holding sanitaristas to undertake such institutional changes arose from a deepening of the Sanitarist Movement's subnational regulative institutions in Curitiba. More specifically, it was Raggio's previous mobilizations that had established core movement principles such as universalization and democratization of access to primary care as broadly accepted goals for public health policy among a range of powerful subnational elites in a variety of political parties. The continued support of Lerner and his IPPUC allies for the sanitarista state-building agenda clearly mattered as well, especially with Lerner's first electoral victory as Curitiba's mayor in 1989. There is little support for the exaggerated view that Lerner and his network of close associates in the IPPUC controlled major changes to the subnational state so narrowly that they superseded parties. Paraná's political-party organizations were less forceful gatekeepers of state reforms in the public health sector than was the case with the PSDB in Ceará, as the next chapter shows. But expanding the primary health sector in this context required sanitarista translation of their agendas into state-building proposals that dovetailed with Lerner's emerging architecture of planning institutions. The earlier support that sanitaristas extracted turned out to matter greatly in the post-1988 period, when Lerner dominated Curitiba's electoral landscape through four years as mayor (1989–1992) and eight years as Paraná's governor (1995–2002). Furthermore, Curitiba's mayors during and after Lerner's two gubernatorial terms were his former advisors, Rafael Greca (PDT, 1993–1996) and Cassio Taniguchi (PDT/PFL, 1997–2003; Irazabal 2009, 214), lending further continuity to the planning process onto which sanitaristas had grafted their project for implanting and expanding their programmatic primary health model.

Curitiba's health-sector state-building between 1989 and 1993 arose from a process of institutionalizing the SUS manager's office at the municipal public health state's nonbureaucratic top in a way that favored sanitarista occupants of the office. After legal codification of the SUS manager's responsibility for universalizing and equalizing access to primary health and before a moment in the late 1990s when the federal health ministry routinized the process of transferring federal financing for the primary-care sector, the process of generating financing to enact the primary-care model involved raising local resources and negotiating with the federal MS for such resources in a largely ad hoc fashion. Office-holding sanitaristas in this period used the office to attract new resources for expanding cities' primary-care networks, and Raggio enjoyed such success in Curitiba. Although Raggio was clearly driven by the very SUS principles of universality and equity in access to care that he fought to codify in the first place through the crystallization of Article 196 of the Constitution and Laws 8,142 and 8,080 creating the SUS, his movement pedigree also made him a logical choice for appointment to the nascent SUS manager's office, if only because mayors recognized his practical ability to build new state capacities that would otherwise have been more difficult or impossible to construct. But if appointing sanitaristas to SUS directorships made good practical and political sense for mayors from all but the most rigidly antiprogrammatic parties, occupying those posts also reinforced both the normative grounding of sanitaristas in ideologies of sanitary reform and their activist reputations.

It was thus hardly incidental that Curitiba's founding occupant and arguably most influential occupant of the SUS manager's office was also among the Sanitarist Movement's most articulate and boisterous advocates for the normative responsibilities inherent within this regulative institution. Beyond just serving as a SUS manager, Dr. Armando Raggio has also been a long-standing articulator of the office's normative responsibilities, sometimes by publishing his writings in the journals of key communicative institutions such as CEBES, the Sanitarist Movement's most important nationwide association (Raggio 1992). He has also argued for these responsibilities even more clearly in *Consensus*, a magazine of the CONASS. In a didactic article called "The Challenge of Being Health Manager in Brazil," Raggio perhaps most clearly echoes Alexander's understanding of political office as a regulative institution of civil society when propagating the "sacred mission" of serving in the office of SUS manager as one requiring normative commitments and tangible acts to advance the right to health. Particularly observable in his moralizing words in this chapter's epigraph, such stances help reproduce the normative claims on the individual actions of sanitarista managers. Raggio's institution-building efforts atop Curitiba's SMS, for example, went well beyond simply hiring new primary-care workers, constructing new clinics, and developing capacities to better direct both toward regions facing the greatest epidemiological risks. In addition, efforts to instantiate the norm of public responsibility to uphold the SUS's principles of universality and equity were clearly observable in his development of early training programs for health professionals, which partly aimed to inculcate workers in Curitiba's network of primary clinics with a sense of public responsibility for upholding such principles.

In sum, sanitarista-driven state-building in Curitiba's primary health sector between 1989 and 1993 involved sanitaristas establishing regulative institutions of the movement such as the SUS manager's office, which they wielded to construct crucial new state capacities for reducing IMR. These interventions included Raggio's signing of official agreements with the state and federal government to formally municipalize the primary public health sector in 1992, an early moment for urban Brazil. Just as important were his earlier efforts to implant and reorient the city's network of public health facilities around a primary-care model. The immediate consequences of these episodes were considerable, with Curitiba doubling its network of primary-care facilities during this part of Raggio's tenure, the largest such expansion during any four-year period of the capital's history. Further, the primary-care model already installed in many such clinics paved the way for subsequent adoption of the PSF model. Ultimately, this sustained pattern of sanitarista-driven state-building in the municipal public health sectors helps explain how Curitiba not only began the SUS era with an already low IMR of 39.96 but also reduced that rate by nearly 40% over the next five years.

3.3. NONSANITARISTA SMS DIRECTORS, WEAK STATE-BUILDING,
AND TEPID IMR REDUCTION, 1993–1998

After Rafael Greca (PDT) began his first term as Curitiba's mayor in 1993, the city experienced a somewhat anomalous five-year period in which sanitaristas did not control the SMS. Raggio completed his time as Curitiba's SMS secretary in 1993, although he continued supporting Curitiba's ongoing municipalization of the public health sector during his eight years as Paraná's SES director under Lerner's governorships (1995–2002). Nevertheless, the five years following Raggio's 1993 replacement as Curitiba's SMS director by Dr. João Carlos Gonçalves Baracho, a geriatric physician and surgeon with no strong ties to the Sanitarist Movement, coincided with a period of relatively weak IMR reduction. Indeed, Curitiba reduced IMR nearly twice as much during Raggio's four years in office than it did between the even longer five-year period from 1994 to 1998, when IMR fell by only 4.65, from 22.74 to 18.09. Furthermore, given that IMR reductions are more difficult to achieve at lower levels, it is even more telling that, during the following five years of sanitarista successors to Baracho as SMS director, Curitiba again witnessed a larger reduction of 6.47, from 18.09 in 1998 to 11.62 in 2003.

To be sure, the mid-to-late 1990s presented difficult nationwide conditions for building municipal capacity to expand primary public health care. The passage of the so-called Kandir Law of 1996 imposed serious practical constraints on the ability of subnational governments to hire public employees. The SMSs of major capitals, in particular, began facing the daunting task of municipalizing entire networks of hospitals located within their jurisdictions, as Curitiba did in 1996. They also typically had to grapple with the administrative challenges of receiving federal funding for service provision in new forms specified by SUS Basic Operating Norm of 1996 (NOB-96). Initially segmented into parcels according to levels of attention and types of services delivered, these multiple funds posed new administrative burdens that necessitated adjustments in planning, even in capitals such as Curitiba with relatively strong capacities in this regard. Furthermore, Curitiba in 1998 assumed the category of full management status specified by the SUS, creating enormous administrative demands for managing an entire network of primary care as well as more complex services.

Nevertheless, Baracho's term as SMS director also featured several unsuccessful managerial and administrative experiments, which were largely of the agency's own making and contributed little in the way of observable contributions to actual capacity-building for primary-care delivery. Some of these interventions later had to be discontinued due to perceived ineffectiveness in accomplishing their objectives as well as their lack of popularity among SMS workers. For instance, the SMS introduced a bonus program in 1994 known as the IDQ to encourage staff to take assignments working in less accessible city regions perceived to subject workers to greater risks of violence and other threats to personal safety. But repeated disputes arose among staff regarding a lack of transparency and accuracy in the criteria used to assess and compare the dangers of various city regions, leading the SMS to quickly end the program (World Bank 2006). Additionally, in 1995 the SMS instituted a bonus scheme program called the Quality Incentive Program (PIQ), which placed health workers at non-PSF primary-care clinics in the SMS in competition with one another for a 30% salary bonus that was intended to reward 10% of clinics for high-quality service provision. Beyond drawing objections from PSF workers who were ruled out of competing for the bonus, the PIQ drew staunch criticism from non-PSF workers for assessing poorly chosen performance targets, such as health outcomes, that they regarded as largely beyond their control, highly subjective, and subject to being gamed by workers. After criticizing the bonus system for undermining the teamwork dynamic inherent to the city's primary-care model, senior SMS administrators abandoned the PIQ in 1997 (World Bank 2006).

These experiments echoed a greater focus during Baracho's directorship on performance-based management of the larger public health system for which Curitiba became responsible during the era, and they signaled a shift away from his directorship's earlier, single-minded focus on primary care.[8] This is not to say that these administrative reforms were all unneeded or unwarranted. On the contrary, Curitiba's SMS established more general but essential capacities for a city that began administering secondary and hospital-based care during this period. For example, the SMS in 1994 established a centralized appointment system for specialized care, which streamlined the referral of patients from clinics into other health care facilities in the capital. These and other improvements in the informational technology systems of Curitiba's SMS facilitated its launch of small programs such as *Carteira de Saúde da Criança* (Children's Health Card) and *Nascer em Curi-*

tiba, Vale a Vida (Born in Curitiba, Value Life), whose stated purposes were improved registration of births in the capital and IMR reduction (SMS-Curitiba 2016). In 1995, it also introduced a management training course (GERUS) for occupants of the newly created position of health clinic director that was intended to foster strategic planning and development of information systems and performance targeting schemes (World Bank 2006, 52). Yet the 1993 to 1998 period was also a phase in which the well-known predilection of Curitiban political society for top-down strategic planning began taking precedence over other objectives such as primary-care expansion, in contrast to the earlier period in which office-holding sanitaristas had made such expansion dovetail with the larger planning apparatus.

One deficit in the programs introduced during the period was that they often favored technocratic approaches to improving performance and correspondingly struggled to embed health worker teams in social relations with one another and the communities they served. Subsequent iterations of such programs introduced by sanitarista SMS directors like Luciano Ducci and Michele Caputo Neto, however, took a different tack by refining and repurposing such programs in ways that emphasized relationship-building and teamwork between care providers and clinic managers. For example, Caputo Neto introduced softer "terms of agreement" that more explicitly fostered teamwork and collaboration among primary-care teams and discouraged absenteeism (World Bank 2006, 49–52). Thus, it was not purely the technical background of sanitarista officeholders atop Curitiba's SMS that explains their relatively successful state-building interventions. On the contrary, the example of Baracho's SMS directorship illustrated how it was more often Curitiba's nonsanitarista SMS directors who exhibited some of the well-documented shortfalls of the archetypal Brazilian técnico. Indeed, although sanitaristas also made problem-solving interventions in the realms of administration and management, these were often focused more on enacting core ideologies of sanitary reform such as universalizing and equalizing access to service provision than they were on more technically oriented performance management schemes like the IDQ and PIQ.

But whatever the other gains of Baracho's administration in laying administrative and managerial groundwork for later expansions to Curitiba's primary-care network, his tangible record of adding primary-care clinics and workers was more mixed than that of his sanitarista predecessor. In terms of physical infrastructure, whereas Raggio's four years in office had increased Curitiba's network by forty-three, from forty-two to eighty-five health clinics by 1993, Baracho's five-years in office raised the total only by thirteen, to ninety-eight, all at a time in which the capital continued to witness sizable population growth in peripheral regions (SMS-Curitiba 2016). These modest expansions were associated mostly with the SMS's unofficial 1995 launch of the PSF, which allowed for the opening of three new health clinics, and Curitiba's movement into the SUS's category of full management status, which allowed for the establishment of eighteen PSF clinics. Still, many of these clinics represented either full conversions of preexisting ones that were not previously observing the PSF model or partial conversions of preexisting ones to simultaneously accommodate care provision through the new PSF regime and preexisting work regimes. In terms of personnel, by 1996, Curitiba had hired 393 PSF health professionals, including doctors, nurses, nurses' assistants, orthodontists, dental hygienists, and dental assistants (Ribeiro 2009: 137), although it is likely that this hiring wave reflected transfers of already existing public employees out of similar positions within clinics observing Curitiba's then more dominant, non-PSF work regime. Additionally, data availability constraints make it difficult to assess when these new hires were made, since the federal MS only began collecting systematic data from all municípios on their PSF staffing and coverage rate in 1998.

What is clear, however, is that the actual service-provision outcomes achieved during Baracho's term were relatively modest in comparison to previous and future episodes. The primary-care model previously installed by sanitaristas such as Raggio remained firmly embedded, even amid the addition of new and more technocratic changes that did relatively little to expand the reach of the model itself. But by the end of 1999, its first full year of official operation in Curitiba and the year after Baracho resigned the SMS directorship, the PSF amounted to only forty-two teams covering an estimated 144,900 residents in a município of over 1.5 million. Curitiba's resulting populational coverage of less than 10% mirrored other capitals, such as Fortaleza, that experienced slow starts with the PSF. Compared to five years earlier in 1993, when Baracho began replacing his predecessors' emphasis on primary-care expansion with the pursuit of what became a series of often ill-fated managerial reforms, IMR in 1998 had perhaps unsurprisingly declined by only a modest 4.65 deaths to 18.09.

3.4. SANITARISTA OFFICE HOLDING, RENEWED STATE-BUILDING,
AND ROBUST IMR DECLINE, 1999–2016

The return of sanitaristas to Curitiba's SMS directorship in mid-1998 pre-cipitated a renaissance in state-building that appreciably expanded munic-ipal capacities to deliver primary health care and other services even more specifically targeted at IMR reduction. In addition to undertaking unprec-edented expansions of the PSF, two office-holding sanitaristas—Dr. Lu-ciano Ducci and Michele Caputo Neto—added new municipal state ca-pacities for lowering IMR, such as improved prenatal and neonatal care for mothers and infants. In particular, Ducci and Caputo Neto deepened existing programs like the PSF and introduced others such as the PMC, whose widely recognized effect led it to become a blueprint for a similar federal program, *Rede Cegonha* (Stork Network). The human consequences of this sanitarista-driven state-building episode were considerable.[9] Com-pared to the beginning of the episode in 1998, Curitiba by 2003 had re-duced IMR 34% (by 6.17) to 11.92. And after nine years of sanitarista of-fice holding, Curitiba had halved IMR to only 9.13 by 2006, becoming the first major capital in urban Brazil to record an IMR below the 10 deaths per 1,000 live births threshold. By 2016, Curitiba was still urban Brazil's top performer in minimizing premature death, with an IMR of 7.95.

Here again, a deeper analysis of this episode illuminates how Curitiba's sanitaristas drove the institution-building processes at the heart of such robust reductions, in part because of their accumulating reputations for both practical effectiveness and normative fidelity to the public responsibil-ities of the SUS manager's office atop state and local government in Paraná and Curitiba. The central protagonist of the episode's municipal reforms was Dr. Ducci, the PUC-Paraná-trained sanitarista physician and veteran of the Brazilian student movement's socialist-oriented LIBELU current. Ducci began his medical career in 1988 working as a municipal public ser-vant in the Cajuru neighborhood clinic after winning a competitive con-curso for the job that his fellow sanitarista, Armando Raggio, had previ-ously opened. As a pediatrician with training in infant pneumology, Ducci thus began his professional career working on the frontlines of Curitiba's ongoing efforts to combat infant mortality through its emerging clinic-based primary-care model. While later holding the municipal posts of san-itary vigilance director and health-service director during the early 1990s, he held two municipal offices that institutionalized two of sanitary reform's most communitarian ideological tenets. Between 1995 and 1998, after Jaime Lerner won his first governorship of Paraná, he appointed Raggio as the SES's director and Ducci as his director general in a clear signal of intent to pursue the same primary-care agenda on a statewide basis that they had previously begun implementing in Curitiba.

In July 1998, however, Ducci transitioned back into working for the municipality, this time as its highest appointed officeholder in the SMS directorship. In doing so, Ducci occupied the office vacated by Baracho, who had resigned at the request of then mayor Cassio Taniguchi amid inquiries by Curitiba's city council into alleged financial improprieties in the administration of Curitiba's new Municipal Health Fund (Folha de Londrina 1998). Established in 1998 as part of the capital's graduation into full SUS management status, the fund became a mechanism for partially financing federal programs such as the PSF that had been relatively deemphasized under Baracho's previous administration. Although Ducci would subsequently refocus attention on expanding the PSF, his first move involved deepening more specific capacities of the SMS to diminish infant and maternal mortality, especially those resulting from avoidable causes. In September of 1998, a team within Ducci's SMS began designing a new program called the Curitiban Mother Program (*Programa Mãe Curitibana*, PMC) that would aim to do so by creating an integrated suite of preventative and more complex health services for mothers and infants at all stages before, during, and after pregnancy.[10] The impetus to create a more consolidated intervention for explicitly targeting infant mortality emerged from ongoing discussions that managers of Curitiba's decentralized health clinics and their encompassing health district managers had already been having with one another, in part through the context of the capital's Municipal Health Council (CMS). Only with the 1998 entry of Ducci into the SMS directorship did a commission of these managers, who had been reviewing statistics and other evidence regarding frequent causes of child and maternal mortality in their jurisdictions, begin collaborating with the highest planning levels of Curitiba's SMS to explicitly design the PMC to address particular causes. The commission's findings were of relatively little surprise to many on-the-ground service providers and managers but pinpointed multiple eminently fixable problems. Among them were that the municipal public health network delivered low proportions of prenatal consultations during critical early stages of pregnancy and that pregnant women experienced consistent difficulties in gaining access to public hospitals for their deliveries (Jiménez et al. 2001).

Launched relatively quickly in March of 1999, the PMC aimed to connect pregnant women, mothers, and infants with a more integrated, hierarchically organized, and risk-oriented regime of publicly delivered prenatal, perinatal, and postpartum health services. The program thus built upon Curitiba's decentralized model of clinic-based care by making the capital's by now considerable network of local health centers the entry points for pregnant women with higher risks of mortality. The program also explicitly aimed to connect pregnant women and mothers to a more integrated, fuller array of health services from conception to infancy, beginning in neighborhood clinics closest to their residences. In this sense, the PMC's design dovetailed with that of the PSF, whose deployment of roving family-health teams could at a minimum help identify pregnant women and spread awareness regarding the expanded range of care available to them earlier than might otherwise be the case. Further, upon confirming pregnancies, health centers immediately created files for each patient, provided an identification card, scheduled (optional) educational and counseling services regarding pregnancy, made a referral to a maternity hospital in the catchment area of the clinic, and scheduled a series of prenatal exams. Crucially, the program also adopted a more systematic, epidemiologically informed approach to formulating an individualized plan of care for pregnant women based on gestational health risks assessed during initial and ongoing prenatal appointments (Curitiba, Prefeitura Municipal 1999, 2012). Even by 2004, the fruits of the PMC were becoming evident, with Curitiba taking the lead among all major capitals in the percentage of live births by mothers with seven or more prenatal appointments (77.9%). The capital was also unsurpassed in the percentage of nonfetal deaths attributed to undefined causes (1.1%; World Bank 2006, 39).

Alongside the pathbreaking implementation of the PMC, Ducci's SMS also considerably expanded the number of PSF teams and clinics delivering primary services during his term. By the end of 1999, Ducci's first full year as director, he had inherited a network with only forty-two PSF teams deployed to serve an estimated 144,900 residents. Although its PSF coverage was among the highest for urban Brazil during this early moment of the program's nationwide introduction, it still managed to cover less than 10% of the capital's population. Following disputes within Ducci's management team regarding the relative benefits of expanding the PSF versus keeping Curitiba's similar but longer-standing model of delivering primary care within basic health units (UBS), the SMS ultimately adopted a dual strategy of expanding both models (Ribeiro 2009, 155; Ducci et al. 2001). The results of this capacity expansion by 2002, when Ducci resigned from the office to run for state deputy, were obvious. The SMS had nearly tripled its number of PSF teams to 114, raising its coverage to 393,300 residents, or over 24% of the population. And compared to 1998, when Ducci entered the SMS directorship, Curitiba's IMR had fallen 34% to 11.92 by 2003, the year after he left the office to successfully run for a state deputy seat.

From late 2002 to 2004, the sanitarista ally Michele Caputo Neto succeeded Ducci in Curitiba's SMS directorship and generally preserved the major expansions that Ducci had made to the PSF. Although Caputo Neto focused less explicitly on capacity-building to further reduce IMR, his SMS added crucial new competencies such as an ambulance service (SAMU) and the *Mulher de Verdade* program, the latter of which focused on serving female victims of physical, sexual, and domestic violence. It also refocused on improving the quality and performance of service delivery in the city-managed health system through new incentives and a system of management contracts between health units, district managers, and the SMS (SMS-Curitiba 2016). Nevertheless, during these three years, the PSF's most decisive inputs plateaued, with the SMS reporting approximately the same number of teams, clinics, and levels of populational coverage at the end of 2004 as it had in 2002. And while marginal gains in mortality reductions at such relatively low levels are considerably more difficult to achieve than at the higher levels Curitiba recorded in the 1990s, IMR reduction slowed during this period of focus on management reforms, falling by just over one death to 10.51 by 2005. This makes it difficult to sustain the argument (Shepherd 2010; World Bank 2006) that discreet administrative instruments such as management contracts and other performance-based incentives mattered as much as the sheer physical and human resources that capitals like Curitiba added for combating IMR during this episode.

Curitiba's next major PSF expansion came when Ducci himself returned as SMS director from 2005 through March 2010. He came to occupy the office again in 2005 by winning the city's vice mayorship twice (2005–2008, 2009–2010) as the PSB running mate of PSDB Mayor Carlos Alberto Richa. Despite assuming the vice mayorship, he also continued directing the

SMS, lending continuity to the expansionary impetus he initiated at the beginning of the decade. It was only in early 2010, when Ducci assumed the mayorship that Richa vacated to run for Paraná's governorship, that he stepped aside from direct control of the SMS to govern the city as mayor. But even during these two years, he elevated the former chief planner and architect of Curitiba's evolving primary-care model during Ducci's SMS directorship, Eliane Regina de Veiga Chomatas, to occupy his vacated position. Perhaps not surprisingly—given Ducci's occupation of Curitiba's SMS directorship as well as the city's second-highest and highest democratically elected offices—the expansionary trend in the primary health sector continued. The level of primary health care briefly plateaued during Caputo Neto's directorship, but the result of Ducci's five years as SMS director and vice mayor and his two years as mayor was another doubling of PSF teams to a total of 229 covering 814,200 residents, or 44% of the population by 2014, where these levels remained until 2015. And by 2016, Curitiba had further reduced IMR below the 9 deaths per 1,000 threshold, remaining urban Brazil's top-performing capital in this regard.

Ducci's tenure demonstrates how repeated episodes of expansion in state capacities for IMR reduction were effective, if not novel. More important than novelty or participatory-democratic deliberations about how to address premature mortality was the consistent advocacy of office-holding sanitaristas for piecemeal but sustained expansion of an already effective model. For instance, building on its territorialized model of primary-care provision, Curitiba was well prepared to incrementally expand the PSF, which required the municipality to absorb at least 75% of the costs associated with each additional team it added (H. M. Magalhães, interview, 2010). Further, Ducci's tenure shows how a focus on improving system-wide performance in an increasingly complex municipal public health system that delivered more sophisticated health services could be complemented with continued efforts to proactively advance core ideological tenets of sanitary reform such as universal and equal access to more basic services. Although Ducci and Caputo Neto continued focusing on performance-management interventions first prioritized during Baracho's SMS directorships, they did so with critical modifications. For instance, the IPQ program instituted by Ducci created incentives for high-quality service provision, but his program prioritized collaboration among health professional teams and between their managers rather than emphasizing zero-sum competitions between teams in different units, as Baracho's ill-fated version had inadvertently done. In this sense, Curitiba's office-holding sanitaristas built other capacities of the SMS to deliver more sophisticated services while continuing to translate the communitarian ethos of sanitary reform into actual programs and processes for reducing premature deaths.

These episodes also illustrate how important it was that Curitiba lacked anything like the excessively protracted and clientelist hegemony of Bahia's Antônio Carlos Magalhães (ACM), which remained so extreme as to effectively preclude meaningful electoral competition well into the mid-2000s. Compared to the Bahian capital of Salvador, Curitiba's electoral landscape was defined by candidates and subnational party organizations that actively competed with one another for the mayorship; this competition was often based on public policy agendas and claims about their records of delivering on them (de Quadros 2013). In this context, it mattered far less that Cassio Taniguchi, Curitiba's mayor during the beginning of the episode, had won election after switching from the PDT into the PFL. Although the PFL had a more center-right orientation on a nationwide basis, ideologies of party organizations often vary dramatically by state in Brazil,[11] and the social policies pursued by elites in Paraná's variant suggest that it was far more centrist in this respect than its counterpart in Bahia, for example. Indeed, Paraná's more progressive PDT mirrored the PFL in its reliance on a small number of high-profile members such as Taniguchi, Lerner, and Greca, as was observable when the PDT's influence in Curitiba largely collapsed after all three left it in 1999 to join Paraná's PFL. In this regard, the PFL's organization in Paraná was not rigidly right leaning or necessarily antiprogrammatic, particularly not after Taniguchi, Lerner, and Greca all joined it and brought along their general interest in public policy planning and their more specific receptivity to health-sector reform. Thus, far from indicating any obvious pattern of clientelist or rigidly conservative rule in Curitiba, Taniguchi's mayorship was more notable for extending the ongoing openness of the executive to the problem-solving interventions of office-holding sanitaristas.[12]

It is also notable that the pattern of Workers' Party rule often credited with IMR reduction on a nationwide basis was completely absent throughout Curitiba's history. Indeed, Curitiba achieved the overwhelming share of its IMR reductions without ever having had a PT mayor or governor of Paraná and before the social policies, particularly Bolsa Família, of national-level PT presidents began taking effect in 2004. This also underscores how even though PT mayors elsewhere typically cultivated sanitarista-driven planning in the primary health sector, openness to proactive interventions by high-profile sanitaristas was no privileged domain of the PT. On the contrary, such sustained openness among a series of Curitiban mayors from several parties ranging from center left to center right was most often engineered by Curitiba's sanitaristas amid rule by executives with no strong convictions or independently formulated plans of their own for the health sector. More specifically, sanitaristas such as Raggio and Caputo Neto did so by consistently commanding local democratic offices, through which they established a central place for a primary health model within the capital's larger planning apparatus. In sum, lacking mayors from Brazil's most renowned left party did not impede office-holding sanitaristas from gaining the support of less overtly progressive mayors from the PDT, PMDB, PSDB—and even the center-right PFL—for their relatively modest and cost-effective proposals to better equip the city for IMR reduction.

Additionally, the absence of influential participatory publics capable of successfully demanding a Participatory Budgeting (OP) process did not stop Curitiba from robustly shrinking IMR, because sanitaristas used the distinct channel of the SMS director's office to introduce new IMR-reducing capacities. Although such institutionalized mechanisms of influence for participatory publics had other benefits in terms of monitoring the public health sector—as the previous chapters about Porto Alegre and Belo Horizonte illustrated—they were not necessary for robust development when sanitaristas controlled the democratic offices that most concentrated their power over mortality-reducing state-building. Ultimately, it mattered relatively little that Curitiba lacked an OP or even a sufficiently empowered CMS, because health reformers controlled the key offices that most impacted the hiring of new primary-care workers, the building of new clinics, and the rollout of programs such as the PMC, which streamlined health care provision to mothers and children most at risk of premature mortality. In sum, even amid the absence of other potential drivers of IMR reduction, office-holding sanitaristas had already carved out a central place for their primary-care-focused, state-building agenda for the health sector among a variety of influential Curitiban political elites, and this perpetuated growth in municipal competencies for IMR reduction well into the 2010s.

The episode also reinforces how the movement lineages of these office-holding sanitaristas mattered for their motivation and ability to secure support for new capacity-building, the content of those capacities, and their mortality-reduction consequences. Further, these actors' experiences as care providers were hardly disconnected from the actual modifications they made to the structure of Curitiba's public health system. Together, the combination of movement lineages and front-line work in Curitiba's early primary public health clinics helped crystallize a communitarian-inspired set of state-building proposals that emphasized neighborhood-based service provision and health vigilance. More specifically, these experiences informed central design features of the state capacities that—as high-level democratic officeholders atop Curitiba's public health state—these sanitaristas added to the capitals' evolving institutional model of IMR-reducing public health care. Clearly, the consequences of these actors were visible not just in the individual work of frontline health care givers, as emphasized in seminal works like Tendler's account of "barefoot doctors" in rural Ceará (1997). Just as importantly, office-holding sanitaristas atop Curitiba's public health state constructed the overarching context of public health politics that led to more than just the hiring of such workers in other domains of municipal politics. More generally, the city's office-holding sanitaristas established an enduring programmatic approach to expanding the municipal public health state that maximized IMR reduction for nearly two decades afterward.

4. Conclusion

This chapter argued that office-holding sanitaristas propelled an early and sustained pattern of state-building by which programmatic health democratization in Curitiba widened access to primary health care and helped reduce IMR to an unprecedented low for urban Brazil. The agency of these actors thus helps explain how—despite entering the health-democratization period with only middling IMR outcomes—Curitiba had become urban Brazil's top performer in this regard by the mid-2000s, while otherwise similar cities that lacked such consistent patterns of sanitarista office holding achieved weaker outcomes. More specifically, the main mechanism by which sanitaristas fostered these impressive strides in Curitiba was through more sustained episodes of office holding in the city's SMS directorship than those in any other capital throughout the period. During this impressively consistent period of office holding, Curitiba's sanitaristas repeatedly wielded municipal state-building levers that were at the fingertips of such officeholders to construct new municipal state capacities required for enacting the municipal state's legal and constitutional responsibilities to universalize and equalize access to health services. From within these positions of power atop the municipal public health state, Curitiba's office-holding sanitaristas propelled nearly all the capital's most significant expansions of municipal capacity in the primary public health sector.

The chapter also illuminated how Curitiban sanitaristas did not succeed in this regard merely because of their reputations as technical experts and public problem solvers of the strictly material problems of missing service-provision capacity in the public health sector. To be sure, these backgrounds mattered, not least because they qualified sanitaristas for SMS directorships on technical grounds in the eyes of the mayors and governors who appointed them. In addition, however, their efforts to iteratively expand the municipal public health state in such a sustained fashion reflected the normative authority that—as movement veterans with long histories of mobilizing to institutionalize principles of universal and equal access to health in the Constitution, laws, and the democratic office of the SUS manager itself—individual sanitaristas commanded as advocates for the very principles crystallized into that office. The ability of Curitiba's sanitaristas to command and wield the office of SUS manager owed much to these individuals' dual status as both prime advocates for the universalistic principle of a right to health and seasoned professionals who had generally demonstrated their commitments to such principles by working as caregivers within the city's earliest primary public health clinics.

Thus, well beyond their mere proficiency in technical matters of disease prevention, mortality reduction, and public health planning, the combined movement pedigrees and practitioner backgrounds of Curitiba's sanitaristas helped establish them as normatively legitimate occupants and agents of the SUS manager's office. Insofar as their activist and professional pedigrees embodied and personified the public responsibilities enshrined in the office itself, individual sanitarista occupants commanded disproportionate access to SUS directorships and marshaled considerable civil power in wielding the office for associated state-building aims in Curitiba. Individual sanitaristas such as Armando Raggio, Luciano Ducci, and Michele Caputo Neto not only embodied normative principles of universalizing and equalizing access to health care among local circles of Sanitarist Movement activists and broader publics with the city but also used these reputations to help transform those principles into a modest but actionable state-building agenda that was well matched to the planning orientations of multiple mayors and governors, who largely adopted it as their own. Ultimately then, the construction and wielding of this new democratic office by local sanitaristas constituted both a defining feature of Curitiba's health-democratization period and a principal cause of the city's robust social development outcome by the mid-2010s.

SEVEN

Fortaleza

> I would say that within the strategy of the PSF resides all our
> anxieties, desires, dreams, and utopias that we accumulated
> over the years of Brazilian sanitary reform. I believe this—
> that the strategy underlying the PSF mirrors that which we
> dreamed of. The possibility of having community-based health
> based on a team of doctors, nurses, and community health
> agents constructing holistic, universal access and seeking
> solutions . . . For us sanitaristas, this is the realization of a
> utopia.
>
> —*Dr. Luiz Odorico Monteiro de Andrade, sanitarista director of*
> *Fortaleza's SMS (2005–2009; my translation from interview in*
> *de Miranda Gondim [2011, 587])*

Given its deeper history of clientelism and lower initial development levels, the northeastern capital city of Fortaleza might initially seem an odd
candidate for comparison to more obvious cases of programmatic health
democratization such as Curitiba. For one, subnational politics in dictatorship-era Fortaleza and its encompassing state of Ceará epitomized the
decidedly antiprogrammatic mode of *coronelismo* for which Brazil's northeastern region was infamous, whereas Curitiba's encompassing state of
Paraná experienced nothing comparable.[1] And although it was never as
central to the Portuguese empire as the territories that encompassed other
northeastern cities such as Salvador or Recife, Fortaleza bore more damaging institutional legacies of colonialism than erstwhile peripheries like Curitiba (Mahoney 2010, 242–49). Fortaleza entered the health-democratization period still bearing these scars: in 1985, its per capita GDP (R$4,783)
ranked last among the major Brazilian capitals examined in this study, and
its 1988 IMR of 64.74 was 60% higher than Curitiba's and ranked among

urban Brazil's worst.[2] It is thus all the more notable that two similarly sized capitals with such different initial levels of social, economic, and political development had achieved roughly similar social development outcomes only thirty years later. For instance, Fortaleza's IMR of 10.68 in 2015 rivaled Curitiba's (8.44) and that of other top-ranked capitals such as Porto Alegre (second at 9.87), Recife (third at 10.17), and Belo Horizonte (fourth at 10.34).[3]

The chapter traces this robust development outcome in Fortaleza to a trajectory of programmatic health democratization that was defined by the state-building interventions of office-holding sanitaristas in the primary-care sector. Although less sustained across the entire period than was the case in Curitiba, interventions by sanitaristas in Fortaleza's SMS and Ceará's SES directorship propelled two especially consequential state-building episodes: one from 1987 to 1992 and a post-2004 episode. During these periods, Fortalezan sanitaristas such as Dr. Anamaria Cavalcante e Silva (1992–1994), Dr. João Ananias Vasconcelos Neto (2007–2009), and Dr. Raimundo José Arruda Bastos (2010–2013) all held the SES directorship, whereas Dr. Luiz Odorico Monteiro de Andrade (2005–2009), Cavalcante e Silva (1989–1990), and Dr. Abner Cavalcante Brasil (1990–1992) held the SMS directorship. All told, sanitaristas occupied Fortaleza's SMS during ten (55%) of the eighteen years between 1995 and 2012 and over half of an earlier episode between 1988 and 1995. It is particularly notable that Fortalezan sanitaristas held the office of SMS director—and propelled sizable IMR reductions and expansions in municipal capacity-building for primary-care expansion—during the earlier episode, which predates the city's period of PT mayors (2005–2012), its post-2005 experience with Participatory Budgeting, and its post-2003 implementation of Bolsa Família. The earlier episode most clearly demonstrates how sanitaristas established sanitary reform's principles of universal and equal access to health services as a widely embraced set of state-building objectives, even among an otherwise centrist group of Fortalezan political elites. That episode shares this characteristic with the post-2005 period of PT rule, however.

A defining feature of Fortaleza's programmatic trajectory of health democratization was the early and outsized role of office-holding sanitaristas in equipping the subnational public health state with formidable new capacities to lower IMR. Particularly important was how these actors constructed a formidable network of primary health clinics, hired considerable numbers of municipal primary-care professionals, and redistributed exist-ing health professionals to clinics in city regions facing higher epidemio-logical risks of premature mortality. Despite not creating more innovative new programs, such as the PMC in Curitiba, office-holding sanitaristas in Fortaleza nevertheless added crucial new capacities to the municipal pub-lic health state that maximized the reach of primary-care provision through the PSF and its programmatic precursors and counterparts. In short, the subnationally focused state-building efforts of sanitaristas were both a de-fining feature of programmatic health democratization in Fortaleza and a central cause of its robust development outcomes.

Thus, the chapter argues that Fortaleza's robust development outcomes can be fully attributed neither to Brazil-wide factors such as its left-party presidents, health-policy diffusion, and Bolsa Família nor to localized ones such as participatory-democratic institutions and left-party mayors. Al-though such factors had a clear bearing on the city's post-2005 improve-ments, most of them arrived too late to explain the city's earlier strides in IMR reduction. As such, much of the analytic challenge in explaining the city's impressive outcomes rests in accounting for the rather dramatic IMR reductions that predate this later phase. Indeed, Fortaleza had already be-come among Brazil's leaders in IMR by the mid-2000s, before the arrival of Bolsa Família, the 2006 advent of Participatory Budgeting (OP), the 2005 beginning of two consecutive PT mayorships, or other such factors.[4] And although the growing institutionalization of Fortaleza's Municipal Health Councils (CMSs) ran apace of its IMR reductions, actual state-building in-terventions in the primary health sector rarely emanated from the coun-cil itself. Further, it is also not possible to attribute the city's robust devel-opment outcomes to the mere presence of a sanitarista network in the city, a factor that was constant throughout a period characterized by fits and spurts in state-building for health. To better explain Fortaleza's robust de-velopment outcomes, it is instead necessary to address more deeply consti-tutive elements of its programmatic trajectory. To begin doing so, the chap-ter next addresses the initial conditions from which this trajectory emerged.

1. Initial Conditions of Civil and Political Society in Fortaleza

Curitiba and Fortaleza entered the health-democratization period exhibit-ing important differences and similarities in their politics and conditions of social and economic development. Among their important differences were that Fortaleza's mayors and governors had long been the patriarchs of conservative, traditional families generally opposed to economic and political liberalism, while subnational executives in Curitiba exhibited a comparatively stronger orientation toward generating new industries and markets through state-directed planning. In this sense, Fortaleza echoed larger patterns of clientelist rule throughout Brazil's Northeast, with just three colonels in Fortaleza's encompassing state of Ceará—Virgílio Távora, César Cals, and Adauto Bezerra—dominating its politics throughout the dictatorship and into the 1980s. Among the associated maladies of their regimes was rampant, selective distribution of state jobs, public funds, and other sources of patronage to political supporters, especially other coronels (Gondim 2004, 68–72). In other words, Fortaleza's politics entailed a decidedly nonprogrammatic approach to public governance that rivaled other northeastern cities such as Salvador and Recife in how it precluded the pursuit of any sustained vision or goals for public governance. But while subnational political societies in both Fortaleza and Curitiba were necessarily allied with powerful military elites during most years of the dictatorship, this translated into a far more antiprogrammatic approach to politics in Fortaleza.

Yet in other dimensions, Fortaleza shared important features with Curitiba and with most other major capitals in Brazil. Both capitals featured similarly large and rapidly expanding populations, with Curitiba growing from over 1.2 million residents in 1988 to over 1.8 million by 2015, and Fortaleza expanding from over 1.6 million to over 2.5 million during the same period. As capitals of their encompassing states of Paraná and Ceará, respectively, Curitiba and Fortaleza both constituted industrial, political, and social hubs within larger metropolitan regions. As such, they also hosted the largest and most important public and private universities in their respective states. In Fortaleza, these included the Federal University of Ceará (UFC) and the State University of Ceará (UECE). The fact that such major universities featured medical and public schools would prove especially important for future trajectories of health democratization, in part because these schools provided incubators for a range of social movement activists, including sanitaristas, during the dictatorship.

In Fortaleza, influential sanitaristas also emerged from university campuses in the capital, where they created and mobilized within key civil-society associations that joined other groups in demanding the restoration of democracy, particularly toward the end of Brazil's dictatorship. In emphasizing the professional backgrounds of high-level political appointees who exercised power as Brazil crystallized a right to health and established the SUS, existing accounts of transformation in Ceará's public health sector have tended to overlook how these actors first laid a seminal foundation of civil-society institutions for advancing future public health reforms (Tendler 1997, 155). For instance, particularly during later phases of the dictatorship, sanitarista associations in Fortaleza such as the *Centro Médico Cearense* (CMC) mirrored nationwide counterparts like CEBES and ABRASCO in doubling as health professional organizations through which activists mobilized in larger prodemocracy struggles. The CMC (later renamed the Associação Médica Cearense, AMC) was initially founded by Dr. Paulo Marcelo Martins Rodrigues, the UFC Medical School professor for whom the university's public health school is now named. Doctors associated with the group became increasingly involved with the *Diretas Já* movement for immediate, direct elections for the president of Brazil. The prominent Cearense sanitarista Antônio Carlile Holanda Lavor described how the cross-fertilization of Fortaleza's CMC members with its *Diretas Já* mobilizations preceded sanitaristas' articulation of more democratically oriented strategies for local health-sector reform: "In Ceará, there weren't large rallies like there were in São Paulo, but there was a coming together of people who wanted a change in the capital and in the interior" (Paranaguá de Santana and Lima de Castro 2016, 25, my translation).

Such sanitarista associations gave rise to a less radical generation of activists such as Holanda Lavor, who nevertheless prized the democratic principle of accountability as a guideline for health-sector reform when he later became state health secretary of Ceará. Despite entering professional worlds of general and public health practice and research at a time when considerable repression sometimes rendered militant organization a life-and-death proposition, sanitaristas in Ceará still mobilized within the prodemocracy struggle of the time and generally envisioned a democratic regime as the most conducive platform for realizing their ambitions for universalizing access to health. Indeed, many in this earlier generation of Ceárn sanitaristas mirrored their nationwide counterparts in supporting pro-democracy struggles they believed would lead to autonomous municipal governments with stronger control over the public health sector and thus more degrees of freedom to locally pursue central tenets of sanitary reform. Cavalcante Brasil, for example, took great pride in signing one of urban Brazil's first agreements to transfer health clinics from state to municipal control in November 1992 (Mota 1997, 64–74). Holanda Lavor, who would later design and roll out Ceará's trailblazing Community Health Agents (ACS) program as SES secretary during the first year of Tasso Jereissati's governorship in 1987, finished his medical education at UFC in 1964 at a moment in which seizure of power by Brazil's military posed dire threats to militant social protest. Lavor thus mirrored other public health professionals of his generation by receding into the academy as a medical professor at the University of Brasília (UnB), where he began designing basic features of the ACS. By 1989, however, he had cofounded Ceará's state branch of the federal, public health–focused Oswaldo Cruz Foundation (FIOCRUZ), initiated the state's rollout of the ACS, and served as nationwide president of CONASEMS (SES-Ceará 2006). Other UFC-trained physicians from the earlier generation such as Dr. Anamaria Cavalcante e Silva, who had more specialized pediatrics training than did Cavalcante Brasil and Holanda Lavor, assumed Fortaleza's SMS directorship in 1988 at moment of rising power for municipalization struggles. Regardless of their training, a unifying feature of UFC-trained physicians such as Cavalcante e Silva and many of those she hired into the secretariat was a shared primary goal of developing programmatic strategies for reducing infant mortality in the capital (Mota 1997, 69–71).

Arising from student and prodemocracy movements of the late 1970s and 1980s, a second wave of sanitaristas in Fortaleza entered politics through more radical pathways of militancy, although they too eventually pursued intra-institutional repertoires of mobilization. For example, Dr. Luiz Odorico Monteiro de Andrade, future SMS secretary in Fortaleza and CONASEMS, initially organized student mobilizations in the small Ceará city of Icapuì before enrolling at UFC's medical school in 1982, where he earned a medical degree and master's degree in public health. After mobilizing within the Sanitarist Movement at UFC, Monteiro de Andrade continued his activism at the State University of Campinas in São Paulo state, where he earned a doctorate in public health. In 1986, after serving as a delegate of the National Student Union (UNE) at the Eight National Health Conference in Brasília, he emerged as a nationally recognized leader in the movement. Monteiro de Andrade describes his own transition into "the institutional movement" of sanitaristas as one in which assuming the position of SMS secretary offered the opportunity to reconcile discussions about sanitary reform with the reality of everyday people living with little or no access to health care (de Miranda Gondim 2011; Machado 2013). Other Fortalezan sanitaristas such as João Ananias Vasconcelos Neto and Raimundo José Arruda Bastos, who both later served as SES directors, followed roughly similar trajectories. As a student at UFC, where he finished his medical degree in 1980, Vasconcelos Neto also organized in the sanitarista, student, and prodemocracy movements in multiple venues. Initially, he helped both to establish sanitarista associations within UFC such as the Academic Center of Medicine and to reestablish broader student associations targeted by the dictatorship such as the Central Student Directorate (DCE).

As Brazil's dictatorship weakened and the country moved toward declaring a nationwide right to health in the mid-1980s, Fortaleza mirrored every other city in this study in that it featured a considerable local community of sanitaristas who were active in civil-society networks and organizations then pursuing democratization struggles and a right to health. Even before Brazil's Constitution codified a right to health, these capitals' sanitaristas had already begun influencing the local public health system in nontrivial ways as primary health workers, activists, and public health managers. But it was not the mere presence of a local sanitarista network that accounted for early expansion of the public health state in these capitals, although such networks were clearly essential. Rather, it was through their various forays as officeholders atop the SMS and SES that sanitaristas began to propel early institutional changes that helped reduce premature mortality in the capital. Sanitaristas earned reputations as qualified and competent holders of such positions, not just because of their technical qualifications and training in relevant medical fields but also because of their previous civil-society activism for the new rights-based SUS. Their activist pedigrees prefigured a future pattern of intra-institutional activism that had overtly political rather than just technical or administrative contours and ramifications for future efforts to reduce childhood mortality and improve public health outcomes more generally. Although sanitaristas' better-documented efforts in codifying the right to health clearly epitomize such political struggles, their subnational mobilizations to control the

SMS and SES directorships proved similarly consequential for local state-building and health outcomes in Fortaleza.

2. *Fortaleza's Programmatic Trajectory of Health Democratization*

As in Curitiba, Fortaleza's programmatic trajectory of health democratization featured both locally specific qualities as well as local reflections of more or less uniform, nationwide dynamics. The subnational state-building achievements of Fortaleza's office-holding sanitaristas rested in part on other, Brazil-wide dimensions of democratization addressed in earlier chapters. First, these achievements would not have been possible without the crystallization of more fundamental, Brazil-wide regulative institutions of civil society, such as elections, laws, and the local autonomy of subnational states arising from the country's far-reaching decentralization processes. Fortaleza's sanitaristas built new capacities of the subnational public health state atop an impressive foundation of nationwide regulative institutions that included the 1988 Constitution—with its declaration of state responsibility for enacting a universal right to health—and 1990 laws establishing the SUS to practically realize that right. Furthermore, the extensive decentralization of the new SUS transformed municipalities—already influential polities after the 1988 Constitution established them as "state-member" counterparts of the federal and state governments—into sites of considerable local autonomy that became uncommonly responsive to civil-society activism.

Further, few could dispute how nationwide dynamics helped transform subnational health politics in Fortaleza by restoring free and fair direct elections—first for Ceará's governorship in 1982 and then for Fortaleza's mayorship in 1985. Not surprisingly, this process generally replaced old-guard political elites in the subnational executive with candidates chosen through more thoroughgoing democratic processes. The localized incarnation of this more general process in Fortaleza and much of the Northeast generally weakened previously dominant coronels, though not immediately. Indeed, Ceará's first free and fair gubernatorial race since 1964 led to the election of Luis Gonzaga Mota (1983–1987), who had previously served as a planning secretary (1979–1982) during the second governorship of Virgílio Távora, a coronel notorious for patronage and corruption. Despite cultivating an image as a modern technocrat, Gonzaga Mota's administration proved decidedly nonprogrammatic, with the governor distributing large numbers of state jobs and public funds among other coronels and his campaign supporters, regardless of qualifications or competency (Gondim 2004: 69). But the pattern soon shifted, first with the 1985 election of PT candidate Maria Luiza Fontenele as Fortaleza's mayor and then with the 1986 election of Tasso Jereissati as governor. Both candidates won competitive elections featuring campaigns that emphasized an end to the endemic patronage associated with coronelismo (Barreira 1998; Gondim 1998, 2004; Ribeiro 1995). Although future mayors and governors in the capitals were hardly immune to criticisms of patronage-oriented management of the public health sector, free and fair direct elections through universal suffrage and party competition played a pivotal role in diminishing coronelismo and making more programmatic modes of governance possible in Fortaleza.

Second, Fortaleza mirrored the rest of urban Brazil in that sequential processes of political, fiscal, and administrative decentralization between 1982 and 1988 bequeathed its state and municipal governments with sweeping new responsibilities in the public health sector. Especially for a northeastern capital better known for minimal, ineffective, and unequal service provision in many public sectors, the mere assignment of Fortaleza's municipal government as the local body chiefly accountable for the primary health sector after 1988 marked a watershed moment in the capital's democratization. This decentralization of formal legal responsibility for managing the public health sector dovetailed with a third feature of health democratization: namely, normative and legal requirements that Fortaleza's SMS assume responsibility for the sector in a manner that fostered universality, integration, and equality in access to health (among other requirements). Manuel Dias de Fonseca Neto, a sanitarista whom Fontenele appointed as SMS director in 1986, alluded to the legal and material importance of this normative shift in establishing the SMS and the city's mayor as locally chosen "sanitary authorities" for realizing public health policy in Fortaleza (Mota 1997, 60). That Fonseca Neto embraced such principles even before their formal codification in Article 196 of the Constitution speaks to their weight as normative anchors that grounded later formal specifications.

Far from merely reflecting homogenous nationwide dynamics, however, other dimensions of health democratization varied considerably across urban Brazil and in Fortaleza. A fourth, subnationally variable dimension of

Fortaleza's programmatic trajectory involved how subnational executives, who replaced the erstwhile political elites destabilized by elections and growing political competition in the capital, varied from their predecessors. Although some proved to be more ideologically progressive in their actual governance of public-service sectors than did others, one unifying feature of most subnational executives in Fortaleza was a general embrace of political and economic liberalism. Thus, when compared to cases of minimalist health democratization such as Rio de Janeiro and especially Salvador, Fortaleza's electoral politics featured a relative absence of rule by the same traditional clientelist politicians who dominated the capital during the dictatorship. With the exception of Luis Gonzaga Mota's victory in the first direct gubernatorial election, the politicians who captured governorships and mayoralties in Fortaleza were democratic liberals of various stripes who hailed from the left-leaning PT and PSB as well as the more centrist PSDB and PMBD. And whereas Tasso Jereissati, Ceara's three-time governor (1987–1991, 1995–2002), typified the class of young entrepreneurs who first captured gubernatorial power as successful businessmen and lawyers, other governors and most of Fortaleza's mayors initially emerged from public-service-oriented professional classes that included university professors, journalists, and doctors (Gondim 2004, 68–72).

Although some Fortalezan mayors and Cearán governors embraced more progressive political ideologies than others, subnational executives in the capital generally managed the state in less overtly clientelist ways than they did in cases of minimalist health democratization such as Salvador. Rather, Fortalezan mayor from parties with a surprisingly wide array of political ideologies remained open to the state-building proposals of pragmatically inclined civil-society actors, especially its sanitaristas. Indeed, such openness was not limited to the PT mayorships of Fontenele (1986–1988) and Luziane Lins (2005–2012) or the PSB (and later PTB) administration of sanitarista mayor Roberto Cláudio (2013–), although such leaders harbored especially progressive ambitions for health-sector and public governance reform. The PSDB (and later the PSB) of Ciro Gomes and Tasso Jereissati, the PMDB of Juraci Vieira de Magalhães, and the PSB of Cid Gomes all feature a similar openness. Although the more centrist of these parties embraced liberal economic principles more fully, they drew upon civil society in complex ways that were distinct from other, clear cases of cooptation in these cities.[5] Probing these patterns offers a fruitful ground for more clearly explaining Fortaleza's trajectory, especially since the PT held its mayorship only during a brief period (1986–1988) that preceded municipal control of the public health sector and during a subsequent period (2005–2012) that followed its most significant improvements in IMR.

In this regard, it is notable that Fortaleza's sanitaristas proved capable of forging alliances with mayors from more centrist parties, such as the PSDB of Ciro Gomes (1989–1990) and the PMDB of Juraci Viera de Magalhães (1990–1992, 1997–2000) and Antônio Cambraia (1993–1996), rather than just with PT and PSB mayors. Among their other consequences, such connections contributed to a pattern in which Fortaleza's mayors rarely excluded sanitaristas from health-policy-making and management in the consistent manner that occurred in Rio de Janeiro and Salvador. Indeed, Viera de Magalhães appointed the sanitarista Dr. Abner Cavalcante Brasil as SMS secretary during his first term, and Gomes appointed a pediatrician, Dr. Anamaria Cavalcante e Silva, whose stated priorities revolved around both expanding primary preventative health care for pregnant women and children and ending the patronage-oriented approach to public health policy of coronelismo (Mota 1997, 69, 72). In short, ruling parties of the center and center-left in Fortaleza generally shared an openness to integrating sanitaristas in part because of their qualifications as problem solvers with actionable proposals for accomplishing relatively uncontroversial public goals such as the reduction of infant mortality. Thus, although Fortaleza lacked the more extended pattern of mayoral rule by left parties observable in distinct cases of participatory-democratic democratization of health like Porto Alegre, Belo Horizonte, and Recife, its mayors shared with these other cities an openness to empowering civil-society actors with programmatic schemes for improving the effectiveness of the primary public health sector in addressing vexing public problems such as rampant infant mortality.

Thus, the newly competitive terrain of local electoral politics was not just salient for the health-democratization period because it created chances for Brazil's most progressive parties to contest and win power, although this undoubtedly helped where it occurred. Rather, the restoration of democracy mattered greatly because of how it undermined the electoral prospects of certain parties—particularly clientelist and right-wing parties. Such parties differed from a range of center and center-left parties that generally mirrored left parties such as the PT in welcoming the problem-solving interventions that sanitaristas offered for addressing public health crises like rampant childhood mortality. Especially when contrasted with cases of minimalist health democratization in cities featuring far weaker party institutionalization (for example, Salvador), subnational executives in Fortaleza hailed from a surprisingly diverse array of left and centrist parties that entertained early and sustained public problem-solving interventions by pragmatist publics such as the city's sanitaristas and often embraced the policy proposals of such actors as their own. Not merely confined to the PT—Brazil's most renowned and successful programmatic party throughout the period—such openness was essential for the ability of sanitaristas to precociously and consistently establish public health as a sustained priority of the cities' most important reformist mayors and governors in Fortaleza. In this regard, the city fundamentally differed from other capitals such as Salvador and Rio de Janeiro, in which clientelist mayors and governors almost uniformly blocked similar sanitarista proposals until a comparatively late moment and instead governed the public health sector in a generally patronage-based fashion that was nonprogrammatic by definition. Among other manifestations of these underlying dynamics, mayors and governors in Fortaleza generally embraced and sought to maximize the reach of programmatic, nationwide interventions, beginning especially during the 1990s with openness to the PSF and forerunners of Brazil's CCT, Bolsa Família.

A fifth, related quality of Fortaleza's programmatic trajectory was that nationwide antipoverty programs such as Bolsa Família (BF) achieved a breadth of coverage that was among the widest in urban Brazil. For instance, Fortaleza was among urban Brazil's top performers in its targeting rate, or the proportion of eligible families who actually received transfers through the program. With an average targeting rate of 88.84% between the program's inception in 2004 and 2016, Fortaleza was surpassed in this regard only by other cases of robust development such as Belo Horizonte (93.57%), Porto Alegre (96.78%), and Recife (89.91%). Additionally, Fortaleza's record appears even more impressive when considering that the proportion of enrolled families to total families, or the coverage rate, also ranked highly among major Brazilian capitals. Indeed, Fortaleza's average coverage rate of 69.8% was unsurpassed by any other city addressed in this study, suggesting that the program had an especially far-reaching significance for a large proportion of residents. Extensive access to social programs such as Bolsa Família epitomizes another dimension of programmatic health democratization beyond statistical evidence from this and other studies about the effects of BF coverage on infant mortality rates: it indicates how Fortalezans have increasingly shifted toward accessing state benefits in an institutionalized manner that is comparatively freer of clientelism than in the city's very recent history.

Sixth, Fortaleza shared with Curitiba a pattern of early and sustained expansion of the subnational public health state's service-delivery arms. In terms of primary public-health-care facilities per capita, Fortaleza ranked among urban Brazil's top performers with 119 primary-care-focused health units (US) for its approximately 831,524 exclusive SUS users. Furthermore, the municipality organized service provision largely according to the PSF model, achieving a ratio of approximately 5,358 exclusive SUS users per PSF team (311). During the 2005 to 2012 period, these capacities included an average of 9,385 exclusive SUS users per PSF team and an impressive 311 PSF teams that by 2015 had lowered this ratio to nearly 5,000. In these respects, Fortaleza ranked among other top performers such as Belo Horizonte, Porto Alegre, and Recife. I return shortly to the step-by-step construction of these capacities in Fortaleza. But when tracing the sources of major expansions in staff, clinics, and other municipal capacities for delivering basic health care through the PSF, the most salient point is that office-holding sanitaristas were never far from the state-building action.

To mold the public health state in decisive ways, Fortaleza's sanitaristas established and fortified communicative and regulative institutions of the movement. Crucially, their mobilizations to equalize and universalize access to primary health care predated—and even helped to precipitate—crystallization of both the right to health and new democratic offices for realizing it. After 1988, sanitaristas increasingly sought to infuse the politically appointed positions of Municipal Health Department (SMS) director and State Health Department (SES) director with new normative responsibilities of the SUS manager, a new democratic office that became publicly accountable for the pursuit of universality and equity in access to health. To be sure, sanitaristas buttressed these efforts by cultivating communicative institutions of civil society, including local chapters of sanitarista associations such as CONASEMS and CEBES. Yet regulative institutions of democratic office became increasingly important for sanitarista efforts to not only enact laws that enshrined a universal right to health but also influence subnational executives who projected an openness to involving civil society in public problem solving.

Particularly given this impressive record of access to mortality-reducing primary public health care, it is notable that Fortaleza's programmatic trajectory of health democratization unfolded despite only weak and late-breaking experiences with participatory democracy. Analysts of its Participatory Budgeting process note that even the electoral campaign of Luzianne Lins, the PT mayor who introduced OP in 2005, characterized Fortaleza as generally lacking any previous culture of participatory politics (de Sousa Arão 2012, 60).[6] In this sense, Fortaleza could hardly be compared to capitals such as Porto Alegre or Belo Horizonte in which, even before the introduction of OP, neighborhood associations and community groups had long demanded participatory institutions for more directly channeling civil-society inputs into public-service-related policy making, including the health sector. Indeed, Fortaleza mirrored Curitiba far more in the inability of participatory publics to win the support of political society for new and more radically devolutionary modes of public policy making such as OP. Furthermore, for the purposes of this study's primary project of explaining robust development, it is difficult to argue that OP was a central cause of robust development in Fortaleza, if only because its seminal experiences with OP and other participatory institutions began well after the capital's most sweeping reductions in infant mortality rates rather than alongside or before them.

Similarly, Fortaleza's Municipal Health Council (CMS), which was created in 1990 by Municipal Decree #8,417, has long struggled to influence or even consistently monitor major state-building processes in the primary health sector. The CMS of Fortaleza exhibits the basic features legally required of it as an autonomous body that deliberates about local implementation of the SUS. For example, Articles 1 and 2 of the CMS's constitution outline its purpose as contributing to the formulation and control of health policy in its economic, financial, and technical administrative dimensions. Additionally, members of the body choose their own president (as opposed to the city SMS secretary also serving as its president automatically), internally formulate its agenda, and reach decisions, through open votes of all members, that require majorities to pass (Faria 2007, 119–21). Furthermore, the most prevalent decisions of CMS-Fortaleza during a brief period in 2003–2004 concerned public health programs, whereas the body regularly addressed health-policy-making and attempted to guide associated state actions.[7] Still, there is little to suggest that the state-building that propelled Fortaleza's most important, mortality-reducing interventions in the primary health sector emanated from the council itself. As was also the case in Curitiba, Fortaleza's health council initially faced a slow institutionalization throughout the 1990s and hesitancy on the part of mayors and municipal health secretaries to fully integrate it into actual public health planning and decision-making. Even sanitarista secretaries of the SMS such as Dr. Abner Cavalcante Brasil, who were generally sympathetic to the council's goals of infusing civil-society preferences into municipal health-policy-making, described the process of working with community organizations and neighborhood health councils as a difficult one that required bounding the power of such entities (Mota 1997, 68–69). Furthermore, when tracing major state-building shifts in the primary health sector, it has more often been the case that participatory institutions supported proposals that were initiated and carried to fruition by office-holding sanitaristas. Overall, Fortaleza's most important participatory-democratic bodies for influencing the public health sector generally mirrored those of Curitiba in suffering from an only distant proximity to the state-building levers that matter most for IMR reduction, reflecting how the city's participatory publics struggled to transform the CMS into an actual cogoverning body in practice.

Yet the absence of such stronger democratic controls on the state, the likes of which defined trajectories of participatory-programmatic health democratization in Belo Horizonte and Porto Alegre, were not necessary for robust expansions in access to primary health care or for reductions in infant mortality. As such, Fortaleza offers another crucial case for this study's core argument that sanitarista-driven expansion of new programmatic capacities onto the subnational public health state was the core mechanism by which health democratization affected robust development outcomes. Next, I turn to the unfolding of these dynamics in Fortaleza.

3. Sanitarista Office Holding and Expansion of Fortaleza's Public Health State

Even before national-level sanitarista mobilizations helped codify a nationwide right to health and establish the SUS, sanitaristas in Fortaleza were propelling some of Brazil's most important state-building initiatives for the primary health sector. Indeed, Brazil's highly publicized public health achievements in Ceará began during the late 1980s with an impressive reduction of infant mortality achieved by expanding primary public-health-care delivery through its trailblazing Community Health Agents (ACS) program. These impressive statewide reductions in mortality, documented by the seminal work of Judith Tendler (1997), garnered the state government considerable global recognition in policy circles.[8] Yet long-standing accounts of this canonical intervention emphasize the program's design elements and the motivations of on-the-ground service providers while focusing less on the civil-society agents who architected the program and successfully advocated for state government to adopt it by occupying offices atop the subnational health state. As such, existing accounts overlook how such major expansions in state capacity reflected underlying shifts in the civil-society institution of democratic office that can regulate such interventions given favorable circumstances. In other words, Fortaleza's pre-SUS reforms offer insights into how the capacity-building efforts of civil societies in democratic office can translate ideologies of universal access to health into tangible interventions by states that help materialize such otherwise abstract notions.

3.1. CONSISTENT SANITARISTA OFFICE HOLDING, STATE-BUILDING, AND ROBUST IMR DECLINE, 1987–1992

Between 1987 and 1992, sanitaristas helped build subnational regulative institutions such as political parties and new democratic offices of the SUS that played a major role in fostering the mortality-reducing capacities and interventions of Fortaleza's municipal public health state. Although they involved distinct actors and contours that were particular to the politics of Fortaleza's municipal polity, these state-building efforts were initially linked to sanitarista propulsion of the impressive infant mortality reductions for which Ceará's state government became globally renowned. In describing how he won political-party support for the introduction of the ACS in Ceará, the program's main sanitarista architect, Antônio Carlile Holanda Lavor, described the process of seizing opportunities presented by the nascent electoral strategy of the PSDB and its gubernatorial candidate in 1986, Tasso Jereissati, as one that involved careful strategic calculations. Yet Holanda Lavor's intervention was also one that sought to mobilize such parties to advance the solidary principles of universality and equality so central to sanitary reform.

> I was an early proponent that our group join the PSDB, thinking that this new party was the most coherent and attuned to the project that we had in

mind for Ceará. . . . Tasso's initial group was very business oriented and largely saw government as an instrument for Ceará's economic modernization. But we brought a social weight to the group. Without many previous ties, the group met Tasso only very soon before the election, but he recognized how our group supported the message of governmental modernization that he had in mind. And we made a strong and enduring alliance (Paranaguá de Santana and Lima de Castro 2016, 43, my translation).

In this sense, the reformist health-sector interventions for which Ceará's politicians became famous in nationwide and global development circles depended, at least in part, on sanitarista molding of priorities within the key political party that would hold gubernatorial power for the next twenty years. More specifically, sanitarista mobilizations such as those described by Holanda Lavor infused ideological tenets of sanitary reform into the political priorities of ruling party elites within Ceara's PSDB, which otherwise lacked any programmatic plans for addressing the public health crisis of rampant infant mortality in the state.[9] Importantly, however, political-society elites in control of the party proved open to the modest state-building proposals of sanitaristas, who offered to serve as their architects and chief enactors. Yet such openness was generally reserved for the proposals of cohesive civil-society actors such as Fortaleza's sanitaristas, particularly during opportune moments such as election years and natural disasters that infused new sources of emergency funding.

Still, Fortaleza's impressive 55% reduction in infant mortality in only four years—from 64.74 in 1988 to 29.15 in 1992—cannot be attributed to the state government's ACS, if only because Fortaleza was the lone município in Ceará that did not operate the program by the end of this period (Tendler 1997, 173). How is it possible that Fortaleza's municipal government reduced infant mortality by a roughly similar degree as that which occurred statewide[10] despite lacking the main programmatic cause typically credited for Ceará's statewide achievements? In short, the same kinds of sanitarista-driven capacity-building processes that expanded state-level health institutions also built similar new capacities of Fortaleza's municipal public health state to reduce mortality. But the particular sanitarista agents of this expansion and the specific programmatic guises that this process generated were different in Fortaleza than in the rest of Ceará. On the statewide level, it was Holanda Lavor who leveraged the state-level office of SES director and infiltrated the highest levels of Ceará's PSDB to first translate sanitarista proposals for universalizing primary health care via the ACS.

Within Fortaleza itself, a different set of office-holding sanitaristas sought from an early moment to build basic institutional capacities of Fortaleza's SMS for expanding primary health care delivery, initially outside the framework of Ceará's famous experiment with the ACS. Although the earliest efforts between 1986 and 1988 were particularly constrained by a lack of basic administrative control over public health facilities and the health professionals who worked in them,[11] the pattern changed significantly in 1989 with the advent of the constitutionally mandated local control of the public health sector. The capital's first SMS secretary of the SUS era was a UFC-trained pediatrician, Dr. Anamaria Cavalcante e Silva, who had previously directed the Dr. Albert Sabin Infant Hospital in the capital and held positions coordinating primary health care delivery in the capital's Porgangbassu neighborhood (SES-Ceará 2006). During the mid-1980s, Cavalcante e Silva had become an increasingly active participant in the discussions that Holanda Lavor convened to crystallize a strategy among sanitaristas for reforming the state's public health sector (Paranaguá de Santana and Lima de Castro 2016, 43). Before later serving as Ceará's SES director (1991–1994), Cavalcante e Silva first served as Fortaleza's SMS director in 1989 and 1990 under the mayorship of Ciro Gomes, then also a member of the PSDB organization that Ceará's sanitaristas had successfully mobilized to pursue movement goals surrounding primary health care expansion.

Although she served as SMS director for less than two years, Cavalcante e Silva pursued a similar approach to building new capacities of the municipal state as the one that Holanda Lavor pursued on the state level. Her first major step was to sign an agreement with both the federal health ministry and Ceará's SES specifying terms of Fortaleza's municipalization of health-service provision and formalizing its takeover of nearly all primary-care clinics within the município's geographic boundaries (Mota 1997, 65). One of the first of its kind in all of Brazil, the agreement dramatically expanded the network of health care facilities under municipal control in a manner that would not be matched in other major northeastern capitals, such as Salvador, until nearly a decade later. It also opened the way for her and subsequent SMS directors to pursue a variety of avenues for building new municipal state capacities to deliver primary public health care. The particularly cohesive manner in which Cavalcante e Silva took these initial steps mirrors the relatively assertive, decisive, and nonconsultative approach that Holanda Lavor exhibited in enacting the statewide ACS program and that Curitiban sanitaristas such as Luciano Ducci demonstrated when enacting the Curitiban Mother Program (*Programa Mãe Curitibana*, PMC). Upon assuming the SMS directorship, she developed no immediate, explicit agenda for her tenure and initially maintained distance from institutional bureaucrats on the secretariat's planning team before iteratively pursuing a series of small reforms aimed at enhancing capacities for service delivery to children, mothers, and pregnant women.

Among the multiple initial interventions that Cavalcante e Silva made in this regard was the reassignment of municipal health professionals previously working at SMS headquarters to geographically dispersed, neighborhood-based health units located throughout the city. The ranks of these reallocated employees included pediatricians specializing in infant respiratory care and other personnel with experience in prenatal and postnatal care. Additionally, Cavalcante e Silva's administration created a new department within the SMS, the Engineering Service, which began during her tenure to renovate parts of municipal clinics dedicated to infant care. These initiatives included the opening of new treatment rooms for administering vaccinations and oral rehydration therapy to infants as well as the renovation of treatment rooms for infants suffering from acute respiratory infection and malnutrition. Alongside this initiative, Cavalcante e Silva opened nutrition centers that operated through community partnerships with residents of the poorest peripheral regions in the city. More generally, Cavalcante e Silva vertically integrated programs for providing services to mothers, children, and pregnant women throughout all stages of pregnancy. Additionally, she initiated the process of opening new concursos for municipal positions within the SMS for three clinical doctors, three gynecologists, and associated teams of obstetricians and pediatricians, all of whom were trained in the theory and practice of delivering primary health services in the city's public clinics (Mota 1997, 69–74).

The state-building and mortality-reduction consequences of Cavalcante e Silva's interventions were considerable. By the end of her administration, the SMS had signed agreements to take over five hospitals and seventeen health posts and had begun undertaking major renovations to these facilities (Mota 1997, 74). Local control and a new focus on targeting primary-care delivery in these municipally run facilities to pregnant women, new mothers, and infants was reflected in unprecedented rates of IMR reduction. Specifically, when Cavalcante e Silva entered office in 1988, Fortaleza's IMR was 64.74 deaths per 1,000 live births, but by 1992, the year after she exited the office, the rate had fallen by a considerable 55% to only 29.15. Amid Ciro Gomes's resignation as mayor in 1990 to run what became his successful campaign for Ceará's governorship, Cavalcante e Silva's tenure as SMS director came to an end. But her work in pursuing infant mortality reduction was hardly complete. On the heels of her recognized success in this regard within the boundaries of Fortaleza, Gomes subsequently appointed her as Ceará's SES director in 1991. Among its other effects, the appointment opened a political space for continuing the state-level pattern of subnational capacity-building that Holanda Lavor initiated in 1987.

After Gomes's vice mayor, Juraci Vieira de Magalhães, assumed the mayorship vacated by Gomes and subsequently won reelection to the office in 1990, he appointed a fellow doctor and another sanitarista, Dr. Abner Cavalcante Brasil, as SMS director. Although Cavalcante Brasil aimed to continue expanding the municipal public health state in the manner begun by Cavalcante e Silva, he enjoyed an even less conducive environment for doing so. In part, this was reflected in how sanitaristas had not infiltrated the new mayor's PMDB party to the same extent that they had Ceará's PSDB, the PSDB's local branches in other capitals such as Belo Horizonte and São Paulo, or the PSDB's nationwide organization, for that matter. Further, diverse observers of Magalhães's administrations agree on the view that the successful electoral strategy that eventually won him three mayoral elections generally was rooted in a populism that prioritized highly visible public works projects, including major roads and viaducts located in Fortaleza's city center, over less conspicuous improvements such as reductions in infant mortality rates (Bruno, de Farias, and Andrade 2002; Gondim 2004; Mota 1997). Despite this context, Cavalcante Brasil still secured mayoral support to municipalize seventeen health posts and five regional hospitals from federal and state governments while undertaking further infrastructural improvements to existing facilities (Mota 1997, 73–74).

Importantly, these sanitarista-led state-building achievements between 1988 and 1992 reflected national-level health-sector reforms that would not have emerged locally or assumed the progressive features they did in Fortaleza without local sanitarista interventions. To be sure, national-level changes such as the codification of both a right to health and creation of the SUS for enacting that right had an indisputable influence on Fortaleza's achievements, in part by enshrining long-standing sanitarista demands for the SUS and SUS manager's office as the law of the land. But the subnational state-building processes that practically narrowed the gulf between these laws and their enactment in Fortaleza ultimately depended as much on changes that sanitaristas such as Holanda Lavor, Cavalcante e Silva, and Cavalcante Brasil made to subnational democratic institutions. More specifically, Fortaleza's sanitaristas helped translate the normative principles of sanitary reform on which nationwide laws were predicated into the actual practice of locally ruling political elites and their party organizations and of subnational offices of the SUS manager.

Thus, expansive state-building resulted from initial sanitarista interventions that paved the way for a continuous stream of later ones. Indeed, Fortaleza's highly organized sanitaristas did not manage to infuse the organizations of all major ruling political parties with a deep or abiding embrace of core movement principles. They also did not wait for the Organic Health Laws' formal establishment of subnational SUS manager offices to begin wielding the SMS directorship as the "sanitary authority" that these laws specified it to be. Rather, the enactment of modest but consequential state-building projects first emerged from sanitaristas infusing select tenets of sanitary reform into the political parties of subnational political elites. Additionally, sanitaristas leveraged the SMS directorship to secure executives' support for small and iterative changes that simultaneously advanced their electoral goals and better aligned the public health state with such principles.

In this sense, Fortaleza's precocious, sanitarista-driven municipalization of the primary health sector accomplished two major feats. Cavalcante e Silva's initial interventions in 1989 to sign the official agreements with state and federal government induced the practical compliance of Fortaleza's municipal government with the new legal responsibility for managing an entire service-provision sector, all at a comparatively early moment for urban Brazil. The immediate consequences of this intervention were considerable, with Fortaleza officially making the single largest expansion of the city's primary health care network of facilities and workers in its history. But the intervention also triggered a subsequent repurposing of the municipality's service-delivery institutions to better advance sanitary reform ideals of universality and equity in access to health and of IMR reduction. Although the initial moment of municipalization in 1989 had brought five hospitals and seventeen primary health clinics under the control of the SMS, iterative expansions during the following four years left Fortaleza with a total of ten hospitals, eighty-nine outpatient health clinics, and nineteen laboratories of some kind. By the year after Cavalcante Brasil's departure, the SMS had become a bureaucracy with 1,246 doctors, 117 dentists, 355 nurses, 115 pharmacists, 135 other high-level personnel, and 2,947 low- or mid-level workers.[12] Ultimately, these far-reaching sanitarista interventions go a long way toward explaining Fortaleza's robust reduction of nearly 35 deaths per 1,000 in only the first five years after the capital's return to democracy.

3.2. SIDELINED SANITARISTAS, MINIMAL STATE-BUILDING, AND TEPID IMR REDUCTIONS, 1993–2004

If Cavalcante e Silva and Cavalcante Brasil had previously added new IMR-reducing capacities, Fortaleza's next decade illustrates how deleterious the absence of office holding by sanitaristas in the SUS directorship was for such processes. Indeed, sanitaristas rarely held the municipal or state-level offices of SUS manager during these twelve years, and IMR reduction initially backslid before recovering some of its earlier gains to post a weak overall degree of change throughout the phase. Especially for a phase that witnessed much greater gains across urban Brazil's other major capitals, Fortaleza's 2002 IMR of 23.32 had improved relatively little from its starting point of 29.15 a decade earlier. In fact, IMR actually worsened during initial years of this phase, increasing from 29.15 in 1992 to 40.11 in 1996 under the PMDB mayorship of Antônio Cambraia (1993–1996) before restabilizing at a level of 29.56 in 1998 during Magalhães's second mayorship. Although one of the few programmatic interventions during this time was Fortaleza's delayed implementation of the Community Health Agents Program (PACS) previously rolled out to every município in Ceará by sanitaristas such as Holanda Lavor, the program achieved only 38% coverage of city regions deemed to be at risk for premature death (Ramos Batista et al. 2005, 26). And by 2004, when Fortaleza concluded its fifteen-year period of uninterrupted PMDB rule, the previous years of sanitarista office holding accounted for the lion's share of the episode's IMR reductions.

Among its other insights, this phase illustrates how relationships between the absence of sanitarista office holding and weak mortality reduction are not just associations but have causal links as well. A major reason for the flatlining in IMR reduction during this period was that the absence of office-holding sanitaristas in the SMS directorship effectively removed the single most important source of both political pressure and problem-solving competency necessary to expand state capacity for primary public-health-care delivery. Although the sequence of SMS directors during this period included physicians such as Dr. Raimundo Coelho Bezerra de Farias, Dr. José Adelmo Mendes Martinsk, and Dr. Galeno Taumaturgo Lopes, it also included individuals such as Renato Parente Filho, who possessed neither public health training of any kind nor experience in the medical profession. What all these directors shared, however, was a relative lack of experience in prior civil-society mobilizations to crystallize sanitary reform principles of universal and equal access to health, particularly when compared to their sanitarista predecessors and successors. Additionally, few had training or experience working in primary-care provision, as their sanitarista predecessors had in spades. Thus, even though IMR reduction becomes more difficult to achieve at lower levels, the near flatlining of IMR reduction that occurred in Fortaleza during this phase was below average even for urban Brazil at the time, although that is unsurprising from the standpoint of this study's central hypothesis about pragmatist movement office holding. Ultimately, insulating sanitaristas from the state-building powers of the SUS manager's office contributed to adverse outcomes by effectively sidelining their continued proposals for expanding Fortaleza's municipal health workers and primary health clinics.

Seen in this light, the minimal IMR reductions that were achieved during this phase can be partially attributed to nationwide qualities of health democratization that affected nearly every other major capital in Brazil, including Fortaleza. In response to federal health ministry encouragements to adopt the PSF via its SUS Basic Operating Norm of 1996 (NOB-96), Magalhães in 1997 named a technical commission to assess needs for implementing the program, which Fortaleza adopted in 1998 (Ramos Batista et al. 2005, 27). Although the reasons for Fortaleza's ultimate adoption are many and complex, Magalhães's rift with his former ally Tasso Jereissati, then governor of Ceará (Bruno, de Farias, and Andrade 2002, 19; Gondim 2004, 72), was not insignificant. Like other mayors of major capitals at the time, Magalhães did not balk at the opportunity that PSF adoption presented to effectively redirect a modicum of federal public health funding around the governor and directly into municipal coffers.

Yet unlike its previous phase, when office-holding sanitaristas in administrations with similarly centrist parties had robustly expanded human and infrastructural resources for mortality-focused primary-care delivery, Fortaleza introduced the PSF in only a very limited way that served relatively few city neighborhoods. During the first full year of the program (1999), for example, the município hired only fifty PSF teams, a number that had grown relatively little for a city of its size to a total of seventy-seven in the year after Magalhães left office. And while coverage rates never exceeded 16% during the remainder of Magalhães's mayorships (1999 to 2004), they actually contracted to under 12% immediately after his departure. Furthermore, the number of PSF teams that had been working during these initial years of the program fluctuated widely, from as many as 101 teams for parts of 2001 and 2002 to as few as 32 in late 2004. In part, this was due to the precarious, temporary contracting of PSF workers using six-month-long "emergency" contracts, typically justified by the administration's claims that the SMS could not afford to hire PSF workers as actual municipal employees. Both the SMS and COOPSAÙDE, a contracting agency it hired as an intermediary, used such practices to hire all levels of PSF workers, including doctors. PSF workers during this period unsurprisingly complained of delayed payments and that they lacked firm connections to the municipal bureaucracy or any other permanent state agency (Coelho 2006; de Oliveira Viana Esmeraldo 2009).

Considering its comparatively weak performance during the 1993 to 2004 phase, it is interesting that the decade did not lack for an official discourse of supposed attention to building the primary public health sector and reducing infant mortality. Indeed, Cambraia's government published a Pluri-Annual Plan for the 1994–1997 quadrennial that named infant mortality reduction, health care for children, and improvements in the quality of health services among its priorities (Ramos Batista et al. 2005, 26). Furthermore, the administration overhauled the municipal bureaucracy through Law 8,000 of 1997, which stipulated that municipal government would be organized for the purposes of guaranteeing citizens' access to services, information, and participation in official decisions regarding urban space where they live (Ramos Batista et al. 2005, 27). Among the implications of this reform for delivery of public health services was the division of city regions into service-delivery jurisdictions called Sanitary Districts, a requirement generally made by the federal health ministry at the time for cities to be given deeper responsibilities for the health facilities within their boundaries. Additionally, these measures subjected some aspects of managing neighborhood-based health clinics to consultation by community groups within center-based health councils.

But despite its discourse, the material record of Magalhães's administration speaks for itself, with few detectable additions of meaningful new state capacities necessary for maximizing the reach of primary health care. In this regard, decentralization measures emanating from the federal level—rather than from any detectable municipal-level agency—for building the primary health sector had the most bearing on Fortaleza's municipal capacities for primary-care delivery during this phase. For instance, a series of the federal health ministry's SUS Basic Operating Norms (NOBs) instituted a new system for transferring federal resources for health into municipal control. The norms changed how transfers were made, first by instituting general block grants for health (NOB-93), then by establishing parcels that separated out the primary health sector (NOB-98), and then by specifying programmatic uses such as costs of administering the PSF (NOB-2001/2002; Carvalho de Noronha, Dias de Lima, and Vieira Machado 2008, 459–60). For an administration whose patronage-based, populist approach came to be associated with the derisory trademark of "works, friends, and votes," these NOBs could only have improved the possibility for channeling federal health funding toward its intended uses (Bruno, de Farias, and Andrade 2002, 19; Gondim 2004, 72). But such changes were instituted relatively contemporaneously across urban Brazil, rendering it difficult to argue that they had any special relevance for hiring primary service providers and for constructing or renovating primary health facilities in Fortaleza relative to other major capitals. Not surprisingly, Fortaleza ended this interstice between episodes of more consistent sanitarista office holding with only mediocre gains in IMR reduction.

3.3. SANITARISTA OFFICE HOLDING, EXTENSIVE STATE-BUILDING, AND ROBUST IMR DECLINE, 2005–2016

The decade between 2005 to 2016 witnessed a return of influential sanitaristas to the SMS directorship as well as a correspondingly elaborate phase of state-building that catapulted Fortaleza into the ranks of urban Brazil's highest-performing reducers of IMR. During these twelve years, sanitaristas occupied both the municipal and state-level offices of SUS manager in a nearly uninterrupted fashion, and IMR reduction was continuous and robust. Specifically, despite entering this phase with an IMR of nearly 19.88, Fortaleza had again nearly halved IMR by 2015 (to 10.68). To be sure, other dimensions of programmatic health democratization in the city contributed to these impressive gains, including sustained rule by left-party mayors, the introduction of participatory-democratic institutions, and consistently high average levels of Bolsa Família's targeting (88.84%) and coverage rates (69.8%). A less-noted driver of these improvements, however, was the modest but sustained state-building that office-holding sanitaristas pursued in their efforts to further expand primary health care delivery. In this sense, the post-2005 period demonstrates that a central, causal link between sanitarista office holding and robust IMR reduction was a resumption and deepening of the sanitarista-driven state-building that had previously launched Fortaleza's initial trend of primary-care-fueled IMR reductions nearly three decades earlier.

One of the most important sanitarista agents of this state-building phase was Dr. Luiz Odorico Monteiro de Andrade, who served as Fortaleza's SMS director from 2005 to 2009 under PT mayor Luzianne Lins. Before assuming this role, Monteiro de Andrade had a long history of activism in the Sanitarist Movement, spanning from extra-institutional mobilizations for the right to health and democracy during the 1980s to eventually occupying the prestigious CONASEMS presidency. In 1988, Monteiro de Andrade became one of Brazil's first SMS directors to implement the ACS program in Icapuí, the first of four Ceárn cities in which he held the post.[13] In 1993, Monteiro de Andrade drew on such direct implementation experiences to both codesign the PSF and help convince the federal health minister to adopt it on a nationwide basis (Borges Sugiyama 2012, 139–40). This advocacy helped induce the MS's absorption of the ACS into a revised PSF model that deployed doctors, nurses, and nurses' assistants alongside community health agents in larger, more highly trained teams. Thus, when Monteiro de Andrade assumed the post of SMS director in Fortaleza, he did so not only as one of the most powerful and broadly recognized sanitaristas in all of Brazil but also as someone intimately familiar with the PSF's design and the need for aggressive municipal support to effectively implement it.

In 2005, the first year after Magalhães's last mayoral term ended, Monteiro de Andrade orchestrated just such support at a moment in which the SMS possessed only minimal inherited capacities for delivering primary health services through the PSF model. Fortaleza's SMS began the year before Monteiro de Andrade's appointment with only seventy-seven precariously contracted PSF teams in place. Given Fortaleza's low economic development levels and correspondingly below average proportion of residents with access to the private sector marketplace for health services, these seventy-seven teams only translated into a ratio of approximately 24,829 exclusive SUS users for every PSF team, a level that ranked worse during 2005 than did all other capitals in this study except Rio de Janeiro. Furthermore, the SMS controlled relatively few (eighty-eight) primary health clinics, only twenty-seven of which the PSF teams used for delivering services (de Oliveira Viana Esmeraldo 2009, 89). As a result, populational coverage through the PSF languished at only 11.77%, a level that also ranked next to last, in front of only Rio de Janeiro. Furthermore, the precarious contracts through which most PSF workers labored undermined consistency and stability in the actual services delivered by Fortaleza's PSF teams, in part because of the SMS's persistent difficulties in retaining doctors, nurses, and nurse's assistants, who frequently left their positions to pursue other, more stable job prospects with longer time horizons.[14]

Strongly motivated to advance what he viewed as a programmatic expression of sanitary reform principles such as universality and equity in access to primary health, Monteiro de Andrade immediately launched a dramatic expansion of the program. The core of this expansion involved radically increasing the ranks of Fortaleza's PSF teams and clinics, the results of which were striking. In 2010, the year after Monteiro de Andrade left the office, the SMS had tripled both the number of PSF teams it implanted, to 258, as well as the program's populational coverage, which reached 35.53%. Although Monteiro de Andrade had initially envisioned an even larger expansion—to 460 teams—the actual increases that were made still dramatically reduced Fortaleza's ratio of exclusive SUS users to PSF teams to 6,891.[15] In addition to these sheer quantitative expansions in coverage, several qualities of these gains were also notable.

Specifically, Monteiro de Andrade's interventions promoted longer-term sustainability of PSF teams, improved training for the health professionals that constituted them, and adopted more sophisticated, epidemiologically and territorially based means of targeting these teams to city regions facing the most serious health risks. First, Monteiro de Andrade regularized the status of the newly hired workers in ways that mirrored the interventions of his sanitarista counterparts in SUS directorships of other cities, including Porto Alegre's Dr. Lucio Barcelos. In 2006, he effectively ended the practice of contracting PSF workers through precarious six-month contracts and instead hired all new workers for the program using public concursos that observed meritocratic, competition-based recruiting standards.[16] The results of this hiring wave were impressive, with the SMS offering positions as municipal employees to 850 health professionals in one of its largest ever expansions. These professionals included 300 doctors, 300 nurses, and 250 dentists.[17] By the end of 2010, Fortaleza's PSF had correspondingly tripled its populational coverage to 35.53% on the strength of 258 total PSF teams. Further, coverage would eventually increase to 50.23% in 2015 after the SMS executed an additional set of hiring plans crystallized by Monteiro de Andrade and his sanitarista successors in the directorship.[18]

Additionally, the SMS under Monteiro de Andrade developed newer technical capacities to target clinics and health workers to city regions facing the gravest epidemiological risks. The core of the new targeting strategy adopted under Monteiro de Andrade's directorship was a territorially based approach that first divided the capital's territory into 2,849 micro-areas and then ranked each on a four-point scale that differentiated various levels of risk faced by their residents. The SMS characterized nearly all (2,627) as facing risks that necessitated at least some degree of PSF presence. Residents of areas classified as Risk 1 were deemed to face the greatest risks, due to poverty, insufficient access to public health care and other public services, and the threat of environmental hazards such as floods and landslides. This category mostly included areas already catalogued by the Civil Defense Agency of Fortaleza's Citizen Security Secretariat for the 1998 PSF rollout. The SMS sought to achieve the lowest ratio—500 residents per PSF team—of all in these areas. Risk 2 areas included many favelas characterized by similarly high degrees of poverty, irregular housing, and low levels of access to sanitation, running water, and basic living conditions. Here, the SMS aimed to achieve a ratio of 750 residents per PSF team. In Risk 3 areas, deemed to be populated by middle-class residents living in established housing and generally good living conditions, the SMS aimed to deploy one PSF team for every 1,000 residents. This left 222 as Risk 4 areas that—by virtue of being populated by generally upper- and middle-class residents living in luxury condominiums and large homes within areas that were well served by public services—were not targeted for PSF coverage (de Oliveira Viana Esmeraldo 2009, 88). By 2010, the new territorialization strategy adopted under Monteiro de Andrade had brought PSF teams into contact with over 890,100 residents, according to the federal health ministry's Basic Attention Department (MS-DAB).

Monteiro de Andrade also implemented a far more systematic and institutionalized process of "permanent education" for training PSF professionals in both technical dimensions of care provision and in the normative origins and political-institutional history of the SUS. A central institutional mechanism he founded for doing so was the SMS's Municipal Health School (*Sistema Municipal de Saúde Escola*, SMSE), which Monteiro de Andrade created in 2006 through Municipal Decree #160 (de Oliveira Viana Esmeraldo 2009, 87). The pedagogy of the school drew from a deep playbook of educational tools developed by Monteiro de Andrade and other sanitaristas during more than a decade in civil-society organizations and municipal health departments that fostered adoption of the PSF model. These experiences included Monteiro de Andrade's 1998 publication of a journal issue in *SANARE: Revista Sobralense de Políticas Públicas*, which highlighted the approach to permanent education he instituted for PSF workers while serving as SMS director in the Ceará city of Sobral (Borges Sugiyama 2012, 140). One dimension of the SMSE focused on orienting teams in contextually specific dimensions of providing health care to populations in the generally less affluent city regions targeted by the PSF. Others, such as its *Ciranda da Vida* program, which doubled as Fortaleza's approach to enacting the National Humanization Policy (PNH) for strengthening the SUS locally, created dedicated spaces within PSF clinics for dialogues intended to connect health practitioners and activists from health-focused and other community-based social movements (de Oliveira Viana Esmeraldo 2009, 87).

Crucially, office-holding sanitaristas such as Monteiro de Andrade understood PSF expansions as a natural extension of their lifelong efforts to codify and otherwise advance sanitary reform tenets of universality and equity in the realm of community health. Monteiro de Andrade's own descriptions of the PSF in this chapter's epigraph convey this dedication to enacting such universalistic principles through a paradoxically discreet and circumscribed but ultimately quite tangible programmatic model for making them more than just grandiose promises. It is particularly notable that he understood the PSF model of creating community-based health teams of doctors, nurses, and community health agents as a piecemeal step toward instituting the "utopia" of a more holistic, universal, and solution-oriented health system (de Miranda Gondim 2011, 587). This understanding of the PSF epitomizes how pragmatic publics such as Brazil's sanitaristas view the work of universalizing and equalizing access to basic public services as a normative project as well as a material one to be executed through local state-building. And despite the PSF's inability to meet the changing preferences of a Brazilian population that increasingly demands higher-quality and more sophisticated health services, such perceptions of the program among its sanitarista creators exemplify how such normative motivations can help transform otherwise impersonal state structures with little prior connection to even the narrow understanding of health universalism embodied by the PSF.

Although a string of Monteiro de Andrade's nonsanitarista successors held Fortaleza's SMS directorship after he left in 2010, all preserved his expansions, and some continued the city's sanitarista-initiated pattern of expanding municipal state capacities to broaden the PSF's reach. Indeed, Dr. Maria de Pepétuo Socorro Martins Breckenfeld, a UFC-trained physician who had previously directed several hospitals in the capital and served as SMS director from 2013 to 2016, continued the fortification of state capacities for PSF expansion that Monteiro de Andrade initiated in 2005. During her directorship, the SMS opened new concursos that brought its total PSF teams to 363 by the end of 2015. Owing to the expanded capacity of these new teams to more fully penetrate city regions not previously served by the program, the PSF had reached approximately 1,255,800 residents that year and achieved a populational coverage rate of approximately 50.39%, which amounted to an average of one PSF team for every 4,417 SUS-dependent residents. Additionally, by the end of 2015, Fortaleza's network of basic health units had expanded to 120. While neither is especially innovative or particularly sizable relative to their precursors, the previously established programs that Breckenfeld expanded had become a largely uncontroversial way for governing political-society elites from the PSB and PT to expand primary health care after 2005.

In this sense, Monteiro de Andrade's major 2006 expansion of the PSF did more than just materially expand the program's reach. It also solidified political elites' acceptance of the PSF model as the central strategy for universalizing access to primary care. Breckenfeld's post-2014 PSF expansions were neither exceptionally large nor unexpected, but they reflected how the program's expansion had become a central expectation of those occupying the SUS manager's office in Fortaleza. As such, proposals to expand the PSF carried with them the normative weight of fulfilling a responsibility of the office to pursue sanitary reform principles such as universality and equity in access to health services. Thus, the depth of Fortaleza's earlier phases of state-building helps explain how state-building subsequently persisted, occasionally even in the absence of sanitaristas themselves in the SMS directorship. Ultimately, the work of establishing core regulative institutions such as the SUS manager's office atop Fortaleza's SMS had sustained and extended the state-building process that transformed the capital into one of contemporary Brazil's least likely but most impressive urban providers of primary health care delivery and reducers of infant mortality.

4. Conclusion

This chapter argued that Fortaleza's office-holding sanitaristas propelled an early and sustained trajectory of programmatic health democratization that widened delivery of primary public health care and correspondingly helped reduce IMR to unprecedented lows in the city. Despite entering the health-democratization period with an IMR that ranked nearly last among major Brazilian capitals, Fortaleza finished the period ranked among the country's highest performers. With a trajectory that mirrored those in other cities such as Curitiba, which began the period with far superior conditions of social, economic, and political development, Fortaleza's path shows how programmatic health democratization improved the human condition even in "least-likely" northeastern contexts that suffer from Brazil's most severe colonial legacies. Especially given the profoundly illiberal and clientelist starting point of public health politics in Fortaleza, baseline features of health democratization played an important role in fostering the city's robust social development outcomes. The restoration of local elections and full party competition for elected office were especially notable because they helped end the dominance of Fortaleza's coronels, who were notoriously immune to public ills such as widespread premature mortality.

But if elections established palpable electoral incentives for aspiring sub-national executives to address rampant public problems such as endemic childhood mortality, they hardly offer a full accounting for Fortaleza's robust development outcomes vis-à-vis other capitals that experienced comparatively weaker changes in this regard. Similarly, the mere codification of a right to health, the 1990 passage of the Organic Health Laws, and the creation of the SUS all offer little explanatory leverage since they were nationwide features that altered public health politics across all cities examined in this study. Rather, this chapter's within-case analysis suggested that defining features of Fortaleza's distinctly programmatic trajectory of health democratization were at the heart of its robust development transformations. Specifically, sanitarista construction of civil-society regulative institutions such as the municipal SUS manager's office and sanitarista infusion of sanitary reform ideology into the otherwise antinormative state position of SMS director helped expand service-delivery arms of the municipal public health state in developmentally consequential ways. Here, the very ability of individual sanitaristas such as Dr. Luiz Odorico Monteiro de Andrade and his predecessors to occupy the SUS manager's office and then fulfill the office's public responsibilities for enacting a right to health owed much to the normative legitimacy they enjoyed as movement veterans who had helped to establish the nationwide office in the first place. And, as in Curitiba, these efforts also relied on no small amount of careful political strategizing by Fortaleza's sanitaristas to crystallize relatively narrow, affordable, and actionable state-building proposals that appealed to ruling political elites. In the end, however, tangible enactment of this state-building project required sustained intra-institutional mobilization by Monteiro de Andrade and office-holding sanitaristas atop the subnational public health state.

Ultimately then, a major difference between Fortaleza and other capitals that witnessed only minimalist trajectories of health democratization and nonrobust development outcomes was that sanitaristas gained more sustained access to the office of SUS manager by establishing sanitary reform proposals as a dominant agenda among a wide range of ruling party executives. In this sense, the remarkably sustained period of sanitarista office holding in Fortaleza's SMS directorship enabled these actors to leverage the office in ways that established crucial new service-provision capacities of the municipal public health state by the mid-2000s. Further, such factors continued to matter considerably even alongside other post-2004 drivers of IMR reduction such as the full institutionalization of Bolsa Família, the establishment of Participatory Budgeting, and a wider range of social policies implemented by Fortaleza's progressive PT mayors. As in Curitiba, sanitarista control of the SUS manager's office not only maximized the state-building processes that defined Fortaleza's trajectory of programmatic health democratization but also mediated the effects of this historic period on the city's impressive social development outcomes by the mid-2010s.

EIGHT

Movement-Driven Development
in Comparative Perspective

This study has documented and sought to explain urban Brazil's historic improvements in human health and well-being during the three decades following the country's return to democracy. During this period, the country's largest cities witnessed a profound democratization in access to basic forms of health care and a monumental reduction in premature death beginning in the mid-1980s. Largely unexpected and unsurpassed by any other large democracy in the contemporary world during the same period, this transformation in human capabilities defied Brazil's previous reputation for widespread infant and child mortality. Yet some cities achieved greater progress than others, and this study's theory of movement-driven development (MDD) traced these patterns of higher performance to a period of democratization in access to health through which programmatic and participatory-programmatic configurations of civil-society and state actors animated the municipal politics of the primary public health sector. A defining feature of both configurations was a consistent pattern of democratic office holding atop the municipal public health state by pragmatist publics, a set of previously untheorized civil-society actors whom Brazil's sanitaristas epitomize. Alongside two other factors—localized success in implementing nationwide antipoverty programs and an infrequency of sustained local rule by mayors from right-leaning political parties—consistent democratic office holding by pragmatist publics was sufficient to maximize growth in social development and access to basic forms of health care.

This chapter first briefly extends this overarching argument to additional cases beyond Brazil's primary public health sector. Then I crystallize several implications of the analysis for theories of civil society and civil society–state relations as well as for theories of how social development can improve over time in democratic settings. In reflecting on its limitations, the chapter concludes by reconciling the theory of MDD and pragmatist publics with more recent setbacks to democracy in Brazil.

1. MDD Beyond Urban Brazil's Primary Health Sector

Does this book's argument that pragmatist publics mobilized an ideologically diverse array of locally ruling political parties to build the IMR-reducing state capacities needed for basic health care expansion also help explain similar outcomes beyond Brazil's primary health sector? Systematically answering this question would require a substantial amount of fieldwork and analysis that transcends the scope of this study. But clues in existing scholarship suggest that such a prediction holds considerable potential for explaining similar outcomes in other Brazilian public-service sectors and in those of other similarly large and highly decentralized democracies of the Global South such as India and Indonesia.

1.1. BRAZIL'S LEGAL, ANTIPOVERTY, AND PUBLIC EDUCATION SECTORS

Whereas Brazil's public education sector offers a cautionary tale of how the state-building needed to broaden the reach of social policies can falter without pragmatist publics, the evolution of its legal sector and the now famous Bolsa Família program are generally consistent with previous chapters' findings from the primary health sector. Particularly fertile grounds for extending this study's theory of how pragmatist publics can advance progressive and democratically oriented state-building can be found in the pattern of activism by which lawyers reformed Brazil's multilevel prosecutorial office, the *Ministério Público* (MP). Sometimes likened to a fourth branch of government because of its far-reaching powers to investigate a wide variety of legal infractions, the MP includes thirty state- and federal-level prosecutorial agencies throughout Brazil. Its approximately 12,000 prosecutors exercise the exclusive authority to initiate criminal proceedings and dismiss allegations in a wide range of legal realms that include human rights, environmental and labor statutes, consumer protections, and political corruption (Coslovsky and Nigam 2015). In 2014, MP prosecutors based in Curitiba initiated the highest-profile corruption case in Brazilian history, an investigation of the infamous Car Wash (*Lava Jato*) scheme that ensnared sitting politicians from multiple parties, including the PT and PMDB, for accepting billions of dollars in illegal payments. The investigation was extraordinary for the enormous scale of corruption it revealed as well as for its nearly unprecedented ability to eventually secure the conviction, sentencing, and actual serving of prison sentences by several current and former politicians. Although journalistic accounts of Brazilian legal activists suggest a near missionary-like zeal for legal reform and self-understanding among many as defenders of Brazil's Constitution and laws (Watts 2017), social scientists have only begun to reconcile the role of MP prosecutors with theories of civil-society and state-society relations. The most sophisticated studies of the MP nevertheless demonstrate how prosecutors reformed the agency in ways that mirror the basic "inside out" approach through which office-holding sanitaristas remade the subnational public health state across urban Brazil (Coslovsky and Nigam 2015).

Distinct from Brazilian judges and other legal officials who have seized upon and sometimes misrepresented their investigative findings for political purposes that some observers associate with a criminalization of left-leaning politicians, MP prosecutors embody at least some of the qualities that have made pragmatist publics such as Brazil's sanitaristas so effective at health-sector reform. Constituted from an even narrower segment of civil society than sanitaristas were, these legal activists constructed both communicative and regulative institutions that became an influential organizational fulcrum for their advocacy as reformers and later prosecutors. Over a century after its 1889 creation at the dawn of Brazil's republic, the MP witnessed profound changes as a result of this activism. Uncannily mirroring the influence and rootedness of sanitarista framers such as Sergio Arouca in civil-society institutions like CEBES, ABRASCO, CONASEMS, and CONASS, lawyers in Brazil's Constitutional Assembly such as Plinio de Arruda Sampaio drafted passages of the 1988 Constitution that codified the MP's public responsibilities into law and made prosecutors publicly accountable for fostering the Constitution's more equal definition of all citizens under the law (Coslovsky and Nigam 2015, 33). In a country better known for an illiberal political culture codified into pre-1988 laws defining different and unequal categories of citizens (Holston 2008), this monumental shift in public legality would have been unlikely without prosecutors and their associations, especially the powerful Confederation of State Prosecutors (CAEMP, later CONAMP). Further, MP prosecutors followed up this watershed reconfiguration of Brazilian law with a sanitarista-like approach to incrementally solving problems of legal inequity. For instance, by wielding that quintessentially pragmatist tool of democratic reform—legal precedent—prosecutors have incrementally won major decisions in favor of historically excluded groups, including the disabled, children and youth, and Afro-Brazilians (Coslovsky and Nigam 2015; dos Santos 2012).

Additionally, MP prosecutors have often displayed a notable reflexivity and openness to participatory-democratic bodies and more deliberative civil-society actors hailing from beyond their own ranks of the legal profession. For example, state prosecutors in the Rio Grande do Sul office of the MP openly welcomed and facilitated the president of Porto Alegre's health council (CMS) in 2010 when she successfully solicited them to condemn the city's mayor and health secretary for repeatedly shirking their legal responsibilities for incorporating the body into municipal-health-sector budgeting and expenditure reporting (M. O. Garcia, personal communication; O. Paniz and H. Scorza, interviews, 2010). The few existing scholarly accounts of prosecutors' relationships with political-society elites suggest that the use of code-switching could well underlie their advocacy also. At a minimum, beyond just astutely deciphering political opportunity structures for appropriate moments to bring forward investigations and indictments, prosecutors have assiduously maintained alliances with political-society elites in their jurisdictions and have "cast themselves as critical allies of whoever had some power at a given time but needed additional support" (Coslovsky and Nigam 2015, 36). Such qualities roughly mirror how sanitaristas more tangibly enacted an equal and universal right to health care by cloaking their associated state-building proposals in the language of political elites' shorter-term concerns with winning elections and improving their own public-opinion ratings. That said, the MP is hardly impermeable to partisan efforts by elites on both the left and right to manipulate the agency for personal or political gain. Indeed, as with any democratic institution that is vulnerable to control by civil-society actors, the MP is also malleable by social and political elites with particularistic interests that defy principles of universal and equal access to justice. All too frequently, it has been used as a tool for partisan-inspired predation on progressive political elites. But none of this denies the possibility that, when wielded by civil-society actors who prize equal and fair treatment under democratic laws, the MP can be made to resist such meddling by political-society elites. Considered in light of the fact that some prosecutors describe norms of equal treatment under the law as their motivation for legal campaigns to prosecute progressive politicians for corruption, such questions involve a thorny set of considerations far beyond the scope of this book. Nevertheless, such actors constitute an intriguing case for deepening the theory of MDD and pragmatist publics crystallized through this book's analysis of Brazil's sanitaristas.

The historical evolution of Bolsa Família (BF) and its forerunners also poses intriguing questions about the fit of this book's theory to the rise of Brazil's now famous antipoverty program, if only because excellent studies of BF and its predecessors (for example, Bolsa Escola and *Fome Zero*, or Zero Hunger) disagree about what initiated it and propelled its remarkable growth. Whereas some political scientists trace its origins and expansion largely to the electoral incentives of Presidents Cardoso and Lula (Garay 2016, 148–61), others contrastingly emphasize the ideological commitments of subnational political-society elites, suggesting "it is actors' social justice commitments and connections to their peers that mattered most" (Borges Sugiyama 2012, 112). In focusing more squarely on national politics of social policies, the former explanation does not take up the question of why some municipalities have implemented BF more expansively than others and whether such expansions are traceable to local activism by civil society or pragmatist publics, more specifically. The latter account, in stressing that the program diffused downwardly from national to local levels in a wavelike fashion that rendered the origins of local officials' social justice commitments a less important consideration, leaves unaddressed the related questions of whether the commitments of local political-society elites have mattered for BF effectiveness, and if so, whether civil society actors such as pragmatist publics have helped mold such commitments in consequential ways. In short, existing accounts have stopped short of arguing that pragmatist publics and civil society are what initiated and drove the causal chain of events that led to the creation and expansion of BF. Rather, as with many existing accounts of Brazilian public-health-sector reform, they tend to locate such agency more squarely in the hands of national-level political-society elites.

Although it is beyond the scope of this study to systematically assess whether the theory of MDD can help explain BF's origins and expansion, two observations nevertheless emerge from the earlier analyses of robust development in Brazil's largest cities. First, all cities that maximally expanded the PSF (and robustly reduced IMR) also featured consistent office holding by pragmatist publics. In some of these cities, such as Belo Horizonte and Curitiba, the social development ministers, vice mayors, and mayors who most helped to expand the program had important civil-society roots as pragmatist publics. As chapters 4 and 6 showed, Belo Horizonte's mayor Dr. Célio de Castro and social development (and previously health) secretary Dr. Helvécio Miranda Magalhães Jr. mirrored Curitiba's vice mayor and mayor Luciano Ducci in that their deep histories of activism within communicative and regulative institutions of the Sanitarist Movement are what initially molded their normative commitments to a universal citizenship right to health. While overseeing the social development agency that helps operate the BF locally, officials such as Magalhães not only noted that sanitaristas recognize the widely known health benefits of providing cash transfers that are conditional upon receipt of basic medical care but also emphasized that BF and its predecessors were clearly conducive to the long-time sanitarista goal of fostering the right to health (H. M. Magalhães, interview, 2010). In all other positive cases of robust development and maximal BF coverage (Fortaleza, Recife, and Porto Alegre), many of the same office-holding sanitaristas who advocated for primary health care expansion and a right to health also favored BF expansions (L. Barcelos and M. L. Jaeger, interviews, 2010). Although their overlap with PT mayorships more clearly diverges from the episodes in Curitiba and Belo Horizonte, examples of support for BF and its predecessors among office-holding pragmatist publics can be found in Maria Luiza Jaeger's tenure as state health director of Rio Grande do Sul from 1999–2002 and in the municipal health directorships of Henrique Fontana (1998) and Lucio Barcelos in Porto Alegre (1999–2002), Humberto Costa in Recife (2001), and Luiz Odorico Monteiro de Andrade in Fortaleza (2005–2009).

Second, the theory's attention to deeper-level causes of the localized state-building needed to actually enact such programs ultimately suggests that pragmatist publics have likely played an underappreciated role in BF expansion. Simply put, maximal BF expansion has likely depended on greater access to primary public health care among program applicants since recipients must demonstrate proof of regular medical attention to receive transfers. At a minimum, this reality should cast more focus on decisive social-policy sectors such as health and education that must operate with a modicum of effectiveness in order for CCTs like the BF to also be effective. As such, questions about the reach and efficacy of BF may well default back to more fundamental issues of state capacity in both sectors. Given this, it is likely no coincidence that the FSA results in chapter 3 showed that all cities with robust IMR reduction and maximal expansion of the PSF also featured consistent office holding by pragmatist publics. It was these actors who most consistently sought to expand municipal state capacities such as primary health clinics, meritocratically hired health professionals, and the ability to target such public resources toward city regions facing the greatest epidemiological risks. Indeed, if one accepts both this study's argument that frequent office holding by sanitaristas was a deeper-level cause of PSF expansion and the fact that BF expansion has at least partially depended on PSF expansion, then BF expansion must also be at least indirectly traceable to frequent municipal office holding by pragmatist publics. In sum, there are good reasons to expect that BF expansion in these cities has relied upon pragmatist publics and their construction and wielding of both communicative and regulative institutions of civil society to a greater extent than accounts emphasizing political-society elites allow for.

By contrast, other Brazilian social-policy sectors such as public education, which have consistently underperformed in service delivery, reflect a notable lack of office-holding pragmatist publics. Indeed, no known accounts of the sector emphasize administrative positions atop any level of the Brazilian public education state as the site of civil-society efforts to propagate normative responsibilities of democratic office or an ideology of equal access to public education. Put simply, the absence of anything like sanitaristas within the state-society politics of Brazil's public education sector may contrastingly help explain why and how comparatively less institutional change and social progress has occurred in that sector. In 2015, the OECD (2015) ranked the Brazilian public education system in the bottom fifth of all countries, alongside sub-Saharan African nations such as Botswana and historically underperforming Latin American countries like Peru. Although Brazil improved the proportion of fifteen-year-olds in school from 56% in 2013 to 71% by 2015, actual education outcomes have languished, with Brazil's average scores for reading, science, and math ranking above only seven out of seventy-one countries (OECD 2015, 9). One notable exception that may prove the rule of how decisive civil society can be for social development is Brazil's still nascent university-level affirmative action program, which black activists successfully mobilized to institute during the 2000s (dos Santos 2012) but right-leaning politicians increasingly attacked as the 2010s unfolded. Overall, however, the federal-, state-, and municipal-level education agencies responsible for primary, secondary, and higher education in Brazil have consistently underperformed vis-à-vis the marked improvements of the country's health sector. Although likely the product of still other factors, this underperformance reflects the fact that the state-society politics of Brazil's public education system has generally lacked the ideologically motivated but problem-solving protagonists that animated health, CCT, and legal reforms following the country's return to democracy.

1.2. POSSIBILITIES FOR PRAGMATIST PUBLICS AND MDD IN SOUTH INDIA AND INDONESIA

The notion of MDD suggests unexplored but intriguing hypotheses of public-service-sector state-building and social development outcomes in other large federalist democracies of the Global South such as India and Indonesia, which alongside Brazil contain nearly half of the world's population living under electoral democracy. Although these countries are less renowned for nationwide rights-based health movements like Brazil's Sanitarist Movement, their polities assign democratic officeholders on local levels with considerable formal authority to enact citizenship rights in certain public-service sectors. Since India and Indonesia share similar political contexts of highly decentralized but weakly institutionalized federalist democracies with those that Brazil's sanitaristas seized upon in their intra-institutional advocacy, openings for pragmatist publics and possibilities for MDD are perhaps more likely in these countries than elsewhere.[1] At a minimum, these political contexts have allowed for and likely motivated subnational executives and civil-society actors to cooperate with one another in coproducing social development. Yet accounts of how civil society has influenced local social development generally stress two more specific qualities that diverge from this study's emphasis on pragmatist publics and MDD: party-based patronage and ruling left parties that experiment with participatory-democratic allocation of public goods. Whereas explanations for the famously progressive South Indian states of Tamil Nadu and Kerala invoke the former and latter accounts, respectively (Harriss and Törnquist

2017; Singh 2015), scholars of Indonesia trace its lukewarm progress in IMR reduction to a briefer and shallower period of formal democracy (McGuire 2010, 276) that likely precluded either patronage or left-party rule from having similarly positive effects on social development.

Scholars of social development in the southern state of Tamil Nadu commonly trace education, health, and other social-policy reforms to two qualities of democratic political processes: populism (Harriss and Törnquist 2017) and subnationalism (Singh 2015). Such accounts agree on the clear relevance of the Dravidian movement's contributions to impressive growth in social development and the fact that subnational democratic government offered an efficacious venue for orchestrating that growth. As with contemporary Brazil's sanitaristas, Tamil Nadu's Dravidian activists went beyond merely pressuring subnational politicians to address public problems such as widespread illiteracy and malnutrition. They also established regulative institutions of civil society, including political parties such as the DMK and ADMK, for advancing social development agendas. And, at times, they have occupied important democratically elected subnational offices in efforts to address developmental deficits themselves (Singh 2015, 122–29). Cognizant of how weak state capacities left them practically incapable of expanding public-service delivery and fostering social development, Dravidian activists who seized reigns of subnational democratic government shared state-building power with civil-society actors outside the state, particularly public-school teachers with activist profiles. At a minimum, such accounts emphasize how a key feature of pragmatist publics—solidary ideologies and a pragmatist approach to materially advancing them—drove such activists into state-building for development, even if the scope of solidarity with the Tamil nation was not nationwide, as was the case with Brazilian activism for a right to health.

Explanations of Kerala's impressive social development record contrastingly emphasize unionized working classes, left-leaning parties in power, and participatory publics not unlike those in Brazil. Yet other civil-society actors with a striking resemblance to pragmatist publics have rarely been far from the state-building action. For example, the statewide membership of the People's Science Movement (KSSP) was an active contributor to participatory development-planning efforts orchestrated by the Communist Party-Marxist (CPM), Kerala's left-leaning social democratic party (Gibson 2012; Heller, Harilal, and Chaudhuri 2007). But just as Brazil's sanitaristas were not reducible to the political parties or labor unions in which they sometimes mobilized or the participatory-democratic institutions to which they remained connected, KSSP activists may well amount to a qualitatively distinct type of civil-society actor. The identities of KSSP activists not only cross boundaries of class and party but also transcend any passing affinity for specific participatory-democratic experiments such as the CPM's People's Campaign for Decentralized Planning of 1996–2000. Often engineers, teachers, and scientists, KSSP members have generally hailed from professional classes since the organization's 1962 founding but have sometimes sought to win democratic offices as a way to orchestrate the statebuilding needed to advance their aspirations for enacted citizenship rights to education, health, and development (Parameswaran 2005). Although such campaigns have often dovetailed with those of the CPM, they are hardly reducible to it, as was evident when the prominent KSSP activist M. P. Parameswaran was expelled from the CPM in 2004 for his sharply critical views of the party (The Hindu 2004). At a minimum, this book's theory of pragmatist publics suggests that such actors—not unlike those in the Family Welfare Movement that Indonesia's Suharto quashed in the 1970s for demanding greater associational autonomy (Prawiro 1998)—merit additional research into whether and how they exert sources of civil power that deviate from the currencies of political power in left parties and from the mere acts of associating or deliberating within participatory democratic forums.

2. Theoretical Implications of Pragmatist Publics and Movement-Driven Development

The book's findings about how pragmatist publics have advanced MDD in urban Brazil ultimately complement authoritative frameworks of civil society's role in social development, social-movement outcomes, institutional change, and public health in the Global South. First, they complement the "encompassing embeddedness" (EE) framework of social development by demonstrating how practically minded civil societies can offer one solution to a sizable missing-agent problem at the model's core. Second, in contrast to the "state-in-society" perspectives that informed much thinking about industrial developmental states, the theory of MDD instead offers a "civil-society-in-state" paradigm in which pragmatist publics concentrate civil power in democratic offices. Third, MDD informs models of social-movement consequences by showing that pragmatist publics' founding and control of new democratic offices can constitute a salient movement outcome with potential to foster still other state-building and health outcomes. Finally, the theory of MDD moves beyond a mere recognition of how professional expertise can guide the design of effective public-service programs that foster social development. It specifically emphasizes how the deep normative roots of pragmatist publics within civil-society ideologies and institutions ultimately contribute indispensable sources of power for building the new state capacities required to tangibly enact such programs.

2.1. PRAGMATIST PUBLICS AND ENCOMPASSING EMBEDDEDNESS

In suggesting one concrete route by which pragmatist publics can work alongside state actors to pursue development, this book's theory of MDD offers to expand the EE model of the twenty-first-century developmental state (Evans 2010; Evans and Heller 2015). As a metaframework of social development and its origins, the EE model usefully conceptualizes capability focused democratic states in the Global South and addresses the most promising kinds of political agents for helping construct them. It particularly emphasizes two such groups of actors: programmatic left parties and participatory publics. Here, encompassing embeddedness can arise when the programmatic social-policy proposals that ruling left parties highlight in successful election campaigns acquire democratically legitimate mandates for their implementation from voters. Additionally, the EE framework emphasizes participatory publics and related governance institutions as one means for more directly channeling civil-society actors into a selection of community-informed social development projects such as Participatory Budgeting (Baiocchi, Heller, and Silva 2011). The ways that such institutions broaden the social foundations of public-opinion formation (Baiocchi and Ganuza 2016) can clearly foster encompassing embeddedness as well.

In conceptualizing pragmatist publics, however, this book highlights a distinct category of civil society whose democratically mediated influence on social development is not solely dependent on participatory democracy or progressive left parties in power, although it is consistent with both. In this respect, the notion of MDD complements the EE framework and related theories of power constellations that emphasize the programmatic orientations of ruling left parties such as those that dominated national-level Brazilian and Latin American politics during the early 2000s (Huber and Stephens 2012). In one respect, the EE framework helpfully supplements power constellation accounts by additionally focusing on newer, direct democratic institutions that can complement representative democratic ones and ruling left parties in building a wider social consensus to construct humanistically minded developmental states. In part, this shift reflects a core dilemma faced by left parties that seek to foster development by incorporating popularly oriented civil-society actors into capability focused, twenty-first-century analogs of the developmental states (the "21DS") that were so essential for twentieth-century economic development. Specifically, if twentieth-century developmental states sustained interactions with industrial elites that "gave these elites a reason to become a more collectively coherent class," contemporary politicians aiming to cultivate the 21DS instead face a taller task. Namely, they must incorporate a far less coherent array of popularly oriented civil societies in deciding on "shared goals, whose concrete implementation can then be 'co-produced' by public agencies and the communities themselves" (Evans 2010, 49). In response, ruling left parties increasingly pursue social development stratagems by devolving participatory publics the decision-making authority to crystallize public health and social policies through more deeply democratic modes.

Despite its many contributions, the EE framework struggles to fully account for arguably the most important social driver of urban Brazil's transformation in social development: namely, pragmatist publics with sources of power other than those of both participatory publics and left parties. The EE framework largely discounts the possibility that such already cohesive civil societies with greater proximity to state power might instead take the lead in building the 21DS by mobilizing political-society actors from a wider spectrum of ideologies than sometimes thought. In part, this mismatch reflects two interrelated assumptions within the framework. First, the framework suggests that cultivating developmentally effective state-society embeddedness requires state agents to organize disparate, fragmented groups of civil-society actors into more consolidated political actors. Secondly, it tends to assume that such civil societies favor deeply democratic approaches to politics that prize deliberation. Participatory-democracy institutions are correspondingly seen as a desirable way of formulating and incorporating preferences of such participatory publics into public policy making and generally integrating this broader spectrum of actors into monitoring and evaluation of actual service delivery (Evans 2010; Evans and Heller 2015).

Less reliant on such qualities, pragmatist publics like Brazil's sanitaristas act more cohesively in wielding new democratic institutions for the public purpose of universalizing and equalizing access to health. When the movement established a new democratic office of the SUS manager atop the public health state, it effectively created an office whose very purpose and normative underpinnings favored sanitarista candidates for its occupancy for decades thereafter. In this regard, its intent differed from that of participatory institutions that sought to involve broader publics in public policy making. Indeed, founding the office of SUS manager as a "sanitary authority" disproportionately privileged sanitaristas themselves in accessing that office on subnational levels during the decades that followed its legal codification in 1990. Further, beyond narrowing the kinds of publics likely to be considered among its most qualified occupants, the office's fusion to a cabinet-level position availed occupants of remarkably cohesive levers for constructing municipal health bureaucracies with the capacities to widely deliver basic health services. Although codification of the SUS also created a distinct set of more broadly inclusive democratic institutions such as municipal and state health councils, these cohesive qualities of the SUS manager's office differ in unmistakable ways from participatory-democratic institutions such as the CMS or OP. And although participatory publics certainly aimed to use such institutions for influencing health-related state-building, these participatory institutions remained contrastingly insulated from the reigns of concentrated state power routinely at the disposal of SUS managers.

2.2. TOWARD A CIVIL-SOCIETY-IN-STATE PERSPECTIVE

The animation of Brazil's MDD process by pragmatist publics also shows how civil-society actors, and not necessarily the political-society elites whom they sometimes mobilize around their own concerns, can be core drivers of social development transformations. In Brazil, sanitaristas did this by fusing the SUS manager's office to the cabinet-level, executive-branch position of SMS director atop the subnational public health state in a manner that created a new civil-society institution with considerable authority over state-building. Particularly in the first decade after the SUS's founding, a few sanitaristas in each city examined in this book tended to wield the office to greatest effect by consistently holding the SMS director-ship and its precursors themselves. On first glance, such cohesion might seem to faintly echo Kohli's theory of economic development as produced by cohesive capitalist state apparatuses such as the one that propelled Ko-rea's industrialization (2004). But any such echoes should not be overstated. For one, the SMS directorships held by sanitaristas possessed nothing like the degree of sheer repressive capacity, hierarchy, or concentrated power at the apex of the state. Further, there is little in common between, on the one hand, the movement lineages and ideological commitment of sanitaris-tas to democratic freedoms and the citizenship right to health and, on the other hand, the authoritarian bents of rulers who constructed cohesive cap-italist states. Indeed, pragmatist publics more often ground claims to state-building power in universalizing ideologies that emerge from civil-society discourses structured by principles of egalitarianism and universalism that are anathema to authoritarian rulers.

Additionally, sanitarista office-holding episodes in the SMS director-ship rarely exhibited personalistic qualities, in part because individual san-itaristas often entered and exited the office periodically to pursue other en-deavors. And the slightly longer duration of years that sanitaristas held the position (3.0) versus their nonsanitarista counterparts (2.6) was not a sta-tistically significant difference (*t*-test not significant with 90% confidence). Thus, it is difficult to sustain the counterargument that individual sani-taristas wielded power as SMS directors simply by holding the office for ex-tended episodes or because of any personalistic qualities. If anything, such patterns of personalism were far more detectable among nonsanitaristas, who often exploited the office for rent-seeking purposes in negative cases of nonrobust development such as Salvador and Rio de Janeiro. Rather than exerting anything like the coercive force of a cohesive capitalist state, sanita-ristas instead wielded the SMS directorship in part as public servants seek-ing to fulfill the office's underlying responsibility for enacting the promise of a universal and equal right to health. By the end of the period in positive cases such as Porto Alegre, Belo Horizonte, Curitiba, and Fortaleza, even nonsanitarista occupants increasingly viewed the pursuit of such principles as professional tasks required of any one occupant in the position of SMS director. In such cases, the civil-society institution of the SUS manager's office became even more deeply institutionalized and woven into the hierarchical structure of the municipal state.

That the office's responsibilities were not immediately embraced and have not always been internalized by nonsanitarista occupants is neither surprising nor especially damaging to the theory of MDD, given Brazil's relative absence of any long-standing political tradition of universal citizenship rights (Baiocchi 2006; Holston 2008). While its sanitarista occupants have most embodied the office's normative responsibilities to enact health universalism, the SUS manager's office itself began and has remained a civil-society institution that enshrined new public responsibilities in surprising ways. As with any democratic office, the mere normative grounding of the SUS manager's office in core principles of sanitary reform ideology such as universal and equal access to health hardly ensured that the office's individual occupants wielded it for such public purposes or in ways that tangibly brought such norms to material fruition. But cases of nonsanitarista occupants exploiting the SUS manager's office for particularistic purposes of self-interest and rent-seeking, as was commonplace in negative cases of nonrobust development like Salvador and Rio de Janeiro, miss the larger point. Namely, in countries such as Brazil that lack established political traditions of democratic offices and universal citizenship rights, it is remarkable that such norms came to be institutionalized within the civil-society offices of the SUS manager at all. By itself, the mere existence of the office testifies to the considerable, if always fragile, translation that civil society has pursued in seeking to materialize a democratic right to health.

Further, while they proved less cohesive than the positions of authority that programmatic left parties assumed by winning elected offices of the subnational executive such as mayorships, SUS directorships have offered occupants more consolidated access to state-building power than have the participatory-democratic institutions emphasized in the EE framework. Brazil's sanitaristas epitomize how pragmatist publics can orchestrate encompassing embeddedness themselves rather than depending on programmatic left parties or participatory publics to do so. Indeed, sanitaristas capitalized on their own normative legitimacy as living instantiations of the very universalizing ideologies crystallized into the democratic offices they sought to hold as veterans and activists of the movement that established the SUS to begin with. It may therefore come as less of a surprise that, particularly in earlier moments of the SUS's institutionalization, office-holding sanitaristas enjoyed considerable access to the office and wielded it to great effect. This pragmatist public's creation and wielding of the SUS manager's office amounted to the creation of a new civil-society institution for mobilizing political-society elites around the universalistic principle of a right to health.

Such a pathbreaking change for Brazilian democracy also has far-reaching theoretical implications for scholarly understandings of state-society relations in the Global South. Namely, it suggests that a civil-society-in-state paradigm may better capture a distinct route to producing encompassing embeddedness—one in which civil societies can mobilize political societies around their goals as much as vice versa. Of particular relevance in Brazil was that the institutional form created by sanitaristas was a democratic office whose holders assume a public responsibility for tangibly enacting a universal right to health. Among its other effects, this created an influential civil-society institution that favored the efforts of pragmatist publics to take the lead in cultivating encompassing embeddedness and generating solidarity with political-society elites around such normative principles. In this sense, Brazil's pattern of MDD in recent decades suggests not the state-in-society paradigm so well-known to theories of development in the Global South (Migdal 2001) but a civil-society-in-state paradigm in which pragmatist publics consolidate civil power within such democratic offices and then leverage that power to build the state from the inside out. This inversion differs in obvious ways from Kohli's (2004) account of how authoritarian political elites insert themselves into networks of capitalist elites within economic society to induce shared projects of economic transformation. It also clearly diverges from Migdal's (2001) account of how authoritarian states similarly impose themselves on economic society for far less collaborative purposes and often for pure social control.

Yet the civil-society-in-state paradigm suggested by MDD processes also inverts a core assumption in the EE model by arguing that civil society, rather than political society or economic society, can initiate and construct encompassing embeddedness. On the most basic level, the EE framework (Evans 2010; Evans and Heller 2015) addresses how states and especially political elites embed themselves in civil-society networks in ways that can foster collaboration around shared social goals. But the point of origination for constructing embeddedness in such accounts typically involves one of two sources. In the famous case of worker-driven social development transformation in Kerala, India (Heller 1999), economic societies of unionized workers effectively took the lead in cultivating embeddedness. In both of Evans's well-known cases of industrial transformations as well as in the more recent pattern of left-party dominance in national-level Latin American politics (Huber and Stephens 2012), political parties in control of the state are thought to launch and sustain encompassing embeddedness, sometimes using participatory governance institutions as discussed earlier (Baiocchi, Heller, and Silva 2011).

This book's account of MDD instead emphasizes how civil society itself can initiate and sustain the construction of encompassing embeddedness through democratic institutions of office that have sources of power in civil society itself rather than in political parties, unions, or even participatory governance spaces. But in rejecting the Gramscian notion that class and economic organizations constitute the most important foundation of civil society, the MDD paradigm instead embraces Alexander's understanding of civil society as a sphere of universalizing solidarity that can exert control over officeholders atop the democratic state. In this view, civil society in democracies can regulate political power by placing their representatives in the state and by trying to regulate their actions while in office (2006, 133). Here, civil society has considerable potential to install high-level officeholders, who take up reigns of state power but simultaneously enter into "a publicly defined role regulated by ethical and legal constraints on both corruption and self-interest" (2006, 133). Since Brazil's return to democracy, sanitarista efforts in urban areas to control the nonbureaucratic top of the public health state in just such a manner have been the principal lynchpin for building the otherwise missing state capacities to realize the commitments at the core of sanitary reform and its ideology of a universal right to health.

Thus, the notion of MDD suggests that even in democracies of the Global South that lack long-standing liberal traditions of office, civil society can still lead efforts to construct developmentally fruitful ties of embeddedness with political-society elites rather than vice versa. In this sense, the paradigm accounts for how major historic transformations in social development such as those witnessed in urban Brazil could emerge from efforts by pragmatist publics to establish and wield democratic offices that enshrine universalizing ideologies like the right to health. That civil-society elites rather than political- or economic-society elites can initiate and sustain such efforts ultimately suggests that the civil-society-in-state paradigm could help explain a variety of democratically driven transformations in development beyond just Brazil.

The earlier account of MDD also addresses theories of movement consequences by demonstrating how democratic office holding by pragmatist publics can constitute a notable outcome of movements in the eyes of activists and scholarly observers alike. Yet office holding also can influence an outcome often overlooked in existing work: actual implementation of the constitutional principles, laws, and policies that movements often demand. Focusing instead on the previous step of establishing such rights, laws, and politics, sociological debates about movement consequences have tended to oscillate between two poles, with one vein of research arguing that policy impacts of movement are unlikely (Giugni 2007) and others suggesting that movements can exert robust "structural impacts" in politics (Kitschelt 1986). The former vein effectively suggests generally that even movements with otherwise effective organizations, frames, and contextually attuned strategies are likely to fall short of directly inducing state adoption or enactment of policies demanded by such actors. At most, movements are instead thought to exert indirect effects when political parties in state power embrace, internalize, and pursue the demands they articulate.

More closely in line with this study's finding about the effects of movement office holding are two other veins of research, the first of which emphasizes how movements can directly influence policy adoption (Uba 2005). Some scholarship argues that movements can have such effects even in the absence of supportive political actors, as Amenta, Caren, and Olasky (2005) demonstrate with the Townsend Plan's influence on pensions and social security in the United States. Here, uncommonly assertive movements are argued to have consequences for outcomes of interest to them when they successfully adapt their strategies to encompassing political contexts and credibly threaten ruling political elites with the loss of their positions. Although yet another body of research cautions that such approaches can result in the absorption of movements by state actors (McCarthy, Britt, and Wolfson 1991), it identifies a range of outcomes achieved through intra-institutional mobilization by movements. For instance, Bell's work on the black power movement's reforms of social work (2014) and Raeburn's account of the LGBT movement's contributions to firm-level expansion of domestic partner benefits (2004) both illustrate that intra-institutional mobilizations have borne fruit in the US context. More sharply focused on their consequences for state institutions and policies, Banaszak (2009) demonstrates the advancement of second-wave feminism by women's movements inside the US federal government. Katzenstein (1999) similarly shows how feminists have leveraged official positions to internally reform US military institutions.

But while such research suggests that movements can affect policy adoption via intra-institutional mobilization, few studies theorize movement office holding or the mechanisms by which it can improve policy implementation and influence relevant issues. Although Andrews's (2001) seminal work on the US civil rights movement shows how activists in subnational state positions helped deepen implementation of the War on Poverty's signature employment programs and social policies, it stops short of explicitly theorizing movement office holding. Accounts of movement office holding in democracies of the Global South are even rarer (see Klandermans, Roefs, and Olivier 1998), with no known work explicitly examining how it can affect policy implementation. Indeed, with few exceptions (Alvarez 2009; Lavalle and Bueno 2011), studies of movements in the Global South often imply that intra-institutional mobilization tends to oligarchize, co-opt, and depoliticize movements without necessarily advancing their intended outcomes (Alvarez 1999; Petras and Veltmeyer 2011).

There are, however, good reasons to expect that movement office holding can matter for policy implementation and development outcomes. When movements help codify universal rights in laws and policies that democratic governments lack the state machinery to enact, it is hardly unusual for activists to support the construction of such missing capacities in various ways. In Brazil, sanitaristas seized on political opportunities precipitated by such a context to establish and wield new democratic offices with concentrated authority for constructing those missing capacities. Perhaps a less glamorous movement outcome than those emphasized in existing literature, the analysis discussed earlier nevertheless showed that movement office holding was no less important for development than were more canonical factors. That movements should help institute and then hold democratic offices consolidating their own political power to build those new state capacities is, however, neither obvious nor guaranteed.

Thus, far from a general theory applicable to all movements across time and place, the notion of movement office holding instead addresses how pragmatist publics frame demands and exploit opportunities within weakly institutionalized democratic contexts to establish and wield political offices responsible for implementing movement-demanded laws and policies. Though difficult to extract from its historical context, the story of Brazil's sanitaristas nevertheless has important lessons for existing debates. The nearly five-decade-long history of sanitarista struggle for health and democracy suggests that democratic office holding can constitute a modest but nontrivial middle ground through which activists foster the enactment of universal rights by establishing and leveraging democratic offices responsible for their realization. It should therefore be obvious that while movement office holding can have relatively fast institution-building outcomes, effects of such changes on macrosociological outcomes like society-wide development require years or decades to accumulate.

Ultimately then, office holding by pragmatist publics has considerable potential to help construct the otherwise missing state capacities that decentralized democracies throughout the Global South require for fulfilling universal social-policy promises. Thus, even in contexts of weakly institutionalized democracies and fragmented party systems that often conspire against party-led programmatic policy implementation, such publics can wield democratic offices to implement such policies. Movement office holding does so by truncating the distance between activists and tangible levers of state-building power to construct the material state capacities without which realization of core movement ideologies remains elusive. Yet office holding also matters on a symbolic level for movements that see their own success as tied up in the practical ability to tangibly advance otherwise abstract principles that such offices are founded to uphold. In short, even without inducing other outcomes like actual policy implementation or amelioration of the social issues that such policies target, office holding itself constitutes a meaningful stand-alone outcome for pragmatist publics. None of this, however, suggests that office holding renders such actors immune to cooptation, depoliticization, demobilization, or other attendant risks of intra-institutional mobilizations. These risks persist and remain potential pitfalls but involve a separate set of considerations that are addressed later.[2]

2.4. PRAGMATIST PUBLICS AS DRIVERS OF HEALTH OUTCOMES

Finally, this study is the first of its kind to systematically demonstrate that pragmatist publics have mattered for society-wide health outcomes even when considering the separate influences of other factors. More specifically, democratic office holding by activists on subnational levels mattered for more expanded primary public-health-care provision and for society-wide health outcomes such as IMR reduction itself. Thus, the findings complement a growing chorus of literature on the Global South that highlights how factors such as women's office holding and certain types of civil-society organizations can help improve public health outcomes. To be sure, the findings hardly suggest that movement office holding was the only or highest-magnitude predictor of policy implementation and development outcomes, which clearly still respond to more canonical predictors. But they do highlight a promising new hypothesis of such outcomes in other, similar political contexts.

The theory of MDD also addresses a growing body of scholarship on determinants of health outcomes by demonstrating the effects of pragmatist publics on reduced childhood mortality. For instance, emerging research points to the macrodevelopmental contributions of civil-society-related factors, including the mere presence of international NGOs (Shandra, Shandra, and London 2010). Other cross-national studies of democracies in the Global South show that women's legislative office holding—a factor with clear ties to women's movements (Fallon, Swiss, and Viterna 2012)—can matter for child survival outcomes when it reaches a critical-mass threshold of at least 20% (Swiss, Fallon, and Burgos 2012). Still other accounts suggest that the mere presence of health-focused movement networks in a given national or local context can promote social development. Whereas McGuire (2010) argues for the cross-national relevance of health-focused policy networks, Borges Sugiyama (2012) argues that the local presence of a sanitarista network across urban Brazil has helped diffuse mortality-reducing primary health programs like the PSF. Nevertheless, such a hypothesis faces limitations when applied to Brazil's largest capitals, in which childhood mortality and PSF coverage outcomes have varied widely but the mere existence of organized sanitarista networks has not.

This book's account of MDD in urban Brazil differs from other accounts that more overtly consider civil society's contributions but tend to either undertheorize or look past the specific ways in which these actors have mattered for mortality-reducing state-building. For one, existing work has tended to focus on the Sanitarist Movement's agency in the national political struggles that helped codify a right to health in 1988 while de-emphasizing the following three decades in which these actors sought to enact that sweeping promise. Other scholarship has often seen these actors' agency through the lens of political science theories of policy diffusion and policy networks without assessing how civil-society lineages of such actors conditioned their political influence. In emphasizing the various medical and expert backgrounds of its activists, still other accounts have tended to conceptualize these actors as health professionals whose political influence was largely reducible to their technical training in fields of public health and medicine. As a result, efforts to define and analyze Brazil's sanitaris-tas have remained surprisingly insulated from sociological theories of social movements and civil society.

Unlike such other accounts, this study has offered an explanation more firmly rooted in the political sociology of civil society and democracy. In this regard, the pragmatist publics that advanced MDD in Brazil differed from these other hypothesized protagonists in several theoretically conse-quential respects. These differences stem from how pragmatist publics ac-cumulate power to influence state-building by institutionalizing and then wielding democratic offices atop the nonbureaucratic state. Although these offices were sometimes the highest locally elected offices, such as the may-orship (for example, in Belo Horizonte and Curitiba), pragmatist publics were more often appointed to offices atop the public health state such as the SUS manager's office. This is notable in part because it raises the ques-tion of how they gained access to such offices at all without winning com-petitive elections or otherwise conducting campaigns in the full public eye. The answers to such questions lie in the fact that pragmatist publics such as Brazil's sanitaristas were essentially founders of the offices they sought to occupy over multiple subsequent decades. Central to the state-building power they exerted when holding these offices was the lineage of these ac-tivists and veterans in a movement that was publicly recognized as having established the SUS and its highest democratic offices atop Brazil's public health state. Further, these lineages were all the more important for exer-cising state-building power in a democracy as young as Brazil's that gener-ally lacked the political cultures and traditions on which democratic offices were established in long-standing democracies of the Global North.

Additionally, the notion of pragmatist publics as drivers of health outcomes differs from arguments stressing the technical savvy and policy networks of medical and health professionals that design public-health-care programs. Such accounts generally emphasize the technical prowess and connectedness of public health experts to one another as the prime source of their effectiveness in enacting the state interventions they design to solve public problems such as widespread premature mortality. Here, the public problem-solving know-how of the policy networks to which medical and public health professionals often belong can itself become a source of power because of the sheer effectiveness that the programs can ultimately have. And in the case of Brazil, scholars have indeed argued that much social development progress has been achieved thanks to such actors' professional training and expertise in crafting such interventions (Harris 2017).

The notion of MDD, however, emphasizes the sources of pragmatist publics' civil power to enact the state-building proposals they design. It more directly locates this power in civil society and the ability of pragmatist publics to fuse arguments about the practical benefits of the interventions they design with normatively infused justifications for them. More specifically, such arguments become powerful in part because they echo universalizing ideologies produced by regulative and communicative institutions of civil society. Such fusion of normatively grounded claims-making with technical problem solving also differs in important ways from the mere depoliticization of civil-society actors or replacement of them with mere professionals or technocrats. In short, pragmatist publics have helped improve health outcomes by toggling between distinct repertoires of contention while drawing civil power from sanitarista associations and especially the civil-society regulative institution of democratic office.

3. The End of MDD in Brazil

Thirty years after the codification of Brazil's 1988 Constitution, efforts to democratize health languished amid new threats from old sources. Although the Sanitarist Movement had begun demobilizing long before the political crisis of 2016 and resulting impeachment of President Dilma Rousseff, these events cast additional darkness over the future of the SUS. In April of that year, Michel Temer replaced Rousseff in the office of president following what many observers called a parliamentary coup mounted by conservative political adversaries fearing the continuation of corruption investigations she had allowed to proceed. In November of 2016, Ricardo Barros, the federal health minister appointed by Temer, formed a high-level work group to study prospects for revising and possibly rolling back the Organic Health Law that created the SUS (Folha de São Paulo 2016). Later that year, Temer's government secured adequate congressional support to pass Constitutional Amendment 95, freezing all government spending at current, inflation-adjusted levels for twenty years. Few could deny the grievous blow that this draconian measure dealt to the universalizing ambitions of the SUS and the right to health more generally.

Nevertheless, such events hardly nullify this book's civil-society-based explanation for Brazil's previous quarter century of social development. If anything, the country's 2016 political crisis and impeachment proceedings exposed holes in some of the most dominant accounts of Brazil's impressive social development trajectory. For example, revelations of widespread corruption within Brazil's progressive Workers' Party (PT) presidencies complicate the fit of theories highlighting national rule by left-leaning political parties as the sole or unambiguous driver of Brazil's democratically rooted development pattern. Additionally, the conservative-led impeachment of Rousseff revived questions about how the country achieved so much progress in health outcomes even before national PT rule began in 2003, when such adversaries of equity-enhancing reforms in nationwide politics enjoyed even stronger ties to Brazil's more centrist and right-leaning former presidents. A core premise of this book is that answers to such puzzles lie in the oft-overlooked fact that although health and social development outcomes improved dramatically across Brazil after its return to democracy, they did so much more fully in some major cities than in others. Rather than bracketing such internal diversity, the account presented in this book traced Brazil's social development transformation to the deepening of localized civil-society institutions, not merely to national-level patterns of political party rule or the rise of effective programmatic models for improving health and reducing poverty such as the PSF and Bolsa Família.

At the same time, it is hardly unusual that the Sanitarist Movement and its political project of health democratization had begun an inevitable denouement long before the conservative backlash of the mid-2010s. Sanitaristas were not alone in this regard, with demobilization becoming a fact of life for many social movements that helped restore democracy in Brazil and codify the most progressive features of its 1988 Constitution. Most obviously, this underscores that pragmatist publics are hardly immune to cycles of contention that affect nearly all organized challengers. At the same time, however, it is also notable that compared to other prominent challengers such as the MST, Brazil's sanitaristas were never as dependent on disruptive repertoires of contention that require larger numbers of highly mobilized supporters. Indeed, the sanitarista project of health democratization remained intact through enduring associations such as CEBES, ABRASCO, and increasingly mainstream but nontrivial campaigns of the CONASEMS and its state-level affiliates across urban Brazil.

As the 2000s progressed, many influential sanitarista activists and organizations began more closely emphasizing other dimensions of sanitary reform ideology than just the principles of universality and equity in access to care. As echoed in the case of Belo Horizonte, office-holding sanitaristas and leaders of nationwide organizations such as the CONASEMS began more actively pursuing enactment during the late 2000s of a different constitutional principle secured in Article 196 and the Organic Health Law— the principle of integrality, or wholeness. Such efforts brought greater attention to the right of all citizens to access a full suite of public health care that would attend to medical needs extending far beyond just primary care. Such campaigns ran apace of controversial programs such as the federal health ministry's More Doctors (*Mais Médicos*) program, which seeks to expand the number of physicians that deliver services to SUS users. Needless to say, Amendment 95 posed a dire threat to all such projects as well as to the SUS itself and its core project of universalizing access to health. And more fundamentally, such future prospects remain overshadowed by the fact that Brazil's health-democratization period was largely the product of a remarkable but now waning and likely irreplaceable generation of sanitaristas. Few could doubt the considerable vulnerability of the movement to the same attendant pitfalls of cooptation, depoliticization, and cycles of demobilization faced by all movements.

Such realities point to the fact that pragmatist publics are clearly no panacea for overcoming the challenges of progressively oriented state-building or the construction of health developmental states in the Global South. And MDD is hardly an unceasing process across all times and places, even in Brazil, where conditions for it were long favorable. Still, the MDD processes that defined the remarkable era of health democratization in Brazil show that civil-society protagonists of progressive social change can take many forms, often in unlikely places and in ways that few anticipated beforehand. As such, they are testament to both the finite constraints as well as the surprising advances that democratic politics makes possible for improving the human condition.

Notes

Chapter 1

1. Author's calculations using data from the Brazilian Statistics and Geographic Institute (IBGE), downloaded from http://ibge.gov.br/. Last accessed June 2013.

2. Sen's *Development as Freedom* (1999, 14–15) offers the definitive statement of this notion of development as the freedom of all people to pursue the lives they have good reasons to value—something that is impossible without infant survival.

3. See Escorel (2008), Falleti (2010b), and Paim (2007).

4. For instance, although the careful analysis of Touchton, Borges Sugiyama, and Wampler (2017) suggests that participatory institutions, social policies, and state capacity interact with one another to improve well-being, it stops short of assessing whether civil-society occupation of new democratic offices has driven IMR reduction.

5. See Borges Sugiyama (2012), McGuire (2010), and Garay (2016) for exceptions.

6. See especially Lange (2009) and Mahoney (2010, 242–52).

7. See, for example, Bailey (2009) and Telles and Paschel (2014, 867).

8. See, for example, Weyland (2009).

9. Author's calculations using data from IBGE, at http://ibge.gov.br/. Last accessed June 2013.

10. See especially Pritchett and Summers (1996) and Filmer and Pritchett (2001).

11. McGuire (2010, 151–52) persuasively makes this point.

12. Escorel, Giovanella, and Magalhães de Mendonça (2009) compellingly

show how the very notion of the PSF as a policy model is unsettled by local actors' considerable restructuring of the program to fit local contexts.

13. See especially Huber and Stephens (2012), Levitsky and Roberts (2011), and Pribble (2013) for applications to Latin America.

14. See also Baiocchi (2005), Baiocchi, Heller, and Silva (2011, 26), Montambeault (2015), and Wampler (2015).

15. See Evans (2010) and Evans and Heller (2015).

16. In Brazil, Abers and Keck (2013) argue that such capacity gaps leave municipal politicians with little of the "practical authority" they need to implement water management policies.

Chapter 2

1. Authoritative accounts include Escorel (2008), Falleti (2010b), and McGuire (2010, 149–80).

2. See, for example, Sheper-Hughes' account of endemic IMR in Recife (1993). Brazil's 1985 rate ranked in the 65th percentile of 199 countries tracked by World Bank records. Last accessed September 16, 2015. www.data.worldbank.org.

3. Author's calculations using data from www.data.worldbank.org. Last accessed September 16, 2015.

4. As in the rest of book, large capitals refer to all state capitals greater than one million residents in 2010 with the exception of Brasília, which is omitted because of differences in its governance structure attributable to its status as the national capital. Author's calculations use data from IBGE, www.ibge.gov.br (last accessed June 2013).

5. Manaus's 1985 IMR ranked close to the 70th percentile value for all countries globally. See note 3.

6. McGuire (2010, 151–52) persuasively makes this point.

7. Borrowing Mandani's well-known term, Gianpaolo Baiocchi, Patrick Heller, and Marcelo Kunrath Silva (2011) liken Brazil's pre-democratic urban politics to decentralized despotism.

8. See Hagopian's authoritative account of *coronelismo* and its contemporary legacies (2007).

9. See Mahoney (2010, 242–52); and McGuire (2010, 149–80).

10. Escorel (2008) offers a persuasive account of these conflictual politics of health during the 1980s.

11. Mahoney (2010, 242–52) shows that the country's northeast region has experienced the most severe colonial legacies.

12. For exceptions, see Dowbor (2012); and Paim (2008). Most Brazilian scholarship on the movement highlights the movement's precursors in the 1960s,

its rise as a movement in the repressive contexts of the 1970s, and its activists' eventual codification of the right to health in Brazil's 1988 Constitution (Escorel 2008). In earlier work, Sarah Escorel argued that the movement had largely demobilized by the early 1990s, with both its organized labor factions and health scholars and professions refocusing on internal debates about public health within unions and academia (1999). Menicucci (2007) offers a similar argument.

13. Although many sanitaristas began their activist careers in the student movement through mobilizations related to the largest Brazilian student union (UNE), their activist trajectories often migrated into organizations explicitly focused on a right to health and into intra-institutional mobilizations atop the national and subnational public health state.

14. Escorel (2008) and Paim (2007) offer detailed accounts of these multiple approaches.

15. For example, the municipality of Porto Alegre's Law #277 of 1992 specified Laws 8,080 and 8,142 in greater detail. It formally created the city's Municipal Health Council, requiring that at least 50% of its seats be held by representatives of civil-society associations, and codified its cogovernance authorities in the local health sector.

16. Among the many insightful accounts of this nationwide process are Escorel (2008); Falleti (2010a, 2010b); Fleury (1997); Lima et al. (2005); McGuire (2010); and Paim (2007).

17. These programs and systems included the Internalization of Health and Sanitary Actions Program (PIASS) of 1976, the so-called CONASP (Consultative Council of Social Security and Health Administration) Plan of 1982, the Integrated Health Actions (AIS) of 1983, and the SUS's most immediate forerunner, the Unified and Decentralized Health System (SUDS) of 1985. See Falleti (2010b); and McGuire (2010) for excellent summaries of this institutional evolution; and see Escorel (2008) for a more detailed account.

18. See Ansell (2011).

19. Sanitaristas themselves often emphasize the Gramscian qualities of their "parliamentary way" as efforts to occupy trenches of the state. Yet the less-noted pragmatist qualities of their activism emerge more subtly in my interviews with activists such as Maria Luiza Jaeger, Dr. Lídia Tonón, Lucio Barcelos, José Maria Borges, and others; in interviews with other well-known sanitaristas such as José Gomes Temporão, Givaldo Siqueira (UNESCO 2005a; UNESCO 2005b, 81); and in the accounts of scholar-activists such as Paim (2008); Escorel (2008); and Fleury (1997).

20. The Brazilian formulation of sanitary reform differs from its precursors in modern Brazil and in Italy.

21. See Escorel (2008) for an account of the movement's steady increasing support for democratic liberalism.

22. Part of a negotiated transition to democracy spawned by economic and political crisis, the regime's 1980 allowance of multiple political parties catalyzed the formation of Brazil's first mass, programmatic political party, the Workers' Party (PT), and other left-leaning political parties, some of which sanitaristas had helped to establish.

23. José Carvalho de Noronha, Luciana Dias de Lima, and Cristiani Vieira Machado (2008) provide a description of shifts over time in financing.

24. See Dantas Neto (2006a, 2006b) for an account of this dominance.

25. Important exceptions to this rule were university hospitals and clinics that were operated by state governments in some cases.

26. See, for example, Avritzer (2009), Coelho (2006), and Coelho and vom Lieres (2010).

27. The baseline improvements seen in capitals such as São Paulo, Manaus, Goiânia, and Belém testify to such general progress. Although space constraints preclude in-depth, case-study analysis of these capitals, chapter 3's statistical and configurational analysis of them is consistent with this study's overall argument.

Chapter 3

1. Sen's conceptualization of social development (1999) was embraced, for example, in the UN's Human Development Index (HDI).

2. For cross-national studies using similar measures, see Shandra, Shandra, and London (2010) and Swiss, Fallon and Burgos (2012). For Brazil-specific studies, see Gonçalves (2013); Macinko, Guanais, and de Souza (2006); Rasella et al. (2012); and Touchton, Borges Sugiyama, and Wampler (2017).

3. The MS calculations assume that each PSF team on average reached approximately 3,450 residents in a catchment area (Macinko, Guanais, and de Souza 2006).

4. All FSA results are substantively similar when Y_1 membership scores are instead calculated from raw measures of change in IMR over time.

5. The equation I use for standardizing scores borrows from the approach of Longest and Vaisey (2008): $\dfrac{ranked\ variable\ -\ \min(rankedvar)}{\max(rankedvar)\ -\ \min(rankedvar)}$. Although using this standardization procedure breaches the convention of defining all fuzzy sets purely through in-depth, case-based knowledge as Ragin (2008) recommends, the scores used reflect calibrations of all sets using case knowledge from intensive fieldwork.

6. Only y-consistency test results are reported here, because it is not substantively meaningful to also conduct n-consistency tests when analyzing just posi-

tive cases. Also, although the L^*r combination has a consistency score of .919, this configuration represents the best fit for only three of five positive cases. The S^*r combination emphasized here, however, represents the best-fit configuration for all five positive cases.

7. Because Manaus scores .5 on both robust development and nonrobust development, it is not considered a member of either set. As such, it is removed from the analysis of negative cases.

8. The only remaining negative case—Goiânia—exhibits a best-fit combination that suggests an at best ambiguous relationship to nonrobust development.

9. Because none of the elaborated configurations that describe the positive cases of Porto Alegre, Fortaleza, and Curitiba were consistent with robust development more than 80% of the time, their elaborated FSA results offer a somewhat less definitive picture of the combined conditions that produced this outcome in these cases. The within-case analyses in coming chapters qualitatively examines the conditions of robust development in these cities, however.

10. Although interacting two such variables is one approach to doing so that was explored in models not presented here, it does not significantly change the substantive conclusions made here. Further, interaction terms cannot assess the combined effects of three or more variables.

Chapter 4

1. Alves (2015) argues that increased political competition for governorships interacted with other factors in creating electoral incentives that led subnational politicians to more effectively coordinate care provision through the SUS.

2. Wampler's research persuasively shows that Belo Horizonte's CMS councillors themselves are not only aware of these constraints but also avoid exerting vetoes because of their general desire for projects to proceed rather than suffer delays (2015, 136).

3. Health had previously been managed alongside other social service sectors by one agency from which the SMS split. Founded in 1948, the Department of Health Assistance (DAS) was an early, municipally run health care institution in Belo Horizonte whose functions included providing both health services and social welfare. The DAS operated through a single municipal hospital that provided inpatient services as well as dentistry and preventative medicine to indigent populations, municipal employees, their families, and other affiliated state institutions (Veloso and Matos 1998).

4. In contrast, the hospital sector remained dominated by the private sector, which owned seventy-one of eighty-six hospitals in the region, according to IBGE's 1992 AMS Survey.

5. Nevertheless, the SMS's active involvement in creating a proto-CMS may have limited other dimension of the council's self-organizing capacity by founding it on the premise that the SMS director would serve as de facto president of the CMS, an arrangement that remained in place until 1998.

6. This estimate varies from that of Belo Horizonte's SMS, which reports the rate as 34.4 in 1993 due to differences in the calculation method used. This chapter uses annual under-one-year-old death rates calculated from data that permit comparisons to other major capitals. Each annual rate is calculated by multiplying 1,000 times the quotient yielded by dividing the total number of resident births in Belo Horizonte (according to the health ministry's SIM system) by the IBGE's estimate of the under-one-year-old population.

7. See Wampler (2015, 76–86) for a deeper discussion of how political leadership fosters progressive social-policy change not just in participatory politics and social justice arenas but in urban planning sectors as well.

8. Although other analysts highlight other dimensions of its influence (see Avritzer 2009), Wampler's (2015) rich account persuasively argues that even after the city's CMS's gained the power to choose its own president, its members rarely set SMS agendas for health-policy-making or state-building and have typically lacked the power and inclination to veto annual budgets for the health sector that they deemed lacking.

9. The PT and PSB repaired the coalition thereafter, leading to fifteen years of subsequent mayoral victories.

10. Scarcities in systematic statistical data cloud the question of exactly how much of an increase had been achieved by the last year of Patrus's administration in 1996. The federally certified collection of such data (SIOPS 2017) began in 1998. In 1998, the year after Castro became mayor, the proportion was 11.67% (about 88 million reais). Archival evidence from CMS meetings in which councillors debated proposed prospective health budgets and retrospective spending reports of the SMS on September 24, 1996; July 7, 1997; and June 25, 1998, ultimately suggest that the proportion had not risen above 10% by 1997.

11. Castro created two "super-secretariats" that consolidated top-down mayoral control over the SMS and all other social-policy agencies. He correspondingly established a new and cohesive body populated by heads of planning and finance and both super-secretariats, who together coordinated major public-investment decisions to be approved by the mayor. This reorganization also subsumed the SMS beneath one super-secretariat for education, health, human rights, and social services. The intent was largely to concentrate the mayor's authority for allocating public goods and resources while creating new means of collaboration between heads of various departments for coordinating different social policies (Wampler 2015, 87–88).

Chapter 5

1. Barcelos eventually left the PT to help found the more leftist Party of Socialism and Freedom (PSOL, or *Partido de Socialismo e Liberdade*).

2. Of the remaining 2,124 employees, 1,707 worked in either municipally run hospitals or emergency service units (UPAs).

3. Dating from the Vargas era, CLTs (*Consolidação de Leis Trabalhistas*) are Brazilian labor laws that still regulate all private employment contracts today. Among the other benefits they require of employers, they guarantee workers thirteen months of salary per year.

Chapter 6

1. Albertini (2002) documents how Curitiba's Popular Health Forum (FOPS) critiqued what it saw as a top-heavy approach to public health planning in the capital.

2. For instance, Curitiba's pattern of party competition differed significantly from Salvador, where the "Carlista" political machine and clientelist network of Antônio Carlos Magalhães (ACM) effectively dominated the city's politics for a quarter century stretching from ACM's installation into power by Brazil's erstwhile dictatorship until as late as 2007 (Dantas Neto 2006).

3. This metric, analyzed in chapter 3, captures the total number of municipally delivered "basic attention" services processed through the federal health ministry's DATASUS repository (www.datasus.gov.br, accessed February 2016).

4. Studies have documented a tendency for OP participants to emphasize public-health-related infrastructure spending in their budgetary choices. See Marquetti, Ariano de Campos, and Pires (2008).

5. Paraná's SESB also operated another ten health centers in conjunction with the FSCMR that Raggio directed. See Curitiba, Prefeitura Municipal (1983).

6. See, for example, the account of IPPUC's continued dominance of planning in Irazabal's work (2009, 214), and see Cubas's account of IPPUC and its associated agency, the Municipal Institute of Public Administration, IMAP (2002, 42–54).

7. See, for example, Ribeiro's discussion of 1979 mobilizations by Vila São Pedro's neighborhood association, whose demands to then mayor Lerner focused on improvements to, rather than a replacement for, the nascent primary-care model then being pursued by the DS (2009, 110–11).

8. The World Bank (2006, 52) identifies this trend as well but neither links it to nonsanitarista directorships per se.

9. Although 2003 has often been used as dividing line for examining Brazilian social development before and after Bolsa Família, the 1999 to 2016 phase

in Curitiba was a continuous period when examined from the standpoint of sanitarista office holding, growth of the capital's public health state, and IMR reduction.

10. Ducci's own cowritten chapter on the topic (Jiménez et al. 2001) in his coedited book (Ducci et al. 2001) remains an authoritative account of the program's genesis and earliest moments, whereas Vieira Carvilhe (2004) usefully traces its evolution during initial years. The following account of the program draws on these sources and the SMS's special issue on the PMC in its epidemiological bulletin of May 1999 (Curitiba, Prefeitura Municipal 1999) and its 2012 program manual (Curitiba, Prefeitura Municipal 2012) unless otherwise noted.

11. Zucco and Power (2009) rated the national PFL's ideology in 2001 as nearly a seven on a ten-point scale in which ten represented the most conservative measure.

12. It was only the mayorship of Greca (1993–1996), who briefly interrupted this overarching pattern of openness to sanitarista problem solving amid the departure from city government of Curitiba's most influential sanitarista, Armando Raggio, to assume Paraná's SES directorship under Jaime Lerner after 1994.

Chapter 7

1. Scholars of pre-1988 Ceará generally agree on the dominance of local politics by the families of just three coronels. See, for example, Bruno, de Farias, and Andrade (2002); Irazabal (2009); and Tendler (1997, 11). Northeastern coronels were not actually military officers but large landholders and local bosses, who consolidated economic and political power into a long-enduring form of traditional rule (Hagopian 2007).

2. Only Recife (67.07) and Manaus (80.67) recorded higher IMRs than Fortaleza. Fortaleza's per capita GDP was less than half of Curitiba's (R$9,743) and nearly a third that of industrial powerhouses such as Rio de Janeiro (R$12,612), São Paulo (R$12,074), and Porto Alegre (R$11,851). These figures are from IPEA's estimates of inflation-adjusted (Year 2000) currency (www.ipea.gov.br, accessed July 1, 2013).

3. Fortaleza's convergence with Curitiba in social development was even more remarkable, given that the cities remained polarized in their economic development levels: Curitiba's 2012 GDP per capita of $R13,820 ranked second highest behind only São Paulo's, while Fortaleza ($R6,862) ranked second lowest.

4. Although PT mayor Maria Luiza Fontenele held Fortaleza's mayorship during a brief period (1986–1988) that preceded municipal control of the public health sector, crises impeded the administration from enacting meaningful health-sector reforms during its brief rule. The PT had also not captured Paraná's

governorship until 2015, well after Fortaleza had achieved such robust development outcomes.

5. Efforts by Curitiba's political society to incorporate sanitaristas into health planning differ qualitatively from other clear examples of cooptation such as the Agents of Change program of Jereissati, which recruited, trained, and employed neighborhood activists to work under the direction of the governor. See Gondim (2004, 69); and Barreira (1998).

6. Mesquita (2007, 81) generally echoes this assessment. When comparing it to other such bodies within Ceará and in the northeast more generally, he finds that Fortaleza's associational density between 1997 and 2004 was below average in terms of the number of operating participatory management councils across all policy sectors, including health.

7. Cunha (2007, 151, 155–56) argues that CMS-Fortaleza was one of few councils in the northeast with "high deliberative effectiveness," insofar as most its decisions address health-policy-making and attempt to guide state actions.

8. For its achievements in infant mortality reduction, the state won UNICEF's Maurice Pate Award in 1993. See especially Tendler (1997), whose excellent analysis of this period nevertheless emphasizes the professional backgrounds of key sanitarista program designers while generally overlooking their activist trajectories and efforts to infuse public health ideologies into the state's mainstream political parties.

9. Existing accounts generally converge on the view that early Jereissati administrations generally destabilized coronelismo by winning competitive elections, cultivated new and old industries, and imposed various austerity measures that sought in part to limit bureaucratic inefficiencies. See Bruno, de Farias, and Andrade (2002); and Gondim (2004). Aside from the public health programs for which sanitaristas ultimately won support, there is little evidence of interest in or commitment to programmatic interventions in other public-service sectors.

10. Tendler (1997, 11) finds that statewide IMR throughout Ceará fell by roughly the same rate of 36%, from 102 per 1,000 in 1987, to 65 per 1,000 in 1992.

11. Several Fortalezan doctors held the SMS directorship under the first democratically elected mayorship of Maria Luiza Fontenele (PT), including Manoel Dias da Fonseca Neto in 1986, Domingos Leitão Neto in 1987, and Antônio José Silva Lima. Nevertheless, their municipal state-building influence was necessarily constrained by the fiscal crisis that Fontenele inherited, a related inability to deliver sanitation services, and a correspondingly rapid loss of public and party support from the PT, which would eventually expel Fontenele amid pervasive infighting. Perhaps most importantly, the fact that Fortaleza took control of the full network of primary health clinics in its jurisdiction only during Novem-

ber of 1989 severely constrained these secretaries' degrees of freedom for state-building, in any case.

12. These included fifty-nine health centers and twenty integrated health and education centers (Mota 1997, 82).

13. Sobral and Quixadá were the others (Machado 2013).

14. See de Oliveira Viana Esmeraldo's study of PSF workers in Fortaleza (2009).

15. The ratio of PSF teams to exclusive SUS users is based on my calculations, whereas the estimates of residents reached are those of MS-DAB.

16. Monteiro de Andrade did not immediately end the practice of contracting PSF teams on an emergency basis. In June 2005, the SMS used six-month contracts to implant twenty-one PSF teams consisting of five doctors, twenty-one nurses, thirty nurses' assistants, twenty-one dentists, and eleven social assistants. See de Oliveira Viana Esmeraldo (2009).

17. Diário Oficial do Município de Fortaleza Edition #13,344, of September 6, 2006, cited in de Oliveira Viana Esmeraldo (2009, 85).

18. Fortaleza's SMS and the federal MS's Department of Basic Attention (DAB) differ in their estimates of the number of PSF teams implanted and coverage rates achieved between 2005 and 2007. Here, I have used the DAB's estimates, which offer both more conservative estimates and allow for cleaner comparisons across the larger sample of capitals analyzed in the study.

Chapter 8

1. Wong (2004), however, points to the influence of social-welfare activists in more centralized settings of South Korea and in Taiwan, whose status as a city-state nevertheless approximates qualities of high decentralization.

2. Alonso and Mische (2017) argue that a new cycle of protest has emerged more recently in which Brazilian civil-society actors have rejected political parties and sought to avoid such pitfalls.

References

Abers, Rebecca Neaera. 2000. *Inventing Local Democracy: Grassroots Politics in Brazil*. Boulder, CO: Lynne Rienner.

Abers, Rebecca Neaera, and Margaret E. Keck. 2013. *Practical Authority: Agency and Institutional Change in Brazilian Water Politics*. New York: Oxford University Press.

Adler, David. 2016. "Story of Cities #37: How Radical Ideas Turned Curitiba into Brazil's 'Green Capital.'" *The Guardian*. May 6, 2016.

Albertini, Silvia Eufênia. 2002. "Metamorfoses do Fórum Popular de Saúde (FOPS): Participação Política de Saúde—Curitiba, PR, 1991–2001." Master's thesis, PUC São Paulo.

Alexander, Jeffrey C. 2006. *The Civil Sphere*. Oxford, UK: Oxford University Press.

Alonso, Angela, and Ann Mische. 2017. "Changing Repertoires and Partisan Ambivalence in the New Brazilian Protests." *Bulletin of Latin American Research* 36, no. 2: 144–59.

Alvarez, Sonia E. 1999. "Advocating Feminism: The Latin American Feminist NGO 'Boom.'" *International Feminist Journal of Politics* 1, no. 2: 181–209.

———. 2009. "Beyond NGO-ization? Reflections from Latin America" *Development* 52, no. 2: 175–84.

Alves, Jorge Antonio. 2012. "Coordinating Care: State Politics and Intergovernmental Relations in the Brazilian Healthcare Sector." PhD diss., Brown University.

———. 2015. "(Un?)Healthy Politics: The Political Determinants of Subnational Health Systems in Brazil." *Latin American Politics and Society* 57, no. 4: 119–42.

Amenta, Edwin, Neal Caren, and Sheera Joy Olasky. 2005. "Age for Leisure? Political Mediation and the Impact of the Pension Movement on U.S. Old-Age Policy." *American Sociological Review* 70, no. 3: 516–38.

Andrews, Kenneth T. 2001. "Social Movements and Policy Implementation: The Mississippi Civil Rights Movement and the War on Poverty, 1965 to 1971." *American Sociological Review* 66: 71–95.

Ansell, Christopher K. 2011. *Pragmatist Democracy: Evolutionary Learning as Public Philosophy*. New York: Oxford University Press.

Arouca, Sérgio. 2003. *O Dilema Preventista: Contribuição para a Compreensão e Crítica da Medicina Preventiva*. Rio de Janeiro: UNESP/Editora FIOCRUZ.

Arretche, Marta. 2004. "Toward a Unified and More Equitable Health System: Health Reform in Brazil." In *Crucial Needs, Weak Incentives: Social Sector Reform, Democratization, and Globalization in Latin America*, edited by Robert R. Kaufman and Joan M. Nelson, 155–88. Baltimore: Johns Hopkins University Press.

Auer, Peter, ed. 1998. *Code-Switching in Conversation: Language, Interaction, and Identity*. New York: Routledge.

Avritzer, Leonardo. 2002. *Democracy and the Public Space in Latin America*. Princeton, NJ: Princeton University Press.

———. 2009. *Participatory Institutions in Democratic Brazil*. Baltimore: Johns Hopkins University Press.

Bailey, Stanley. 2009. *Legacies of Race: Identities, Attitudes, and Politics in Brazil*. Stanford, CA: Stanford University Press.

Baiocchi, Gianpaolo. 2003. "The Long March through Institutions: Lessons from the PT in Power." In *Radicals in Power: The Workers' Party (PT) and Experiments in Urban Democracy in Brazil*, edited by Gianpaolo Baiocchi, 1–27. London: Zed Books.

———. 2005. *Militants and Citizens: The Politics of Participatory Democracy in Porto Alegre*. Stanford, CA: Stanford University Press.

———. 2006. "The Civilizing Force of Social Movements: Corporate and Liberal Codes in Brazil's Public Sphere." *Sociological Theory* 24, no. 4: 285–311.

Baiocchi, Gianpaolo, and Ernesto Ganuza. 2016. *Popular Democracy: The Paradox of Participation*. Stanford, CA: Stanford University Press.

Baiocchi, Gianpaolo, Patrick Heller, and Marcelo Kunrath Silva. 2011. *Bootstrapping Democracy: Transforming Local Governance and Civil Society in Brazil*. Stanford, CA: Stanford University Press.

Banaszak, Lee Ann. 2009. *Women's Movements Inside and Outside the State*. New York: Cambridge University Press.

Bandelj, Nina. 2009. "The Global Economy as Instituted Process: The Case of Central and Eastern Europe." *American Sociological Review* 74, no. 1: 128–49.

Barreira, Irlys Alencar Firmo, ed. 1998. *Os Desafios da Gestão Municipal Democrá-tica: Fortaleza*. Recife, BZ: Centro Josué de Castro.

Beck, Nathaniel. 2001. "Time-Series-Cross-Section Data: What have we Learned in the Past Few Years?" *Annual Review of Political Science* 4 (1): 271–93.

Beck, Nathaniel, and Jonathan N. Katz. 1995. "What to Do (and Not to Do) with Time-Series Cross-Section Data." *American Political Science Review* 89, no. 3: 634–47.

Bell, Joyce M. 2014. *The Black Power Movement and American Social Work*. New York: Columbia University Press.

Bennett, Andrew, and Jeffrey T. Checkel, eds. 2014. *Process Tracing: From Meta-phor to Analytic Tool*. New York: Cambridge University Press.

Borges Sugiyama, Natasha. 2012. *Diffusion of Good Government: Social Sector Re-forms in Brazil*. Notre Dame, IN: University of Notre Dame Press.

———. 2016. "Pathways to Citizen Accountability: Brazil's *Bolsa Família*." *The Journal of Development Studies* 52, no. 8: 1192–1206.

Brady, David, Jason Beckfield, and Martin Seeleib-Kaiser. 2005. "Economic Globalization and the Welfare State in Affluent Democracies, 1975–2001." *American Sociological Review* 70, no. 6: 921–48.

Brazil, Federal Republic of. 1988. *Constitution of the Federated Republic of Brazil*. Brasília: Senado.

———. 1990a. *Federal Law 8,080 of September 19, 1990*. Brasília: Diário Oficial da União.

———. 1990b. *Federal Law 8,142 of December 28, 1990*. Brasília: Diário Oficial da União.

Bruno, Artur, Aírton de Farias, and Demétrio Andrade. 2002. *Os Pecados Capi-tais do Cambeba*. Fortaleza, BZ: Editora Expressão Gráfica.

Campos, Cezar Rodrigues, Deborah Carvalho Malta, Afonso Teixeira dos Reis, Alaneir de Fátimas dos Santos, and Emerson Elias Merhy, eds. 1998. *Sistema Único de Saúde em Belo Horizonte: Reescrevendo o Público*. São Paulo: Xamã.

Carvalho de Noronha, José, Luciana Dias de Lima, and Cristiani Vieira Ma-chado. 2008. "O Sistema Único De Saúde—SUS." In *Políticas e Sistema de Saúde no Brasil*, edited by Lígia Gianovella, Sarah Escorel, Lenaura de Vas-concelos Costa Lobato, José Carvalho de Noronha, and Antonio Ivo de Car-valho, 435–72. Rio de Janeiro: CEBES & Editora FIOCRUZ.

Cavalcante e Silva, Anamaria. 1999. *Viva Criança: Os Caminhos da Sobrevivência Infantil no Ceará*. Fortaleza: Fundação Demócrito Rocha.

Chorev, Nitsan. 2012. "Changing Global Norms through Reactive Diffusion: The Case of Intellectual Property Protection of AIDS Drugs." *American Socio-logical Review* 77, no. 5: 831–53.

CMS-PA (Conselho Municipal de Saúde de Porto Alegre). 1999. *Meeting Minutes of May 13, 1999*. New York: Mimeo.

———. 2012. *Conselho Municipal de Saúde de Porto Alegre, 1992–2012: 20 Anos de Protagonismo na Defesa do SUS*. Porto Alegre, BZ: Conselho Municipal de Saúde de Porto Alegre.

———. 2017. "Histórico da CMS-Porto Alegre." Last accessed March 21, 2017. http://www2.portoalegre.rs.gov.br/cms/.

Coelho, Márcia Oliveira. 2006. "Humanização das Ações de Saúde na Atenção Básica de Fortaleza-CE: Caminhos e Descminhos." Master's thesis, Universidade Estadual de Ceará.

Coelho, Vera Schattan, and Bettina von Lieres, eds. 2010. *Mobilizing for Democracy: Citizen Action and the Politics of Public Participation*. London: Zed Books.

Conniff, Michael L. 1981. *Urban Politics in Brazil: The Rise of Populism, 1925–1945*. Pittsburgh, PA: University of Pittsburgh Press.

Cortés, Carlos E. 1974. *Gaúcho Politics in Brazil: The Politics of Rio Grande do Sul, 1930–1964*. Albuquerque: University of New Mexico Press.

Cortes, Soraya Maria Vargas. 2002. "Construindo a Possibilidade da Participação dos Usuários: Conselhos e Conferências no Sistema Único de Saúde." *Sociologias* 4, no. 7: 18–49.

Coslovsky, Salo, and Amit Nigam. 2015. "Building Prosecutorial Autonomy from Within: The Transformation of the Ministério Público in Brazil." NYU Wagner Research Paper (2709104).

Cubas, Marcia Regina. 2002. "Planejamento Local de Unidades Básicas de Saúde de Curitiba-PR: Da Teoria à Prática, Aspectos Facilitadores e Limitantes." Master's thesis, UEPG-PR.

Cunha, Eleonara Schettini Martins. 2007. "A Efectivade Deliberativa dos Conselhos Municipais de Saúde e de Criança e Adolescente no Nordeste." In *A Participação Social no Nordeste*, edited by Leonardo Avritzer, 135–65. Belo Horizonte, BZ: Editora UFMG.

Curitiba, Prefeitura Municipal. 1979. *Diretrizes Gerais de Núcleos Comunitários*. Curitiba: Departamento de Desenvolvimento Social.

———. 1983. *Relatorio de Gestão*. Curitiba, BZ: Prefeitura Municipal de Curitiba.

———. 1999. "Edição Especial: Programa Mãe Curitibana." Special issue, *Boletim Epidemiológico de Curitiba* (May).

———. 2012. *Pré-Natal, Parto, Puerpério e Atenção ao Recém-Nascido*. Curitiba, BZ: SMS-Curitiba.

Dantas Neto, Paulo Fábio. 2006a. "O Carlismo para Além de ACM: Estratégias Adaptivas de uma Elite Política Estadual." In *Governo, Políticas Públicas e Eli-*

tes Políticas nos Estados Brasileiros, edited by Paulo Fábio Dantas Neto and Celina Souza. Rio de Janeiro: Revan.

———. 2006b. *Tradição, Autocracia e Carisma: A Política de Antonio Carlos Magalhães na Modernização da Bahia (1954–1974)*. Belo Horizonte, BZ: Editora UFMG.

de Miranda Gondim, Gracia Maria. 2011. "Entrevista: Luiz Odorico Monteiro de Andrade." *Trabalho, Educação e Saúde* 8, no. 3: 587–94.

de Oliveira Viana Esmeraldo, Geordany Rose. 2009. "A Organização de Estratégia Saúde da Família em Fortaleza-CE: Do Processo de Implantação ao Contexto Atual." Master's thesis, Universidade Estadual do Ceará.

de Quadros, Doacir Gonçalves. 2013. "Partidos Políticos e Propaganda Política: As Estratégias Discursivas nas Eleições para Prefeito de Curitiba." *Revista Organização Sistêmica* 4, no. 2: 242–67.

de Sousa Arão, Márcia Regina Mariano. 2012. "Orçamento Participativo em Fortaleza: Práticas e Percepções." Master's thesis, UECE.

Dewey, John. (1927) 2012. *The Public and Its Problems*. University Park: Penn State University Press.

dos Santos, Sales Augusto. 2012. "The Fight for Affirmative Action for Brazil's Public Universities: What Explains Academic and Political Resistance to Quotas for Black Students." Paper presented at UNC-Duke Consortium on Latin American Studies Conference, Chapel Hill, NC, February 17.

Dowbor, Monika. 2012. "A Arte da Institucionalização: Estratégicas de Mobilização dos Sanitaristas (1974–2006)." PhD diss., Universidade de São Paulo.

Ducci, Luciano. 2017. "Biography of Luciano Ducci, Congressional Representative." Brazil's Chamber of Deputies: Get to Know the Deputies. Accessed January 2017. http://www2.camara.leg.br/deputados/pesquisa/layouts_deputados _biografia?pk=178931.

Ducci, Luciano, Maria Alice Pedotti, Mariângela Galvão, and Samuel Jorge Moysés, eds. 2001. *Curitiba: Saúde De Braços Abertos*. Rio de Janeiro: CEBES.

Eakin, Marshall. 2016. *Tropical Capitalism: The Industrialization of Belo Horizonte, Brazil, 1897–1997*. New York: Palgrave.

Emirbayer, Mustafa, and Mimi Sheller. 1999. "Publics in History." *Theory and Society* 28, no. 1: 143–97.

Escorel, Sarah. 1999. *Reviravolta Na Saúde: Origem e Articulação do Movimento Sanitário*. Rio de Janeiro: Editora FIOCRUZ.

———. 2008. "História das Políticas de Saúde no Brasil De 1964 a 1990: Do Golpe Militar à Reforma Sanitária." In *Políticas e Sistema De Saúde no Brasil*, edited by Lígia Gianovella, Sarah Escorel, Lenaura de Vasconcelos Costa Lobato, José Carvalho de Noronha, and Antonio Ivo de Carvalho, 385–434. Rio de Janeiro: CEBES & Editora FIOCRUZ.

Escorel, Sarah, Lígia Giovanella, and Magalhães de Mendonça, Maria Helena. 2009. *Estudos de Caso Sobre Implementação da Estratégia Saúde da Família em Quatro Grandes Centros Urbanos*. Rio de Janeiro: Editora FIOCRUZ.

Estado de Minas. 2000a. "Saúde é Maior Problema do Doutor BH." February 20, 2000. https://www.em.com.br/.

———. 2000b. "Secretária Vai a Brasília Hoje." May 23, 2000. https://www.em.com.br/.

Evans, Peter B. 2010. "Constructing the 21st Century Developmental State: Potentialities and Pitfalls." In *Constructing a Democratic Developmental State in South Africa*, edited by Omano Edigheji, 39–58. Cape Town, SA: Human Science Research Council Press.

Evans, Peter B., and Patrick Heller. 2015. "Human Development, State Transformation, and the Politics of the Developmental State." In *The Oxford Handbook of Transformations of the State*, edited by Stephan Leibfried, Evelyne Huber, Matthew Lange, Jonah D. Levy, and John D. Stephens, 691–713. New York: Oxford University Press.

Falleti, Tulia G. 2010a. *Decentralization and Subnational Politics in Latin America*. New York: Cambridge University Press.

———. 2010b. "Infiltrating the State: The Evolution of Health Care Reforms in Brazil, 1964–1988." In *Explaining Institutional Change: Ambiguity, Agency, and Power*, edited by James Mahoney and Kathleen Thelen, 38–62. New York: Cambridge University Press.

Fallon, Kathleen M., Liam Swiss, and Jocelyn Viterna. 2012. "Resolving the Democracy Paradox: Democratization and Women's Legislative Representation in Developing Nations, 1975 to 2009." *American Sociological Review* 77, no. 3: 380–408.

Faria, Cláudia Feres. 2007. "Sobre os Determinantes das Políticas Participativas: A Estrutura Normativa e o Desenho Institucional dos Conselhos Municipaie de Saúde e de Direitos da Criança e do Adolescente no Nordeste." In *A Participação Social no Nordeste*, edited by Leonardo Avritzer, 111–35. Belo Horizonte: Editora UFMG.

Filmer, Deon, and Lant Pritchett. 1999. "The Impact of Public Spending on Health: Does Money Matter?" *Social Science & Medicine* 49, no. 10: 1309–23.

Fleury, Sonia, ed. 1997. *Saúde e Democracia—A Luta do CEBES*. São Paulo: Lemos.

Folha de Londrina. 1998. "Crise Derruba Secretário de Saúde." *Folha De Londrina*, July 7. http://www.folha.uol.com.br/.

Folha de São Paulo. 1995. "Prefeitos Dizem Investir na Área." *Folha de São Paulo*, June 22, 1995. http://www.folha.uol.com.br/.

————. 1997. "Castro Diz que Saúde É Meta." *Folha de São Paulo*, January 2, 1997. http://www.folha.uol.com.br/.

————. 2016. "Para Frear Gastos em Saúde, Temer Estuda Rever SUS." *Folha de São Paulo*, August 31, 2016. http://www.folha.uol.com.br/.

Frees, Edward. 2004. *Longitudinal and Panel Data: Analysis and Implications in the Social Sciences*. Cambridge, UK: Cambridge University Press.

Galeano, Diego, Lucía Trotta, and Hugo Spinelli. 2011. "Juan César García y El Movimiento Latinoamericano de Medicina Social: Notas sobre una Trayectoria de Vida." *Salud Colectiva* 7, no. 3: 285–315.

Garay, Candelaria. 2016. *Social Policy Expansion in Latin America*. New York: Cambridge University Press.

Gardner-Chloros, Penelope. 2009. *Code-Switching*. New York: Cambridge University Press.

Gibson, Christopher L. 2012. "Making Redistributive Direct Democracy Matter: Development and Women's Participation in the Gram Sabhas of Kerala, India." *American Sociological Review* 77, no. 3: 409–34.

————. 2017. "The Consequences of Movement Office-Holding for Health Policy Implementation and Social Development in Urban Brazil." *Social Forces* 96, no. 2: 751–78.

Giovanella, Lígia, Sarah Escorel, Lenaura de Vaconcelos Costa Lobato, José Carvalho de Noronha, and Antonio Ivo de Carvalho, eds. 2008. *Políticas e Sistema De Saúde no Brasil*. Rio de Janeiro: Editora FIOCRUZ.

Giugni, Marco. 2007. "Useless Protest? A Time-Series Analysis of the Policy Outcomes of Ecology, Antinuclear, and Peace Movements in the United States, 1977–1995." *Mobilization: An International Quarterly* 12, no. 1: 53–77.

Goldfrank, Benjamin. 2011. *Deepening Local Democracy in Latin America: Participation, Decentralization, and the Left*. University Park, PA: Penn State University Press.

Gonçalves, Sónia. 2013. "The Effects of Participatory Budgeting on Municipal Expenditures and Infant Mortality in Brazil." *World Development* 53: 94–114.

Gondim, Linda Maria de Pontes. 1998. *Clientelismo e Modernidade nas Políticas Públicas: Os "Governos das Mudanças" no Ceará, 1987–1994*. Ijuí, BZ: Editora Unijui.

————. 2004. "Creating the Image of a Modern Fortaleza: Social Inequalities, Political Changes, and the Impact of Urban Design." *Latin American Perspectives* 31, no. 2: 62–79.

Gramsci, Antonio. 2000. *The Antonio Gramsci Reader: Selected Writings, 1916–1935*. Edited by D. Forgacs. New York: New York University Press.

Gue Martini, Jussara. 2000. "Implantação do Programa de Saúde da Família em Porto Alegre." *Revista Brasileira De Enfermagem* 53: 71–76.

Habermas, Jürgen. 1981. *The Theory of Communicative Action*. Vol. 1, *Reason and the Rationalization of Society*. Translated by Thomas McCarthy. Boston: Beacon Press.

Hagopian, Frances. 2007. *Traditional Politics and Regime Change in Brazil*. New York: Cambridge University Press.

Harris, Joseph. 2017. *Achieving Access: Professional Movements, Politics, and the Struggle for Health in Thailand, Brazil, and South Africa*. Ithaca, NY: Cornell University Press.

Harriss, John, and Olle Törnquist. 2017. "Comparative Notes on Indian Experiments in Social Democracy: Kerala and West Bengal." In *Reinventing Social Democratic Development: Insights from Indian and Scandinavian Comparisons*, edited by John Harriss and Olle Törnquist, 53–86. Copenhagen: NIAS Press.

Heidrich, Andréa Valente. 2002. "O Conselho Municipal de Saúde e o Processo de Decisãos sobre a Política de Saúde Municipal." Master's thesis, Universidade Federal do Rio Grande do Sul.

Heimann, Sterman L., Ester Do N. Castro, I. J. Kayano, J. Leite Da Rocha, and L. Ferreira Riedel. 1998. *Descentralização do Sistema de Saúde no Brasil: Uma Proposta sobre o Impacto de Políticas, Relatório Final*. São Paulo: Instituto de Saúde, SES-SP.

Heller, Patrick. 1999. *The Labor of Development: Workers and the Transformation of Capitalism*. Ithaca, NY: Cornell University Press.

Heller, Patrick, K. N. Harilal, and Shubham Chaudhuri. 2007. "Building Local Democracy: Evaluating the Impact of Decentralization in Kerala, India." *World Development* 35, no. 4: 626–48.

The Hindu. February 16, 2004. "CPI(M) Expels M. P. Parameswaram." Last accessed July 8, 2011. http://www.thehindu.com/2004/02/16/stories/2004021602610700.htm.

Hochman, Gilberto. 1998. *A Era do Saneamento: As Bases da Política de Saúde Pública no Brasil*. São Paulo: Hucitec/ANPOCS.

Holston, James. 2008. *Insurgent Citizenship: Disjunctions of Democracy and Modernity in Brazil*. Princeton, NJ: Princeton University Press.

Huber, Evelyne, and John D. Stephens. 2012. *Democracy and the Left: Social Policy and Inequality in Latin America*. Chicago: University of Chicago Press.

Hunter, Wendy. 2010. *The Transformation of the Workers' Party in Brazil, 1989–2009*. New York: Cambridge University Press.

Irazabal, Clara. 2009. "Urban Design, Planning, and the Politics of Development in Curitiba." In *Contemporary Urbanism in Brazil: Beyond Brasília*, edited by Vicente del Rio and William Siembieda, 202–23. Gainesville: University Press of Florida.

Jiménez, E. J. B., E. C. X. F. Soares, M. B. G. Simão, M. E. Shimazaki,

L. Ducci, M. B. G. Simão, and S. G. Moisés. 2001. "Avançando na Atenção Materno-Infantil: Programa Mãe Curitibana." In *Curitiba: A Saúde de Braços Abertos*, edited by Luciano Ducci, Maria Alice Pedotti, Mariângela Galvão Simão, and Samuel Jorge Moysés, 201–12. Rio de Janeiro: CEBES.

Jobim, Rita, and Denise Aerts. 2008. "Mortalidade Infantil Evitável e Fatores Associados em Porto Alegre, Rio Grande do Sul, Brasil, 2000–2003." *Cadernos De Saúde Pública* 24, no. 1: 179–87.

Jornal Brasil. 1988. "Invasão Melhora Posto De Saúde no Sul." *Jornal Brasil* (September 15).

Junqueira, Virginia, Umberto Catarina Pessoto, Jorge Kayano, Paulo Roberto Nascimento, Iracema Ester do Nascimento Castro, Jucilene Leite da Rocha, Marcelo Fernando Terence, Roberta Cristina Boaretto, Lauro Cesar Ibanhes, Carlos Tato Corizo, and Luiza Sterman Heimann. 2002. "Equidad en la Salud: Evaluación de Políticas Públicas en Belo Horizonte, Minas Gerais, Brasil, 1993–1997." *Cadernos da Saúde Pública* 18, no. 4: 1087–101.

Katzenstein, Mary Fainsod. 1999. *Faithful and Fearless: Moving Feminist Protest Inside the Church and Military*. Princeton, NJ: Princeton University Press.

Keck, Margaret E. 1992. *The Workers' Party and Democratization in Brazil*. New Haven, CT: Yale University Press.

Kitschelt, Herbert P. 1986. "Political Opportunity Structures and Political Protest: Anti-Nuclear Movements in Four Democracies." *British Journal of Political Science* 16, no. 1: 57–85.

Klandermans, Bert, Marlene Roefs, and Johan Olivier. 1998. "A Movement Takes Office." In *The Social Movement Society: Contentious Politics for a New Century*, edited by David S. Meyer and Sidney G. Tarrow, 173–94. Boulder, CO: Rowman and Littlefield.

Kohli, Atul. 2004. *State-Directed Development: Political Power and Industrialization in the Global Periphery*. New York: Cambridge University Press.

Kristal, Tali. 2010. "Good Times, Bad Times: Postwar Labor's Share of National Income in Capitalist Democracies." *American Sociological Review* 75, no. 5: 729–63.

Lange, Matthew. 2009. *Lineages of Despotism and Development: British Colonialism and State Power*. Chicago: University of Chicago Press.

Lavalle, Adrian Gurza, and Natália S. Bueno. 2011. "Waves of Change within Civil Society in Latin America: Mexico City and Sao Paulo." *Politics & Society* 39, no. 3: 415–50.

Leite Lima, Luciana. 2010. "A Política de Regulação do Setor Privado na Saúde em Perspectiva Comparada: Os Casos de Belo Horizonte/MG e Porto Alegre/RS." PhD thesis, Universidade Estadual de Campinas.

Levcovitz, Eduardo, Luciana Dias de Lima, and Cristiani Vieira Machado. 2001.

"Política de Saúde nos Anos 90: Relações Intergovernamentais e o Papel das Normas Operacionais Básicas." *Ciência e Saúde Coletiva* 6, no. 2: 269–318.

Levitsky, Steven, and Kenneth M. Roberts, eds. 2011. *The Resurgence of the Latin American Left*. Baltimore: Johns Hopkins University Press.

Lima, Nísia Trindade, Silvia Gerschman, Flavia Coelho Edler, and Julio Manuel Suárez, eds. 2005. *Saúde e Democracia: História e Perspectivas do SUS*. Rio de Janeiro: Editora FIOCRUZ.

Lipset, Seymour Martin, Martin A. Trow, James Samuel Coleman, and Clark Kerr. 1956. *Union Democracy: The Internal Politics of the International Typographical Union*. Glencoe, IL: Free Press.

Lobato, Lenaura, and Luciene Burlandy. 2000. "The Context and Process of Health Care Reform in Brazil." In *Reshaping Health Care in Latin America*, edited by Sonia Fleury, Susan Belmartino, and Enis Baris, 79–102. Ottawa: International Development Research Centre.

Longest, Kyle C., and Stephen Vaisey. 2008. "Fuzzy: A Program for Performing Qualitative Comparative Analyses (QCA) in Stata." *Stata Journal* 8, no. 1: 79.

Machado, Katia. 2013. "Entrevista: Luiz Odorico Monteiro De Andrade." Revista Radis. Last accessed June 13, 2013. http://www6.ensp.fiocruz.br/radis/revista -radis/09/reportagens/entrevista-luiz-odorico-monteiro-de-andrade.

Machado, Moisés, Telma Gonçalves Meniucci, and Zoraya Bernadete de Souza. 2009. "A Experiência da Política de Segurança Alimentar e Nutricional de Belo Horizonte: Parcerias, Participação e Controle Social." *Revista do Observatório do Melênio De Belo Horizonte* 2, no. 1: 83–99.

Macinko, James, Frederico C. Guanais, and Maria de Fátima de Souza. 2006. "Evaluation of the Impact of the Family Health Program on Infant Mortality in Brazil, 1990–2002." *Journal of Epidemiology and Community Health* 60, no. 1: 13–19.

Magalhães, Helvécio Miranda, Jr., ed. 2010. *Desafios e Inovações Na Gestão do SUS em Belo Horizonte: A Experiência de 2003 a 2008*. Belo Horizonte, BZ: Mazza.

Mahoney, James. 2010. *Colonialism and Postcolonial Development*. New York: Cambridge University Press.

Mahoney, James, and Kathleen Thelen, eds. 2015. *Advances in Comparative-Historical Analysis*. New York: Cambridge University Press.

Mainwaring, Scott. 1999. *Rethinking Party Systems in the Third Wave of Democratization: The Case of Brazil*. Stanford, CA: Stanford University Press.

Malta, Deborah Carvalho, Leila Maria Ferreira, Teixeira dos Reis, and Emerson Elias Merhy. 2000. "Mudando o Processo de Trabalho na Rede Pública: Alguns Resultados da Experiência em Belo Horizonte." *Saúde em Debate* 24, no. 56: 21–34.

Marquetti, Adalmir, Geraldo Ariano de Campos, and Roberto Pires. 2008. *Democracia Participativa e Redistribuição: Análise de Experiências de Orçamento Participativo*. São Paulo: Xamã.

McCarthy, John D., David W. Britt, and Mark Wolfson. 1991. "The Institutional Channeling of Social Movements by the State in the United States." *Research in Social Movements, Conflicts and Change* 13, no. 2: 45–76.

McGuire, James W. 2010. *Wealth, Health, and Democracy in East Asia and Latin America*. New York: Cambridge University Press.

Menicucci, Telma. 2007. *Público e Privado na Política de Assistência à Saúde no Brasil: Atores, Processos e Trajetória*. Rio de Janeiro: Editora FIOCRUZ.

Mesquita, Erle Cavalcante. 2007. "Participação, Atores Políticos, e Transformação Institucional no Ceará." In *A Participação Social no Nordeste*, edited by Leonardo Avritzer, 65–84. Belo Horizonte, BZ: Editora UFMG.

Migdal, Joel S. 2001. *State in Society: Studying How States and Societies Transform and Constitute One Another*. Cambridge, UK: Cambridge University Press.

Ministério de Saúde (MS). 2017. "Sistema de Informações sobre Orçamentos Públicos em Saúde, SIOPS (online health expenditure data)." Last accessed February 2017. http://portalms.saude.gov.br/repasses-financeiros/siops.

Mische, Ann. 2008. *Partisan Publics: Communication and Contention across Brazilian Youth Activist Networks*. Princeton, NJ: Princeton University Press.

Montambeault, Françoise. 2015. *The Politics of Local Participatory Democracy in Latin America: Institutions, Actors, and Interactions*. Stanford, CA: Stanford University Press.

Mota, Maria Vaudelice. 1997. "Evolução Organizacional da Secretaria da Saúde do Município de Fortaleza." Master's thesis, Universidade Federal do Ceará.

Niedzwiecki, Sara. 2016. "Social Policies, Attribution of Responsibility, and Political Alignments: A Subnational Analysis of Argentina and Brazil." *Comparative Political Studies* 49, no. 4: 457–98.

Nunes Rocha, Marcelo, Sara Cristina Carvalho Cerqueira, and Carmen Fontes Teixeira. 2010. "Planejamento Municipal no SUS: O Caso da Secretaria Municipal de Saúde-Salvador." In *Planejamento em Saúde: Conceitos, Métodos e Experiências*, edited by Carmen Fontes Teixeira, 77–94. Salvador: Editora da Universidade Federal da Bahia.

OECD (Organization for Economic Cooperation and Development). 2015. "PISA Country Report for Brazil." Last accessed January 4, 2017. http://www.oecd.org/pisa/pisa-2015-Brazil.pdf.

Paim, Jairnilson Silva. 2007. "Reforma Sanitária Brasileira: Contribuição para a Compreensão e Crítica." PhD diss., Universidade Federal da Bahia.

———. 2008. "Modelos de Atenção à Saúde no Brasil." In *Políticas e Sistema de Saúde no Brasil*, edited by Lígia Giovanella, Sarah Escorel, Lenaura de Vaconcelos Costa Lobato, José Carvalho de Noronha, and Antonio Ivo de Carvalho, 547–74. Rio de Janeiro: Editora FIOCRUZ.

Parameswaran, M. P. 2005. *Empowering People: Insights from a Local Experiment in Participatory Planning*. Delhi: Daanish Books.

Paranaguá de Santana, José, and Janete Lima de Castro. 2016. *Os Sanitaristas de Jucás e o Agente de Saúde: Entrevista com Antonio Carlile Holanda Lavor e Miria Campos Lavor*. Natal, BZ: Una.

Pedotti, Maria Alice, and Samuel Jorge Moysés. 2000. "A Historia dos 20 Anos de Atenção Primaria a Saude em Curitiba e Outras Estorias." *Divulgação Saúde em Debate* 19: 6–13.

Pereira Lopes, Maria Inês, and Sonia Gesteira e Matos. 2010. "A Construção da Mudança do Modelo da Atenção com Emfâse na Atenção Primária." In *Desafios e Inovações na Gestão do SUS em Belo Horizonte: A Experiência de 2003 a 2008*, edited by Helvécio Miranda Magalhães Júnior, 127–47. Belo Horizonte, BZ: Mazza.

Petras, James, and Henry Veltmeyer. 2011. *Social Movements in Latin America: Neoliberalism and Popular Resistance*. New York: Palgrave McMillan.

Plümper, Thomas, Vera E. Troeger, and Philip Manow. 2005. "Panel Data Analysis in Comparative Politics: Linking Method to Theory." *European Journal of Political Research* 44, 2: 327–54.

Power, Timothy, and Cesar Zucco. 2009. "Estimating Ideology of Brazilian Legislative Parties, 1990–2005." *Latin American Research Review* 44, no. 1.

Prawiro, Radius. 1998. *Indonesia's Struggle for Economic Development: Pragmatism in Action*. New York: Oxford University Press.

Pribble, Jennifer. 2013. *Welfare and Party Politics in Latin America*. New York: Cambridge University Press.

Pritchett, Lant, and Lawrence H. Summers. 1996. "Wealthier Is Healthier." *Journal of Human Resources* 31, no. 4: 841–68.

Putnam, Robert. 2000. *Bowling Alone: The Collapse and Revival of American Community*. New York: Simon & Schuster.

Raeburn, Nicole C. 2004. *Changing Corporate America from Inside Out: Lesbian and Gay Workplace Rights*. Minneapolis: University of Minnesota Press.

Raggio, Armando. 1992. "A Saúde é Mudança: A Direção e o Sentido das Mudanças na Secretaria Municipal da Saúde de Curitiba." *Divulgação Em Saúde Para Debate* 8: 55–58.

———. 2016. "O Desafio de Ser Gestor da Saúde no Brasil." *Consensus* 14: 1–3.

Raggio, Armando, and Carlos Homero Giacomini. 1996. "A Permanente Construção de um Modelo de Saúde." *Divulgação Saúde em Debate* 16: 9–16.

Ragin, Charles C. 2008. *Redesigning Social Inquiry: Fuzzy Sets and Beyond*. Chicago: University of Chicago Press.

Ramos Batista, Fatima Lucia, Maria Irismar de Almeida, Sílvia Maria Nóbrega-Therrien, José Maciel de Sousa, Lucianna Leite Pequeno, and Lucélia Maria Duavy. 2005. "Políticas Públicas de Saúde em Fortaleza: Do Movimento pela Reforma Sanitária à Reforma Administrativa." *O Público e o Privado* 6: 19–33.

Rasella, Davide, Rosana Aquino, Carlos A. T. Santos, Rômulo Paes-Sousa, and Mauricio L. Barreto. 2013. "Effect of a Conditional Cash Transfer Programme on Childhood Mortality: A Nationwide Analysis of Brazilian Municipalities." *The Lancet* 382, no. 9,886: 57–64.

Réos, Janete Cardoso. 2003. "Participação em Saúde na Gerência 5 de Porto Alegre: Glória/Cruzeiro/Cristal." Master's thesis, Universidade Federal do Rio Grande do Sul.

Ribeiro, Elisete Maria. 2009. "Análise da Atenção Primária à Saúde Em Curitiba: Enfoque nos Atributos das Equipes Saúde da Família." Master's thesis, Pontifícia Universidade Católica de São Paulo.

Ribeiro, Francisco Moreira. 1995. "De Cidade a Metrópole." In *Fortaleza: A Gestão da Cidade (Uma História Políticoadministrativa)*, edited by Simone de Souza, Francisco Moreira Ribeiro, Sebatião Rogério Ponte, Ricardo Oriá, and Gisafran Jucá. Fortaleza, BZ: Fundação Cultural de Fortaleza.

Rodrigues Neto, Eleutério. 1997. "A Via do Parlamento." In *Saúde e Democracia*, edited by Sonia Fleury, 63–91. São Paulo: Lemos.

Rodrigues Neto, Eleutério, José Gomes Temporão, and Sarah Escorel. 2003. *Saúde: Promessa e Limites da Constituição*. Rio de Janeiro: Editora FIOCRUZ.

Sandbrook, Richard, Marc Edelman, Patrick Heller, and Judith Teichman. 2007. *Social Democracy in the Global Periphery: Origins, Challenges, Prospects.* New York: Cambridge University Press.

Sant'Ana, A. M., W. W. Rosser, and Y. Talbot. 2002. "Five Years of Family Health Care in São Jose." *Family Practice* 19, no. 4: 410–15.

Santos, Aleneir Fátima, Janete Maria Ferreira, Batista, Maria de Fátima Pereira, and Nayara Souza Lages. 1998. "Criando um Sistema de Informação Estratégico em Saúde: A Experiência do Projeto da Avaliação de Desempenho." In *O Sistéma Único de Saúde em Belo Horizonte: Reescrevendo o Público*, edited by Cezar Rodrigues Campos, Deborah Carvalho Malta, Afonso Teixeira Reis, Aleneir Fátima Santo, and Emerson Elias Merhy, 201–17. Belo Horizonte, BZ: Xamâ.

Sen, Amartya. 1999. *Development as Freedom.* New York: Knopf.

SES-Ceará (Secretaria da Saúde de Ceará). 2006. *A História dos Secretários da Saúde do Estado do Ceará, 1961–2006.* Fortaleza, BZ: SES-Ceará.

Shandra, John M., Carrie L. Shandra, and Bruce London. 2010. "Do Non-Governmental Organizations Impact Health? A Cross-National Analysis of

Infant Mortality." *International Journal of Comparative Sociology* 51, nos. 1–2: 137–64.

Sheper-Hughes, Nancy. 1993. *Death without Weeping: The Violence of Everyday Life in Brazil.* Berkeley: University of California Press.

Shepherd, Geoffrey. 2010. "A Civil Service Which Performs: Primary Healthcare in Curitiba, Brazil." Paper presented at the World Bank Conference, Phnom Penh, Cambodia, April 26–27.

Singh, Prerna. 2015. *How Solidarity Works for Welfare: Subnationalism and Social Development in India.* New York: Cambridge University Press.

SIOPS (Sistema de Informações sobre Orçamentos Públicos em Saúde). 2017. *Statistics on Municipal Health Spending, 2000–2017.* Last accessed January 15, 2017. http://siops-asp.datasus.gov.br/.

Skidmore, Thomas E. 2010. *Brazil: Five Centuries of Change.* New York: Oxford University Press.

SMS-BH (Secretaria Municipal de Saúde de Belo Horizonte). 2008. *Annual Management Report of the SMS, 2008.* Belo Horizonte, BZ: SMS-BH.

———. 2009. *Annual Management Report of the SMS, 2009.* Belo Horizonte, BZ: SMS-BH.

SMS-Curitiba. 2016. *Histórico Da Secretaria.* Last accessed November 16, 2016. http://www.saude.curitiba.pr.gov.br/a-secretaria/historico-da-secretaria.html.

SMS-PA (Secretaria Municipal de Saúde de Porto Alegre). 2016. *Annual Management Report of the SMS, 2016.* Porto Alegre, BZ: SMS-PA.

———. 2017. *Annual Management Report of the SMS, 2017.* Porto Alegre, BZ: SMS-PA.

Snyder, Richard. 2001. "Scaling Down: The Subnational Comparative Method." *Studies in Comparative International Development* 36, no. 1: 96–110.

Souza, Celina. 2005. "Federalismo, Desenho Constitucional e Instituições Federativas no Brasil Pós-1988." *Revista de Sociologia e Política* 24: 105–21.

Souza, Celina, and Paulo Fábio Dantas Neto, eds. 2006. *Governo, Políticas Públicas e Elites Políticas nos Estados Brasileiros.* Rio de Janeiro: Revan.

Swiss, Liam, Kathleen M. Fallon, and Giovani Burgos. 2012. "Does Critical Mass Matter? Women's Political Representation and Child Health in Developing Countries." *Social Forces* 91, no. 2: 531–58.

Tarrow, Sidney. 2011. *Power in Movement: Social Movements and Contentious Politics.* New York: Cambridge University Press.

Telles, Edward, and Tianna Paschel. 2014. "Who Is Black, White, or Mixed Race? How Skin Color, Status, and Nation Shape Racial Classification in Latin America." *American Journal of Sociology* 120, no. 3: 864–907.

Tendler, Judith. 1997. *Good Government in the Tropics.* Baltimore: Johns Hopkins University Press.

Tocqueville, Alexis de. 1945 [1840]. *Democracy in America, Vol. II.* Translated by Henry Reeve. New York: Random House.

Touchton, Michael, Natasha Borges Sugiyama, and Brian Wampler. 2017. "Democracy at Work: Moving Beyond Elections to Improve Well-Being." *American Political Science Review* 111, no. 1: 68–82.

Touchton, Michael, and Brian Wampler. 2014. "Improving Social Well-Being through New Democratic Institutions." *Comparative Political Studies* 47, no. 10: 1442–69.

TSE (Tribunal Superior Eleitoral). 2016. "Previous Elections." Last accessed July 2016. http://www.tse.jus.br/eleicoes/eleicoes-anteriores.

Uba, Katrin. 2005. "Political Protest and Policy Change: The Direct Impacts of Indian Anti-Privatization Mobilizations, 1990–2003." *Mobilization: An International Quarterly* 10, no. 3: 383–96.

UNESCO. 2005a. *Memória e Patrimônio da Saúde Pública no Brasil: A Trajetória de Sérgio Arouca, Relatório de Atividades Sérgio Arouca, 1976–1988.* Rio de Janeiro: UNESCO.

———. 2005b. *Memória e Patrimônio da Saúde Pública no Brasil: A Trajetória de Sérgio Arouca, Relatório de Atividades Sérgio Arouca, 1989–2003.* Rio de Janeiro: UNESCO.

Vaisey, Stephen. 2007. "Structure, Culture, and Community: The Search for Belonging in 50 Urban Communes." *American Sociological Review* 72, no. 6: 851–73.

Vasi, Ion Bogdan, and Brayden G. King. 2012. "Social Movements, Risk Perceptions, and Economic Outcomes: The Effect of Primary and Secondary Stakeholder Activism on Firms' Perceived Environmental Risk and Financial Performance." *American Sociological Review* 77, no. 4: 573–96.

Veloso, Bianca Guimarães, and Sonia Gesteir Matos. 1998. "A Complexa Construção do SUS—Belo Horizonte—Os Desafios que Ele Propôs." In *Sistema Único de Saúde em Belo Horizonte: Reescrevendo o Público*, edited by Cezar Rodrigues Campos, Deborah C. Malta, and Afonso Teixeira Reis. São Paulo: Xamã.

Vieira Carvilhe, Márcia Helena. 2004. "Processes de Gestão do Conhecimento e suas Contribuições para a Geração de Benefícios Intermediários em Programas Públicos: O Caso do Programa Mãe Curitibana." Master's thesis, PUC-Paraná.

Vieira Machado, Cristiani, Luciana Dias de Lima, and Tatiana Wargas de Faria Baptista. 2011. "Princípios Organizativos e Instâncias de Gestão do SUS." In *Qualificação de Gestores do SUS*, edited by Roberta Gondim de Oliveira, Victor Grabois, and Walter Vieira Mendes Jr., 47–74. Rio de Janeiro: EAD/ENSP.

Wampler, Brian. 2015. *Activating Democracy in Brazil: Popular Participation, Social Justice, and Interlocking Institutions*. Notre Dame, IN: University of Notre Dame Press.

Watts, Jonathan. 2017. "Operation Car Wash: Is This the Biggest Corruption Scandal in History?" *The Guardian*, June 1.

Weyland, Kurt. 1998. *Democracy without Equity: Failures of Reform in Brazil*. Pittsburgh: University of Pittsburgh Press.

———. 2009. *Bounded Rationality and Policy Diffusion: Social Sector Reform in Latin America*. Princeton, NJ: Princeton University Press.

Wirth, John D. 1977. *Minas Gerais in the Brazilian Federation, 1889–1937*. Stanford, CA: Stanford University Press.

Wolford, Wendy, and John D. French. 2016. "Deconstructing the Post-Neoliberal State: Intimate Perspectives on Contemporary Brazil." *Latin American Perspectives* 43, no. 2: 4–21.

Wong, Joseph. 2004. *Healthy Democracies: Welfare Politics in Taiwan and South Korea*. Ithaca, NY: Cornell University Press.

World Bank. 2006. *Enhancing Performance in Brazil's Health Sector (Report #35691-BR)*. Washington, DC: World Bank.

Zucco, Cesar, and Timothy Power. 2009. "Data and Estimates: Estimating Ideology of Brazilian Legislative Parties, 1990–2005." Harvard Dataverse. http://hdl.Handle.net/1902.1/11567.

Index

Page numbers followed by *f* or *t* indicate material in figures or tables.

ABRASCO (Brazilian Public Health Association), 35–36, 40, 139, 212, 243, 265

ACM (Antônio Carlos Magalhães), 54, 93–94, 108, 178, 203, 273n2 (ch6)

Acolhimento (Intake project), 120

ACS (Community Health Agents), 125, 185, 213, 223–226, 233

Agents of Change, 275n5

Agosto, Flávio Mouro, 150

AIS (Integrated Health Actions), 46, 112, 138, 148–149, 185

Alexander, Jeffrey C., 17–19, 21, 37, 104–106, 193, 257

Alonso, Angela, 276n2

Alvarez, Sonia E., 259

Alves, Jorge Antonio, 93–94, 271n1

AMC (Associação Médica Cearense), 212

Amenta, Edwin, 258

Amoretti, Rogério, 152

Ananias, Patrus, 88, 108, 109, 119–121, 123–124, 272n10

Andrews, Kenneth T., 259

Ansell, Christopher K., 165

ARENA party, 141, 177

Arouca, Sérgio, 42, 44, 49, 53, 139, 243

Arruda Bastos, Raimundo José, 209, 214

Arruda Sampaio, Plinio de, 243

Avritzer, Leonardo, 16, 34, 162

Azeredo, Eduardo, 89, 108, 132

Azevedo Couto, Tereza de Jesus, 89

Back, Heriberto, 150

Baiocchi, Gianpaolo, 22, 44, 139, 142–143

Banaszak, Lee Ann, 259

Baracho, João Carlos Gonçalves, 181, 194–197, 199, 202–203

Barcelos, Lucio: departure of, 167; "emergency" health care hires, 164–167; jailing of, 138; militancy of, 138, 140, 168; pragmatism of, 269n19; PSF teams under, 158, 160, 166; and PT (Workers' Party), 89, 134–135, 138, 140, 158, 161–168, 170, 246; as SMS director, 161–163, 170; supporting BF expansions, 246

"barefoot doctors," 205

Barros, Ricardo, 264

Barros Carvalho, Paulo Gustavo de, 183

Beck, Nathaniel, 69

Belém, Pará, 75–80 (79t), 84–85

Bell, Joyce M., 259

Belo Horizonte, Minas Gerais, 97; 1940s–1960s, 99–100; 1970s, 101–103; 1980s–1990s, 107–109, 111–117; 1993–1996, 118–122; 2000s, 108–110; 1997–2002, 122–126; 2003–2016, 127–131; Belo Horizonte Doctors' Union, 114; BF

Belo Horizonte, Minas Gerais (*continued*) (Bolsa Familia), 55; CMS (Municipal Health Councils), 109–110, 115, 119–120, 132, 271n2; FSA findings, 87–92; fuzzy-set analysis, 75–80 (79t); health care expansion, 56; health-sector municipalization, 151–152; IMR, 31–32, 65; IMR (1988), 97; IMR (1993–1996), 118–122; IMR (1997–2002), 122–128; IMR (2003–2016), 129–131, 209; Kubitschek, Juscelino, 99; left-party office holding, 32; Mineiro Sanitarista Party (PMS), 35, 103; Neves, Tancredo, 99–100, 111–112; "participatory-programmatic" health democratization, 3–4, 14, 24, 29, 57–59, 85, 87, 107–111, 132; PSF coverage rate, 65, 179; robust development, 78, 84; Sanitarista office holding in, 3, 79, 98, 111, 118–131; Sanitarista primary-care experiments, 111–118; SINDIBEL (Municipal Public Servants Union), 103. *See also* Castro, Célio de

Bezerra, Adauto, 211

Bezerra de Farias, Raimundo Coelho, 230

Bezerra Filho, João da Costa, 89

BF (Bolsa Família/"Family Allowance"): in Belo Horizonte and Porto Alegre, 89, 108–109, 144; as CCT measure, 69; coverage rates for, 72, 73t; in Curitiba, 91–92, 144, 178, 203; in Fortaleza, 209–210, 219, 233, 240; implementation levels of, 84–85, 87; pragmatist public support for, 12; and theory of MDD, 12, 245–247; variations in coverage of, 55–56, 69, 79, 108–109, 144, 178–179, 219–220. *See also* CCT (conditional cash transfer) programs

BH-Saúde (BH-Health), 125–127

BH Vida project, 120–121

Bolsa Escola, 245

Borges, José Maria, 88, 97–98, 101–106, 112–118, 120, 123, 245, 261, 269n19

Borges Sugiyama, Natasha, 11, 120, 178, 245, 261

Breckenfeld, Maria de Pepétuo Socorro Martins, 237–238

Britt, David W., 258

Bueno, Natália S., 259

CAEMP/CONAMP (Confederation of State Prosecutors), 243–244

Cajuru neighborhood health clinic, 176, 182, 184, 189, 198

Cals, César, 211

Cambraia, Antônio, 218, 229, 231

Campos, Cezar Rodrigues, 88, 98, 118, 120, 122–123

capital cities: fuzzy-set analysis, 75–80 (79t); regression analysis, 63–75 (69t, 73t)

Caputo Neto, Michele, 91, 172, 176, 182, 196, 198, 201–202, 204, 206

Cardoso, Fernando Henrique, 12, 245

Caren, Neal, 258

"Carlista" political machine, 54–55, 93–94, 273n2 (ch6)

Carneiro, João Henrique de Barradas, 94–95

Carteira de Saude da Crianca (Children's Health Card), 195

Car Wash (Lava Jato) scheme, 243

Castro, Célio de, 101; as "Doctor BH," 124; versus Genro faction, 168; Magalhães and, 130, 246; mayorship of, 98, 122–128, 272nn10; PSB (Brazilian Socialist Party), 89, 108, 122; and "super-secretariats," 110, 272n11

Cavalcante Brasil, Abner, 209, 218, 222, 227–229

Cavalcante e Silva, Anamaria, 115, 209, 213, 218, 225–229

CCT (conditional cash transfer) programs, 12, 55, 69, 219, 247–248; regression analyses, 69–75 (70t), 90. *See also* BF (Bolsa Família/"Family Allowance")

Ceará, 274n1; ACS (Community Health Agents), 213, 223–225, 233; Anamaria Cavalcante e Silva, 115, 209, 213, 218, 225–229; Antônio Carlile Holanda Lavor, 212–213, 223–229; "barefoot doctors" in, 205; *coronelismo* in, 142, 208, 211; and *Diretas Ja* movement,

212; elections, 215–216; local politics, 274n1; PACS (Community Health Agents Program), 229; Sanitarista associations in, 212–213; Sanitarista office holding in, 3; SES directorship in, 209, 225, 227; student mobilizations in, 213; Tasso Jereissati, 9, 213, 216–217, 223–224, 230, 275nn5; universities, 211. *See also* Fortaleza, Ceará; PMDB (Brazilian Democratic Movement Party); PSDB (Brazilian Social Democratic Party)

CEBES (Brazilian Center for Health Studies): and Armando Raggio, 182–183, 189, 193; founding and purpose of, 35–36, 40; and Maria Luiza Jaeger, 139; sanitarista associations and, 212, 220, 243, 265; *Saude em Debate* journal, 66t, 176; and SESACS forums, 101, 175

CHA (comparative-historical analysis), 23–25, 61, 62, 64, 96

Children's Health Card (*Carteira de Saude da Crianca*), 195

Chomatas, Eliane Regina de Veiga, 202

CIMS, 153–154, 157

CIMS-Porto Alegre, 148–149, 151

Ciranda da Vida, 236

citizen oversight, 3

Citizens Constitution (1988), 53

citizenship right to health, 2, 13, 18, 28, 52–53, 215–216, 265. *See also* Constitution (1988)

city-level case studies, 23–25, 61, 62, 64, 96

Civil Defense Agency/Citizen Security Secretariat (Fortaleza), 235

"civil power," 19, 21, 98, 104–106, 206, 250, 256, 263

civil-society actors. *See* pragmatist publics

"civil-society-in-state" paradigm, 250–251, 253–258

Cláudio, Roberto, 217

clientelist politics: in Belo Horizonte, 107; in Curitiba, 203, 273n2 (ch6); of far right, 13; in Fortaleza, 208, 211, 217–220, 238; and nonrobust development, 75; and pragmatist public, 14; in Salva-

dor, 93; weakening public health state, 55–56, 59

CLIS (local health commissions), 153–154, 157

CMC (Ceará Medical Center), 212

CMR (child mortality rate), 23, 26, 61–62

CMS (Municipal Health Councils): of Belo Horizonte, 109–110, 115, 119–120, 132, 271n2; as comanaging authorities, 7, 157; conflict with SMS directors, 169–170, 272n5; councillor autonomy issues in, 146, 160–161, 173, 180; of Curitiba, 170, 173, 180–181, 199, 204; of Fortaleza, 170, 210, 221–222, 275n7; and infant mortality issues, 199; under Organic Health Laws, 157; and Participatory Budgeting process, 159–160; and participatory publics, 16, 56–57, 98, 109, 131–132, 135–136, 146, 154; of Porto Alegre, 119, 135–137, 143, 145–147, 170, 244; and pragmatist publics, 143; tied to FMS (Municipal Health Fund), 157

code-switching, 13, 21–23, 44–47, 244

"coffee with milk" alliance, 99

Collares, Alceu, 139, 142, 149–150, 152, 155

colonialism, legacy of, 5, 30, 32, 60, 64–65, 78, 208

Community Health Agents Program, 125, 185, 213, 223–226, 233

comparative-historical case-study (CHA), 23–25, 61, 62, 64, 96

CONASEMS (National Council of Municipal Health Secretaries), 117, 129, 176, 213, 220, 233, 243, 265

CONASS (National Council of State Health Secretaries), 103, 105, 176–177, 193, 243

Conceição Hospital Group (GHC), 152, 154

Conde, Luis Paulo, 55

Constitution (1988), 18–19, 265; Amendment 29 (2000), 114; Amendment 95 (2016), 264; Article 196 of, 36–37, 44, 48, 139, 192, 265; Constitutional Assembly, 31, 36, 243; Laws 8,080 and 8,042, 37; Laws 8,142 and 8,080, 39,

Constitution (1988) (*continued*)
192; Municipal Health Council (CMS) in, 180; and Organic Health Laws, 29, 265; private/public-sector issue, 50; ratification of, 30, 53. *See also* citizenship right to health
COOPSAÙDE, 231
coronelismo, 107, 142, 208, 216, 218, 275n9
corporatist rule, 9
Cortes, Soraya, 153, 156
Coslovsky, Salo, 243–244
Costa Lima, Humberto Sérgio, 89, 246
CPM (Communist Party-Marxist), 249–250
CSTS (cross-sectional time-series) data, 23, 62
Cunha, Eleonara Schettini Martins, 275n7
Cunha, Heverson da, 159–160, 211
Curitiba, 31–32, 205–207; 1960s–1970s, 173–178, 182–183; 1980s–1990s, 176–178, 180–181, 184–193; 1993–1998, 194–197; 1999–2016, 178–180, 197–205; Sanitarista office holding in, 3, 79, 181–186; Sanitarista state building, 187–194, 198–205; nonsanitarista state building, 194–197; CMS (Municipal Health Councils), 170, 173, 180–181, 199, 204; colonialism and, 208; FSA findings, 87–92; fuzzy-set analysis, 75–80 (79t); health care expansion, 56; IMR (1988), 171, 186; IMR (1989-1993), 187–193; IMR (1993-1998), 194–197; IMR (1999-2016), 171, 173, 178, 198–205, 209; Municipal Health Conference, 189; Municipal Law 6,817 (1986), 185; programmatic health democratization, 3, 14–15, 24, 29, 87–92, 171–172, 177–181

da Veiga, Pimenta, 89, 108, 112–113, 132
DCE (Central Student Directorate), 214
DDS (Department of Social Development), 183
democratization. *See* health democratization

DEROS (Department of Education, Recreation, and Health), 182
development as freedom, 6, 267n2
Dewey, John/Deweyanism, 13, 21, 122, 165
Dias, Àlvaro, 178
Direct Elections Now! (*Diretas Ja*), 38, 52, 100, 212
"districtization," 189
DMP (Department of Preventative Medicine), 93, 101–103
"Doctor BH," 124. *See also* Castro, Célio de
Doctors Union of Minas Gerais (SINDMÉD-MG), 103
Dr. Albert Sabin Infant Hospital, 225
DS (Health Directorate), 183–185, 188
Ducci, Luciano, 274n10; enacting PMC, 226; and IMR decline, 198; as mayor, 202, 246; and PSF expansion, 199; as SMS director, 91, 172, 176, 182, 196, 199–202, 206
Dutra, Olívio, 143, 145, 151–152, 154, 156, 162, 164

Eighth National Health Conference (Brasília), 36, 213
Emirbayer, Mustafa, 33–34
Escorel, Sarah, 49, 269n12
Evans, Peter B., 116, 251–253, 256–257

Fagundes, Sandra, 135, 168–169
Falleti, Tulia G., 51
Family Health Program. *See* PSF (Family Health Program)
Family Welfare Movement (Indonesia), 250
FAURGS (Fundação da Universidade Federal do Rio Grande do Sul), 164–166, 169
FCMR (Caetano Munhoz da Rocha Foundation), 185
Fernandes de Souza, Luis, 93
Fernandes Tigre, Clovis Heitor, 137
FHEMIG (Hospital Foundation of Minas Gerais), 113

FIOCRUZ (Oswaldo Cruz Foundation), 213
Fischmann, Airton, 137
FMS (Municipal Health Fund), 157–158
Fogaça, José, 169
Fonseca Neto, Manuel Dias da, 216, 275n11
Fontana, Henrique, 89, 135, 161, 167, 170, 246
Fontenele, Maria Luiza, 216–217, 274n4, 275n11
FOPS (Popular Health Forum), 180–181, 273n1 (ch6)
Fortaleza, Ceará: associational density, 275n6; Civil Defense Agency/Citizen Security Secretariat, 235; CMS (Municipal Health Councils), 170, 210, 221–222, 275n7; FSA findings, 87–92; fuzzy-set analysis, 75–80 (79t); health care expansion, 56; health democratization in, 29, 31, 215–222; IMR (1987–1992), 223–229, 275n10; IMR (1993–2004), 229–232; IMR (2005–2016), 209, 232–238; left-party office holding, 32; Luiz Odorico Monteiro de Andrade, 92, 208–209, 213, 233–237, 239, 246, 276n16; Municipal Decree #8,417, 221; Sanitarista expansion in, 212, 222–238; Sanitarista office holding in, 79; SMS director, 209, 220, 225, 233, 236. *See also* Ceará
Freedom and Struggle (LIBELU), 176, 198
French, John D., 117
FSA (fuzzy-set analysis), 23–25, 61–62, 87–92; of configurational consistency, 79, 80–82; and MDD, 75–78, 95–96; negative case of Salvador, 92–95; outcome and causal sets, 77–80 (79t); and overlapping conditions, 74; positive, negative, individual cases, 84–86; of primary health-service, spending outcomes, 86–87; of robust versus nonrobust development, 82–84, 247

Garcia, Hélio, 112
García, Juan César, 49

generality, meso-, micro-, and macro-level of, 8
Genro, Tarso, 143, 152, 155–157, 161–163, 165, 167–168
GERUS training course, 196
GHC (Conceição Hospital Group), 152, 154
Giugni, Marco, 258
Global South, 1–2; civil-society-in-state, 256; democracies in, 24, 248, 259–260; encompassing embeddedness (EE) model and, 251; lack of state capacities in, 20; MDD in, 251, 256–257; measuring social development in, 12, 63–64, 242, 248; and power constellations framework, 12; public health in, 250; scholarship on, 5–7, 250, 256–257, 259–261, 265; SUS and, 41; and women office holders, 261. *See also* MDD; pragmatist publics
Goiânia, Goiás, 63, 75–79 (79t), 84, 270n27, 271n8
Gomes, Cid, 217
Gomes, Ciro, 217–218, 225, 227
Gonzaga Mota, Luis, 215–217
Gouvêa Teixeira, Marcelo, 130
GPLD (Division of Planning and Development), 126–127
Gramsci, Antonio, 13, 19–21, 39–40, 257, 269n19
Greca, Rafael, 178, 192, 194, 203, 274n12
Guimarães Rocha, Fernando José, 94

Habermas, Jürgen, 23
health democratization: in Fortaleza, 29, 31, 210, 215–222, 233, 238, 240; and IMR (infant mortality rate), 58–59, 98, 177–181; "minimalist" health democratization, 4, 14, 32, 52, 87, 142, 156, 177, 217. *See also* MDD (movement-driven development); "participatory-programmatic" health democratization; programmatic health democratization
health units (US), 109, 113, 115, 153, 179, 220

"health vigilance" system, 189, 205
Health Workers Union of Minas Gerais
(SINSAÚDE-MG), 103
Heck, Selvino, 150
Heller, Patrick, 251–253, 256–257
Holanda Lavor, Antônio Carlile, 212–213,
223–229
Hunter, Wendy, 157

IDQ (Index of Service Quality), 195–196
Imbassahy, Antonio, 94
IMR (infant mortality rate), 1, 77–79; in
1980s, 29, 58, 65; from 1997–2002, 59,
65, 122–128; from 2003–2016, 65, 129–
131; Belo Horizonte (1980–1992), 97,
111, 116–117; Belo Horizonte (1993–
2002), 123; Belo Horizonte, Minas Gerais, 31–32, 97; Ceará, 275n10; in Chile
under Pinochet, 9; Curitiba (1988), 171,
186; Curitiba (1989–1993), 187–193; Curitiba (1993–1998), 194–197; Curitiba
(1999–2016), 171, 173, 178, 198–205;
failures of, 14; Fortaleza, 64; Fortaleza
(1988), 208, 227; Fortaleza (1990), 227,
229; Fortaleza (1993–2004), 210, 229–
232; Fortaleza (2005–2016), 209, 210,
232–240; Fortaleza (2015), 209; FSA results, 87–92; and health democratization, 58–59, 98, 177–181; Indonesia,
249; Manaus, 274n2; under nonrobust
development trajectory, 83–84; per
capita income and, 10; Porto Alegre,
64, 151, 170; Porto Alegre (1980s–1993),
134, 147, 151–155; Porto Alegre (1993–
1996), 155–161; Porto Alegre (1997–
2001), 161–167; Porto Alegre (2002–
2016), 134, 167–169; pragmatist publics
and, 242, 247; process tracing of, 25;
and PSF, 246–247; Recife, 64, 274n2;
Rio de Janeiro, 14; Salvador, 14, 92–
95; and sanitarista office holding, 23–
24, 61–62, 98, 111, 118–122, 129–131,
155–169. *See also* CMR (child mortality
rate); PSF (Family Health Program)
INAMPS (National Institute for Medical
Assistance in Social Security), 38, 42,
56, 113, 148–150, 154

Indonesia, 242, 248–250
influential participatory publics, 71–72,
80, 81, 88–92, 204
IPEA (Institute of Applied Economic Research), 103
IPEDASAR (Training and Research Institute for the Development of Rural
Sanitary Care), 102
IPPUC (Institute for Urban Research and
Planning of Curitiba), 173–174, 183,
191
IVS (Health Vulnerability Index), 126–
127

Jaeger, Maria Luiza, 269n19; on CNS
(National Health Commission), 138–
139; cofounding local PT, 140; defeating privatization proposal, 154; and
health-management districts, 153; IMR
increase under, 156; as SES director,
135, 149, 162; as SES worker, 138–139;
as SMS director, 89, 135, 167–168, 170,
246; as SMSSS secretary, 151–154
Jereissati, Tasso, 9, 213, 216–217, 223–224,
230, 275nn5

Kandir Law (1996), 125, 156, 161, 194
Katz, Jonathan N., 69
Katzenstein, Mary Fainsod, 259
Kerala, India, 248–250, 257
Kitschelt, Herbert P., 258
Klandermans, Bert, 259
Kliemann, Joaquim, 140, 167–168
Kohli, Atul, 9, 254, 256
Korea, 254, 276n1
KSSP (People's Science Movement), 249–
250
Kubitschek, Juscelino, 99

Lacerda, Marcio, 108, 130
Lage, Rui, 112
Lava Jato (Car Wash) scheme, 243
Lavalle, Adrian Gurza, 259
Lerner, Jaime: establishing munici-
pal state agencies, 182–184; founding
DDS (Department of Social Develop-
ment), 183; as governor, 192, 194, 199;

as IPPUC president, 174, 183, 191; and PDT, 203; positions held by, 177–178, 187; urban planning processes of, 171

LIBELU (Freedom and Struggle), 176, 198

Lima e Silva, João Paulo, 89

Lins, Luziane de Oliveira, 92, 217, 221, 233

Lipset, Seymour Martin, 105

Lomba do Pinheiro, Porto Alegre, 158

Longest, Kyle C., 24, 77, 82, 85

Lula da Silva, Luiz Inácio, 101, 245

Machado, Cristiani Vieira, 39

Machado, Francisco "Chicão" de Assis, 102, 103, 114, 119–120, 123

Magalhães, Antônio Carlos (ACM), 54, 93–94, 108, 178, 203, 273n2 (ch6)

Magalhães, Juraci Vieira de, 217–218, 227, 229–232, 234

Magalhães Jr., Helvécio Miranda, 88, 98, 110, 117–118, 129–130, 246

Mahoney, James, 64, 81

Maia, César, 55

Malagutti, Marílio, 126

Manaus, Amazonas, 29, 75–80 (79t), 97, 270n27

Martins Rodrigues, Paulo Marcelo, 212

Mata, Lídice da, 94

McCarthy, John D., 258

McGuire, James W., 249, 261

MDB (Brazilian Democratic Movement), 100–101

MDD (movement-driven development), 1, 28, 58–60 (59t), 95–96, 265–266; and civil-society-in-state-perspective, 253–258; and encompassing embeddedness model, 251–253; end of in Brazil, 263–266; fuzzy-set analysis (FSA) of, 75–78; in Global South, 251, 256–257; health democratization pathways to, 14–15; legal/antipoverty/public education sectors, 242–248; meso-level analysis of, 8; and policy diffusion, 8, 10–11, 16; and power constellations framework, 12, 60, 251–252; pragmatist publics and, 12–16, 23–24, 28, 74, 95, 258–

263; in South India, Indonesia, 248–250; theory of, 241–242, 245, 250–263. *See also* "participatory-programmatic" health democratization

MDS (Social Development Ministry), 55, 178

Mendes Martinsk, José Adelmo, 230

Mesquita, Erle Cavalcante, 275n6

Migdal, Joel S., 256

"minimalist" health democratization, 4, 14, 29, 32, 57t, 59t, 87, 142, 177, 217

Mische, Ann, 34, 276n2

mixed-methods research design, 23–26

Monteiro de Andrade, Luiz Odorico, 92, 208–209, 213, 233–237, 239, 246, 276n16

More Doctors (*Mais Medicos*), 265

Mota, Eduardo, 94, 157

Mota, Luiz Henrique de Almeida, 155–160, 162–165, 167

MP (Ministerio Publico), 242–245

MS (Ministry of Health): and AIS (Integrated Health Actions), 112; and Community Health Agents Program, 125; contracting by, 166, 197; formal agreements with, 187–188, 192; paying retirement expenses, 164; and PSF model, 190; and SMS staffing, 128

MS-DAB (Basic Attention Department), 236

MSP/PMS (Mineiro Sanitarista Party), 35, 97–98, 103–104, 117, 122–123, 140

Mulher de Verdade program, 201

multivariate regression analyses, 23, 69–75 (70t, 73t)

Municipal Committee on Maternal Mortality, 188

Municipal Health Conference (Curitiba 1991), 177, 189

Municipal Health Fund, 116, 157, 199

Municipal Law 6,817 (1986), 153

Municipal Law 277 (1992), 153

Municipal Public Servants Union (SINDIBEL), 103, 126

municipal spending on public health, sanitation, 24, 58–59, 61, 71, 74, 78, 124–127, 129

Nascer em Curitiba, Vale a Vida (Born in Curitiba, Value Life), 195–196
National Sanitary Reform Commission (1986), 152
Neto, Domingos Leitão, 275n11
Neves, Tancredo, 99–100, 111–112
Nigam, Amit, 243–244

O Dilema Preventista (Arouca), 49
OECD (Organization for Economic Co-operation and Development), 247
Olasky, Sheera Joy, 258
Oliveira Garcia, Maria Letícia de, 169
Olivier, Johan, 259
OP (Participatory Budgeting), 68, 168, 251; Belo Horizonte, 88, 98, 109–111, 119–120, 131; Curitiba, 91–92, 172–173, 180, 204; Fortaleza, 92, 209, 221; participatory publics and, 56–57; Porto Alegre, 30, 89, 111, 134–136, 140, 145–146, 153, 159–160; Recife, 89
OPAS (Pan-American Health Organization), 114, 188
Organic Health Laws (1990): attempts to revise, roll back, 264; Borges on, 115; cogoverning authority of, 146, 228; enactment of, 28–29; municipal requirements of, 157, 159, 174; and principle of integrality, 265; sanitaristas and, 18; and social code switching, 44
OSs (Health Organizations), 94, 181

PACS (Community Health Agents Program), 229
Paim, Jairnilson Silva, 49, 93
PAMs (urgent-care units), 113, 150–151, 153, 167
Parameswaran, M. P., 250
Paraná, 171–177, 180, 183–185, 187, 191–192; SES/SMS directors, 194, 198–199, 202–203. *See also* Curitiba; Raggio, Armando Marinho Bardou
Parente Filho, Renato, 230
"participatory-programmatic" health democratization, 3–4, 57t, 59, 132, 222; in Belo Horizonte, 97–99, 107–111, 118;

FSA tests, 81, 83, 85–91, 96; in Porto Alegre, 134–136, 141–147, 169
participatory publics, 16, 34; and CMS (Municipal Health Councils), 16, 56–57, 98, 109–110, 131–133, 135–136, 146, 154; influential, 71–72, 80, 81, 83–85, 88–92, 204
PCB (Brazilian Communist Party), 36, 49
PC do B (Communist Party of Brazil), 102, 103, 120, 123, 126, 183
PDT (Democratic Labor Party), 94, 139, 142, 149, 151–152, 178, 192, 194, 203–204
People's Campaign for Decentralized Planning (1996–2000), 250
Perreira, Paulo Cesar, 106, 114, 126–128
Petras, James, 259
PFL (Liberal Front Party), 178, 203–204, 274n11
PIASS (Internalization of Health and Sanitarist Actions), 103
Pimenta Jr., Fabiano Geraldo, 130–131
Pimentel, Fernando, 88–89, 108, 127, 129
Pinochet, Augusto, 9
PIQ (Quality Incentive Program), 195
plano diretor (city master plan), 173, 182, 186
Pluri-Annual Plan (1994–1997), 231
PMC (Curitiban Mother Program), 172, 198–200, 204, 210, 226
PMC (Montes Claros Project), 102, 188
PMDB (Brazilian Democratic Movement Party): Belo Horizonte, 103, 111–112; Curitiba, 178, 186, 204, 243; Fortaleza, 217–218, 227, 229; Porto Alegre, 151, 169
PMS/MSP (Mineiro Sanitarista Party), 35, 97–98, 103, 117, 122–123, 140
PNH (National Humanization Policy), 236
policy diffusion framework, 8, 262; and Curitiba, 173; and Fortaleza, 210; and MDD, 8, 10, 11, 16
policy models, 11, 268n12
political agency, 9, 33, 106

Pompéia Health Center, 188–190
Pont, Raul, 143, 161–162, 166
Popular Health Forum (FOPS), 180–181, 273n1 (ch6)
Portela, Luis Eugênio, 95
Porto Alegre, 29, 31–32; pre-SUS-Era, 136–141; participatory-programmatic democratization, 24, 85, 141–147; Sanitarista public health expansion, 147–148; Sanitarista (1982–1987), 151–155; Sanitarista (1993–1996), 155–161; Sanitarista (1997–2001), 161–167; Sanitarista (2002–2016), 167–169; CMS (Municipal Health Councils), 119, 135–137, 143, 145–147, 170, 244; fuzzy-set analysis, 75–80 (79t), 87–92; health care expansion, 56; left-party office holding, 32
Power, Timothy, 68, 80, 274n11
power constellations framework, 7–8, 12, 60, 68, 251–252
"pragmatist democracy," 165
pragmatist publics, 2, 258–263; civil-society actors as, 2, 18; code-switching by, 21–23; and Gramscian theory, 20–21; and MDD processes, 16–26; molding institutions, 18–20; and radically inclusive ideologies, 17–18; *sanitaristas* as, 33–47; and state-building impulse, 20; as unique source of agency, 16–19; use of associations by, 21; use of democracy by, 13–15. *See also* Sanitarist Movement (*Movimento Sanitario*)
Prais-Winsten models, 24, 61, 69
premature death. *See* IMR (infant mortality rate)
Pritchett, Lant, 9
process tracing, 25
programmatic health democratization: Curitiba, 3, 14–15, 24, 29, 87–92, 171–172, 177–181; Fortaleza, 24, 29, 31, 210, 215–222, 233, 238, 240
Pro-Health (*Pro-Saude*) agreement, 188
PSB (Brazilian Socialist Party): Belo Horizonte, 102, 103, 111, 132–133; Célio de Castro, 89, 98, 108, 122–123, 168; Curi-

tiba, 201; Fortaleza, 217–218, 237; Marcio Lacerda, 130
PSDB (Brazilian Social Democratic Party), 201; Belo Horizonte, 89, 103, 111–113, 123, 126, 130, 132; Curitiba, 178, 201, 204; Fortaleza, 217–218, 223–225, 227
PSF (Family Health Program), 61–62, 261; adaptations to, 11; in Belo Horizonte, 109, 125–126, 128, 130–131; Cardoso and, 12; coverage rate of, 24, 26, 65, 72–74 (73t), 79; creation of, 40, 43; in Curitiba, 179–180, 185, 189–190, 193, 195–202; in Fortaleza, 208, 210, 219–220, 230–238, 246–247; fuzzy-set analysis of, 86; MS (Ministry of Health), 37, 94–95, 112, 125, 128, 164, 166, 187–192, 197, 236; in Porto Alegre, 136, 140, 144–145, 158–166, 169; resistance to, 94; Salvador spending on, 95. *See also* MS (Ministry of Health)
PT (Workers' Party): Car Wash (Lava Jato) scheme, 243; Catholic activists and, 100; corruption within, 264; cost concerns and health care hiring, 157–158, 163–165; in Curitiba, 172–173, 180, 203–204; Dilma Rousseff, 111, 263–264; elections, 30, 54, 80, 89, 91, 113, 123; factionalization within, 162; Fernando Pimentel, 88–89, 108, 127, 129; in Fortaleza, 209, 216–219, 233; Joaquim Kliemann, 140, 167–168; loss of power, 160; Lucio Barcelos, 89, 134–135, 138, 140, 158, 161–168, 170, 246; Luiz Inácio Lula da Silva, 101, 245; Marcio Lacerda, 108, 130; Maria Luiza Fontenele, 274n4, 275n11; Patrus Ananias, 88, 108, 109, 119–121, 123–124, 272n10; in Porto Alegre, 30, 125, 138–139, 142–145, 152; and PSB, 133; in Rio Grande do Sul, 140; and *sanitarista* officeholders, 68, 103, 120, 132, 141, 161, 167; Tarso Genro, 143, 152, 155–157, 161–163, 165, 167–168
PUC-PR (Catholic Pontificate University of Paraná), 174–175

Putnam, Robert, 18
PW-PCSE (panel-corrected standard errors), 69, 70t, 73t

Raeburn, Nicole C., 259
Raggio, Armando Marinho Bardou: "Challenge of Being Health Manager in Brazil," 193; and Curitiba IMR reductions, 187, 193, 194, 197, 204; as FCMR director, 185; international partnerships, 188; more, 206, 274n12; primary-care-oriented model, 189–190; Pro-Health (*Pro-Saude*) agreement, 188; and "sanitary reform" movement, 182–184, 186, 191–192, 198; as SES director, 199, 274n12; as SMS director, 91, 172, 176, 185, 192–193, 194; and SUS mission, 105–106, 171, 188–189, 193, 206
Ragin, Charles C., 24, 75–77, 83, 270n5
Raiz, Saul, 182
Recife, Pernambuco, 31–32; FSA findings, 87–92; fuzzy-set analysis, 75–80 (79t); health care expansion, 56; IMR (infant mortality rate), 64–65, 274n2; left-party office holding, 32; "participatory-programmatic" health democratization, 85; sanitarista office holding in, 3, 79
Rede Cegonha (Stork Network), 172, 198
regression analysis: cross-sectional time series, 23; Prais-Winsten, 23, 61, 69–75. *See also* FSA (fuzzy-set analysis)
Requião de Mello, Roberto, 177–178, 186
Richa, Carlos Alberto "Beto," 178, 201–202
Rio de Janeiro, 29; BF (Bolsa Familia), 109, 144; CEBES, 175; data and regression analysis, 63; FSA analysis, 75, 78, 79t, 84–85, 87; fuzzy-set analysis, 75–80 (79t), 84–85; "minimalist" health democratization, 4, 14, 29, 32, 57t, 58–59 (59t), 87, 142, 217; non-robust development, 254–255; Participatory Budgeting (OP), 109, 145, 170; patronage-oriented politics, 54–55, 219
Rio Grande do Sul, 244; Collares, Alceu,

139, 142, 149–150, 152, 155; INAMPS, 148–150; sanitarista activism, 138–142, 144; sanitarista office holding, 137; SES in, 135, 151, 154–155, 162; SMS denunciation by TCU-RS, 169; TCU-RS (National Accounts Tribunal of Rio Grande do Sul), 169. *See also* Barcelos, Lucio; Jaeger, Maria Luiza; Porto Alegre
robust versus nonrobust development, 4, 31–32; Belo Horizonte, Minas Gerais, 78, 84; clientelist politics, 75; FSA (fuzzy-set analysis) of, 62, 82–84, 247; and IMR, 14, 83–84; process tracing of, 25–26; Rio de Janeiro, 29, 58, 87, 254–255; Salvador, 29, 58, 87, 92–96, 172, 254–255; and sanitarista management, 239
Rocha Silva, Aldely, 94
Rodrigues Neto, Eleutério, 38, 42, 44, 46, 112
Roefs, Marlene, 259
Rousseff, Dilma, 111, 263–264

Sabin Infant Hospital, Dr. Albert, 225
Salvador, Bahia, 29; clientelism, 59; CMS, 170; fuzzy-set analysis, 75–80 (79t), 84–85, 92–95; and "incapacitated states," 58; "minimalist" health democratization, 4, 14, 29, 32, 57t, 59t, 87, 142–144, 177, 217; non-robust development, 172, 254–255; Participatory Budgeting (OP), 109; patronage-oriented politics, 54–55, 219; PSF coverage, 65; sanitary reform mobilization, 93. *See also* ACM (Antônio Carlos Magalhães)
SANARE: Revista Sobralense de Politicas Publicas, 236
sanitarista office holding, 2, 11, 15, 24, 66t; Belo Horizonte, 3, 79, 98, 111, 118–131; as civil-society activists, social-movement veterans, 15; Curitiba, 3, 79, 181–189, 191–194, 207; Fortaleza, Ceará, 212, 222–238; and IMR (infant mortality rate), 23–24, 61–62, 98, 111, 118–122, 129–131, 155–169; Mineiro Sanitarista Party (PMS/MSP), 35, 97–

98, 103, 117, 122–123, 140; municipal health department directorship, 79; Porto Alegre, 79; PT (Workers' Party), 68, 103, 120, 132, 141, 161, 167; Recife, 3, 79; "sanitary authorities," 189–190, 216; SUS directorship position, 15, 65, 94, 106, 192; SUS management position, 15, 40–42, 165, 189, 192, 206, 229, 253; SUS managers, 39, 42, 189–190, 198, 253, 255. *See also* FSA (fuzzy-set analysis)

Sanitarist Movement (*Movimento Sanitario*), 2; anticorporate orientation of, 50; Armando Marinho Bardou Raggio, 182–183, 186, 191–192, 198; in Belo Horizonte, 105–106, 111–118, 133; campus activism, 100; CEBES (Brazilian Center for Health Studies), 212, 220, 243, 265; civil power and, 104–106; in Curitiba, 172, 175, 177, 187–194, 198–207; and end of MDD, 263–264; in Fortaleza, 79, 209, 212–214, 223–224, 228–229, 234–239; key tenets of, 48–50; lacking civil mobilization experience, 230; Luciano Ducci, 198–199, 202; Luiz Odorico Monteiro de Andrade, 92, 208–209, 213, 233–237, 239, 246, 276n16; mobilization in 1970s, 1980s, 35; motivations of, 104–105, 155; National Sanitary Reform Commission, 152; and Organic Health Law, 265; "parliamentary way" toward, 38–39; PMS support of, 104; in Porto Alegre, 147–148, 156, 162, 168; as pragmatist public, 33–47; primary care based on, 117–118; and PT (Workers' Party), 140; and right to health, 13, 117, 262; in Rio de Janeiro, Salvador, 32, 175; in Rio Grande do Sul, 139; sanitarista code-switching and, 47–48; sanitarista motivations, 104–105; Sergio Arouca, 49; SESAC and, 175; at subnational level, 51; and SUS management, 42, 255; tied to infant survival, 122. *See also* Castro, Célio de; IMR (infant mortality rate)

Santa Cecília, 137, 153

Santos, Eliseu, 169

São Paulo, 63, 75–80 (79t), 84–85, 109, 112, 118, 144

Saraiva Felipe, José, 101–102, 104, 112–113, 120, 123

Saude em Debate (CEBES), 66t, 176

Scorza, Humberto, 159–160

Sen, Amartya, 6, 63, 267n2, 270n1

Serra, José, 126

SES (state health department), 155, 220, 225; and AIS (Integrated Health Actions), 112; in Bahia, 93; effectiveness of, 140; in Fortaleza/Ceará, 209, 213–215, 220, 224–227; in Minas Gerais, 102, 112, 120; Murialdo clinic, 138; in Paraná, 171–173, 174, 176, 185, 187, 194; in Porto Alegre, Rio Grande do Sul, 135, 140, 142, 144, 148–155, 156, 162; women's representation in, 80, 89–91, 138. *See also* SES directorships

SESACs (Community Health Studies Weeks), 101, 175

SESB-PA (Secretariat of Health and Well-Being for Paraná), 184

SES directorships, 67t, 135, 194, 209, 214–215; Anamaria Cavalcante e Silva, 115, 209, 213, 218, 225–229; Antônio Carlile Holanda Lavor, 212–213, 223–229; in Fortaleza, 214–215; João Ananias Vasconcelos Neto, 209, 214; José Saraiva Felipe, 101–102, 104, 112–113, 120, 123; Michele Caputo Neto, 91, 172, 176, 182, 196, 198, 201–202, 204, 206; non-PT governors, 68; Raimundo José Arruda Bastos, 209, 214; and SUS managers, 220; women in, 80, 91. *See also* Jaeger, Maria Luiza; Raggio, Armando Marinho Bardou

Sheller, Mimi, 33–34

Silva Lima, Antônio José, 275n11

SINDIBEL (Municipal Public Servants Union), 103, 126

SINDMÉD-MG (Doctors Union of Minas Gerais), 103

SIND-SAÚDE, 126

SINSAÚDE-MG (Health Workers Union of Minas Gerais), 103

SMS (municipal health secretariat), 157; Belo Horizonte, 98, 112, 152; CMS conflict with, 169–170, 272n5; Curitiba, 185, 194; Engineering Service, 226; Fortaleza, 152, 209, 220, 225; participatory publics and, 146–147; Porto Alegre, 145, 149, 151, 156–161; work of, 115–116

SMS directorship, 98, 146, 254; Baracho, João Carlos Gonçalves, 181, 194–197, 199, 202–203; Barcelos, Lucio, 161–163, 170; Bezerra de Farias, Raimundo Coelho, 230; Borges, José Maria, 88, 97–98, 101–106, 112–118, 120, 123, 245, 261, 269n19; Campos, Cézar Rodrigues, 88, 98, 118, 120, 122–123; Cavalcante Brasil, Abner, 209, 218, 222, 227–229; Cavalcante e Silva, Anamaria, 115, 209, 213, 218, 225–229; as de facto CMS president, 119–120; Ducci, Luciano, 91, 172, 176, 182, 196, 199–202, 206; Fagundes, Sandra, 135, 168–169; Fonseca Neto, Manuel Dias da, 216, 275n11; Fontana, Henrique, 89, 135, 161, 167, 170, 246; Fontenele, Maria Luiza, 216–217, 274n4, 275n11; in Fortaleza, 209, 220, 225, 233, 236; Gouvêa Teixeira, Marcelo, 130; Jaeger, Maria Luiza, 89, 135, 167–168, 170, 246; Kliemann, Joaquim, 140, 167–168; Magalhães Jr., Helvécio Miranda, 88, 98, 110, 117–118, 129–130, 246; Malagutti, Marílio, 126; Mendes Martinsk, José Adelmo, 230; Monteiro de Andrade, Luiz Odorico, 92, 208–209, 213, 233–237, 239, 246, 276n16; Mota, Luiz Henrique de Almeida, 155–160, 162–165, 167; Neto, Domingos Leitão, 275n11; Paraná directors, 194, 198–199, 202–203; Parente Filho, Renato, 230; Perreira, Paulo Cesar, 106, 114, 126–128; Portela, Luis Eugênio, 95; Raggio, Armando Marinho Bardou, 91, 172, 176, 185, 192–193, 194; Santos, Eliseu, 169; Scorza, Humberto, 159–160; Silva Lima, Antônio José, 275n11; and SUS management position, 107, 117, 162, 220, 253–254; Taumaturgo Lopes, Galeno, 230; Tuebner, Evilázio, 126–129

SMSE (Municipal Health System School), 236

SMSSS (Municipal Health and Social Service Secretariat), 148, 150–156

Snyder, Richard, 8

social code-switching, 13, 21–23, 44–47, 244

Solla, Jorge, 93–94

"state-directed development" framework, 7, 9–10

"state-in-society" perspective, 250

State University of Ceará (UECE), 211

State University of Paraná (UESPAR), 174

Stork Network (*Rede Cegonha*), 172, 198

subnational analysis, 6–7

Suharto (Indonesia), 250

SUS (Unified Health System): in Belo Horizonte, 120–121, 129; establishment of, 2; NOBs (Basic Operating Norms), 37, 121, 157, 159, 188, 190, 194, 230, 232; in Porto Alegre, 141, 145; *semiplena* ("partial") management status, 121, 157

SUS directorship position, 37; biases of, 42; creation of, 19; in Curitiba, 176, 188–189, 192–193, 198–199, 206; effect of on PSF adoption, 40; in Fortaleza, 228-230, 235, 238–240; as "honorable mission," 105; and IMR/CMR rates, 23–24, 26, 69; lessons learned by, 43; at multiple levels, 2–3, 19; obstructionism toward, 4; and Organic Health Laws, 44, 174, 288; in Paraná, 198; in Porto Alegre, 143; pragmatic approach to, 41, 43–44; pragmatist public and, 256, 262; Raggio on mission of, 171; responsibilities of, 7, 13–14, 39, 42; as "sacred mission," 193; sanitaristas occupying, 15, 40–42, 65, 94, 106, 165, 189, 192, 206, 229, 253; as "sanitary authorities," 39, 42, 189–190, 198, 228, 253, 255; and SES directorships, 220; and SMS directorship, 107, 117, 162, 220, 253–254; and state-building power, 255. *See also* Barcelos, Lucio; Raggio, Armando Marinho Bardou

Tamil Nadu, India, 248–249
Taniguchi, Cassio, 178, 192, 199, 203
Taumaturgo Lopes, Galeno, 230
Tavares, Darilo, 112
Távora, Virgílio, 211, 215
TCU-RS (National Accounts Tribunal of Rio Grande do Sul), 169
Temer, Michel, 263–264
Tendler, Judith, 10, 205, 223, 275nn8
Tocqueville, Alexis de, 18
Tonón, Lídia, 101–102, 106, 113–114, 120–122, 269n19
Trotskyite groups, 102, 117, 120, 176
Tuebner, Evilázio, 126–129
"21DS" (twenty-first-century developmental states), 252

UBS (basic health units), 127, 201, 237
UECE (State University of Ceará), 211
UESPAR (State University of Paraná), 174
UFC (Federal University of Ceará), 211–214, 225, 237
UFMG (Federal University of Minas Gerais), 100–102
UFPR (Federal University of Paraná), 174–175, 183
UNE (National Student Union), 101, 175, 213, 269n13
Unified Health System (*Sistema Unico de Saude*, SUS). *See* SUS
uninsured population, 24, 26, 61, 65

universalizing ideology, 15, 18–21, 35, 104–106, 117, 155, 196, 254–258
Uptake project, 121
US (health units), 109, 113, 115, 153, 179, 220

Vaisey, Stephen, 24, 77, 82, 85
Vargas, Getúlio, 9, 134
Vasconcelos Neto, João Ananias, 209, 214
Veloso, Fernando Megre, 102
Veltmeyer, Henry, 259
Verle, João, 143, 163
Vieira Carvilhe, Márcia Helena, 274n10
Vilaça, Eugenio, 114
Vila Cruzeiro region, 150, 155
Vila São Pedro neighborhood, 189, 273n7

Wampler, Brian, 271n2, 272n8
wars of position, 19, 21, 39
"wealthier is healthier" paradigm, 9–10
Weyland, Kurt, 5, 33, 120
"whole-nation bias," 8
within-case analysis, 23–25, 61, 62, 64, 96
Wolford, Wendy, 117
Wolfson, Mark, 258
Wong, Joseph, 276n1

Zanoni, Luiz Carlos, 183
Zero Hunger (*Fome Zero*), 245
Zucco, Cesar, 68, 80, 274n11

The authorized representative in the EU for product safety and compliance is:
Mare Nostrum Group
B.V Doelen 72
4831 GR Breda
The Netherlands

www.ingramcontent.com/pod-product-compliance
Lightning Source LLC
Chambersburg PA
CBHW020457270326
41926CB00008B/644